Optimizing Women's Health and Training

of related interest

Pilates-Based Movement for Menopause
A Guide for Teachers and Practitioners
Dinah Siman
Foreword by Elizabeth Larkam
ISBN 978 1 91342 667 5
eISBN 978 1 83997 647 6

Menopause Yoga
A Holistic Guide to Supporting Women on their Menopause Journey
Petra Coveney
Foreword by Dr Louise Newson
ISBN 978 1 78775 889 6
eISBN 978 1 78775 890 2

Teaching Yoga for the Menstrual Cycle
An Ayurvedic Approach
Anja Brierley Lange
Foreword by Dr Shijoe Mathew Anchery
ISBN 978 1 83997 247 8
eISBN 978 1 83997 248 5

The Power and the Grace
A Professional's Guide to Ease and Efficiency in Functional Movement
Joanne Elphinston
Foreword by Thomas W Myers
ISBN 978 1 91208 538 5
eISBN 978 1 91208 539 2

OPTIMIZING WOMEN'S HEALTH AND **TRAINING**

Embracing Female Physiology for Performance and Wellbeing

Dr Katja Bartsch

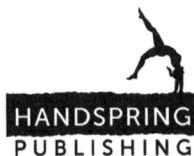

HANDSPRING
PUBLISHING

First published in Great Britain in 2026 by Handspring Publishing, an imprint of Jessica Kingsley Publishers
Part of John Murray Press

2

A CIP catalogue record for this title is available from the British Library and the Library of Congress

ISBN 978 1 91342 675 0
eISBN 978 1 83997 646 9

Printed and bound in the United States by Integrated Books International

Jessica Kingsley Publishers' policy is to use papers that are natural, renewable and recyclable
products and made from wood grown in sustainable forests. The logging and manufacturing
processes are expected to conform to the environmental regulations of the country of origin.

Handspring Publishing
Carmelite House
50 Victoria Embankment
London EC4Y 0DZ

www.handspringpublishing.com

John Murray Press
Part of Hodder & Stoughton Limited
An Hachette UK Company

The authorised representative in the EEA is Hachette Ireland, 8 Castlecourt
Centre, Dublin 15, D15 XTP3, Ireland (email: info@hbgi.ie)

Contents

Part II: Female Flow Throughout the Lifespan

Acknowledgements

I would like to express my gratitude to a number of people who have supported this project along the way. To Sarena Wolfaard, Robert Schleip, Melanie Burns, Jill Miller and David Lesondak, who helped to get this book project started. To Tiffany Cruikshank, Alison Slater and Anja Ippach for contributing their experience and wealth of knowledge. In addition to the females already mentioned, to all the strong and daring women I am lucky to call my companions near and far. I may not get to see them often, but they have impacted this work in one way or another: Tammy Teske, Ulli Sattler, Bernie Landels, Janine Mikolajczak, and many more.

To the editorial team at Handspring Publishing, Sarah Hamlin, Jenny Edwards, Katie Forsythe and Emma Holak who helped to shape the final form of this book.

To my husband Sebastian, my kids Jai and Yoko, and my parents, who enthusiastically support me in all my endeavors and encourage me to bring my dreams to life.

Part I

UNPACKING FEMALE PHYSIOLOGY AND CYCLE-BASED LIFESTYLE

Introduction

While over half of the world's population is female, research on sports, exercise and movement has historically focused on the male population. One major reason: the menstrual cycle comes with fluctuations of sex hormones and changes of physiological processes; this makes scientific investigations on women complex. Considering users of hormonal contraceptives and women with different hormonal profiles across the lifespan (e.g. during pregnancy and breastfeeding/pumping, in peri- and postmenopause) further increases the variability to be considered by researchers. Only utilizing male participants allows meaningful results with fewer subjects and consequently with less funding. Concerns of potentially harming unborn fetuses historically also led to clinical trials solely conducted in men. Consequently, years of excluding females followed, assuming that men were adequate proxies for women (Bruinvels *et al.*, 2017).

Fortunately, research is catching up and the last couple of years have produced a plethora of new research on female physiology and its effects on physical performance and psychology. Notwithstanding, a gender disparity remains in the current sports medicine and exercise physiology research landscape, with females still being under-represented in the literature (Costello, Bieuzen and Bleakley, 2014; Hutchins *et al.*, 2021).

While science focusing on women is advancing, methodological challenges remain. Where research has already examined the special features of female physiology, subtleties of existing research can make it hard to compare studies, extrapolate findings to larger populations, and give general recommendations. Some examples: investigated cohorts between studies are heterogeneous and sometimes small in subject number; time points at which measurements are taken are not standardized; the type and potency of oral contraception pills used in examination vary largely between studies. Fortunately, recommendations regarding methodological considerations for studies in sport and exercise science with women as participants emerge, aiming to enhance future execution of experiments and result in more high-quality publications (Janse De Jonge, Thompson and Han, 2019; Elliott-Sale *et al.*, 2021; Schmalenberger *et al.*, 2021).

As research on women keeps evolving in quantity and quality, an emerging perspective emphasizes the individuality of women's experience related to female hormones: noticeable inter-individual differences in endogenous hormone profiles exist and the sensitivity to hormonal changes differs greatly between women (Schmalenberger *et al.*, 2021). Furthermore, women have to navigate significant individual day-to-day variations in hormone concentrations, which makes it important to track and understand each female's individual menstrual cycle and related body-mind responses (Bruinvels, Hackney and Pedlar, 2022). A growing body of research therefore favors individualized approaches over general recommendations. This, in turn, requires that women and health professionals develop a thorough understanding of female physiology and underpinning mechanisms, and that professionals are hence encouraged to take a deeper look into the research to forge an individualized approach for their clients and patients. I hope this book outlines basic mechanisms as well as highlights from the research in a detailed and rich, yet accessible and enjoyable way. Rather than giving generalized recipes, this work aims to provide a nuanced view, enabling practitioners and female individuals to make empowered decisions that are suitable for the individual body-mind system.

The book focuses on female health and well-being throughout the lifespan. This explicitly includes transgender and non-binary people. Many transgender people use gender-affirming hormone treatment, and understanding the effects and mechanisms of female sex hormones can support these populations to make empowered decisions about their hormone treatment. Health professionals accompanying transgender and non-binary people may use the information to adequately and empathically contribute to their clients' journey. Moreover, recent research considers transgender and non-binary people in the sports and wellness sphere more extensively—related research highlights are included in this book. In large parts, this book discusses the biological mechanisms and effects of sex hormones; please note that in many instances the terms "female," "woman," "male" and "man" are therefore used to refer to the biological sex, rather than gender. Throughout the parts of the book specifically dedicated to research on transgender and non-binary populations, gender descriptors and related pronouns are used to describe individuals' gender identity.

As this book has a focus—but is explicitly *not* limited to exercise-related topics, sports performance, and movement—it is intended for health-related professionals, such as athletic trainers, fitness coaches, movement teachers (e.g. yoga facilitators) and therapists, who want to increase their expertise on female sex hormones and would like to create tailor-made offerings to their clients. The topics covered in this book are also highly relevant for professionals in the realm of manual medicine. It is of note that the offered content is not only of interest to female professionals, but particularly addresses male practitioners as well—the physiology of the female client probably constitutes even more unchartered territory for the latter group. Furthermore, the book may be of interest to athletes, yoga practitioners as well as inclined readers who are interested in aligning their training and lifestyle with their female physiology.

In the first part of the book, female physiology and a menstrual cycle-based lifestyle are unpacked. The first chapter lays the ground for the rest of the book. It gives an overview of the underlying physiological processes related to female sex hormones and the menstrual cycle. Chapter 2 describes symptoms and disorders of the menstrual cycle and reproductive system. Chapter 3 focuses on the effects female sex hormones have on the musculoskeletal system and sports performance as well as on structural tissue adaptations in response to movement and training. Aspects related to thermoregulation, respiration and injury risk of female movers during the ebb and flow of their cycle are also covered in this section. Of high practical relevance for female movers are nutritional aspects, which is why Chapter 4 sheds light on the following questions: Which macronutrients play important roles in the different phases of a woman's cycle? What should females consider regarding fluid and electrolyte balance? What does the current understanding of "RED-S" (relative energy deficiency in sport) entail? Chapter 5 examines important psychological aspects of a woman's monthly cycle. It explains how the stress response and female reproductive hormones are connected. Beyond that, practices influencing the stress response are described, both in general as well as in relation to their application in sports. With many women around the globe relying on hormonal contraceptives, Chapter 6 highlights the impact of oral contraceptives on hormonal status, training and injury risk.

The second part of the book describes the flow of female reproductive hormones throughout the lifespan. It looks at pregnancy and the postpartum period (Chapter 7), peri- and post-menopause (Chapter 8) and sheds light on physical performance, dietary considerations and other important aspects during these times of a woman's life.

Text boxes throughout the book highlight bits of research I find particularly inspiring or thought-provoking. Other text boxes provide a detailed description of mechanisms or methodological research considerations for those who are here for the scientific deep dives.

Discovering what the emerging research has to offer and reconciling these findings with the subjective experience of each woman opens up an exciting journey for practitioners and their female clients. Ideally, both will find that female physiology and the flow of sex hormones throughout the lifespan are no burden—they are a privilege, with boundless potential and capacity waiting to be harnessed!

CHAPTER 1

The Menstrual Cycle: Monthly Flow of Female Sex Hormones

1.1. FEMALE PHYSIOLOGY AS POTENTIAL AND CAPACITY

1.1.1. Why women menstruate

Here is a weighty question to begin with: What is the meaning of life? Many psychological and spiritual concepts will suggest happiness as the objective to align oneself with. When taking a purely biological viewpoint, however, the goal of life is clear—we are to reproduce. At the same time, reproduction for humans is a huge and risky endeavor, since pregnancy places mother and child at odds. One particularly interesting design feature in this context is the placenta, a temporary organ, which connects the fetus to the mother's blood supply and nourishes the fetus while she grows. In most mammals, the placenta is confined behind a barrier of maternal cells, thereby letting the mother take control over the nutrient supply to the growing life. In humans, however, the placenta penetrates into the mother's circulatory system and directly accesses her bloodstream. Through this design, if the fetus is damaged or dies, the mother's health can become endangered. It is therefore important for the mother's body to screen embryos carefully. Here, menstruation is serving a protective mechanism. Each time ovulation doesn't result in a healthy pregnancy, the womb gets rid of the endometrial lining, along with any unfertilized eggs and sick, dying or dead embryos (Jarrell, 2018).

There is only a handful of mammals that menstruate: the common spiny mouse, elephant shrew, some bats, as well as primates and humans (Bellofiore *et al.*, 2018). The shortest menstrual cycle length can be observed in the spiny mouse (8–9 days) and elephant shrews (12 days), while the menstrual cycles of bats, primates and humans range from 21 to 37 days (Catalini and Fedder, 2020). This makes for up to 500 menstrual cycles within a human female's reproductive lifespan (Najmabadi *et al.*, 2020).

For normal ovulatory cycles to occur, a large number of follicles—small sacs of fluid in the ovaries that contain a developing egg—is needed. Follicles are formed while the female fetus is still in-utero during a process starting as early as five weeks into the pregnancy. A mother of a female fetus therefore carries the future eggs of her daughter inside her womb. A female is born with one to two million follicles. At puberty, the number of follicles has declined to about 300,000 to 500,000. During a woman's reproductive years, about 1000 follicles are lost monthly. By menopause few or no follicles remain and the monthly bleeding ceases (Hirshfield, 1997; Macklon and Fauser, 2001a, 2001b; Oyelowo, 2007; Davis *et al.*, 2023).

What happens when women menstruate in space?

Menstruation was part of the argument for why women shouldn't become astronauts in the early days of manned (pun intended) space flight. In the 1960s, researchers still suggested that putting a "temperamental psychophysiologic human" (i.e. menstruating woman) together with a "complicated machine" was a bad idea. Others referred to potential health risks, fearing that microgravity might increase the incidence of blood flowing up the fallopian tubes into the abdomen. And—shockingly—one line of argumentation to actually bring women to space was the "sexual release on a long-duration space mission" for their male counterparts. The past decades of space travel have revealed that menstruation in space microgravity is not related to any problems at all. Periods in space have been normal after all (Cole, 2015).

1.1.2. Embracing the menstrual cycle

Some women, especially athletes, will state something along the lines of "not having a period is a blessing." In fact, over 40% of exercising women have been reported to believe their menstrual cycle negatively impacts their training and performance (Bruinvels *et al.*, 2016). This doesn't come as a surprise. Menstrual disturbances, such as painful periods or premenstrual syndrome (PMS), can go far beyond annoying sensations (see Chapter 2). Besides the physical and mental burden, this can impact one's social life and career (Maity *et al.*, 2022). Studies have even linked severe cases of PMS—termed premenstrual dysphoric disorder—with an increased risk of suicidality (Osborn *et al.*, 2021; Prasad *et al.*, 2021; Yan, Ding and Guo, 2021). Despite this somber outlook, regular, normal-length menstrual cycles are considered a vital sign, indicating a woman's overall health (Diaz, Laufer and

Breech, 2006; Saei Ghare Naz, Rostami Dovom and Ramezani Tehrani, 2020; Itriyeva, 2022). The menstrual cycle is not only indicative of females' reproductive health, but also of the functioning of other body systems. Dysfunctions in the reproductive system and the menstrual cycle have been linked to hypothyroidism, osteoporosis, some forms of cancer, and cardiovascular diseases (Harlow and Ephross, 1995; Mumford and Kim, 2018; Najmabadi *et al.*, 2020). Thus, it is important for a woman to have a solid understanding of her menstrual cycle. In the recent past, a rise in popular media, training concepts and technology has fostered menstrual health literacy and has helped women to actively work with their monthly cycle. Knowing and tracking the menstrual cycle can not only be used as a natural contraception method but can also support females to plan their exercise or nutrition throughout the month (Maijala *et al.*, 2019; Stanford, 2019; Zwingerman, Chaikof and Jones, 2020; Schantz, Fernandez and Anne Marie, 2021; Alzueta *et al.*, 2022; Yu *et al.*, 2022).

While this trend can be seen as very positive, we certainly have not yet reached the end of the road when it comes to normalizing the menstrual cycle and female health education—this holds true for low-, middle- as well as high-income countries (Holmes *et al.*, 2021; Sons and Eckhardt, 2021; Baird *et al.*, 2022; Long *et al.*, 2022). Not only females themselves profit from being experts regarding their menstrual characteristics; therapists, trainers and movement teachers also benefit from a thorough understanding of female physiology and the implications for therapy and training to specifically tailor their offerings to the female demographic.

Menstrual cycle myths

- **Ancient bloodlines:** Many period-related taboos stem from misguided beliefs from the past. Previous teachings were characterized by patriarchal attitudes and echoed through the past 2000 years up until the last century. It was assumed that the touch of a menstruating woman may kill crops, rust metal, turn wine to vinegar or blunt a sword (Quint, 2021). It was hypothesized that menstrual blood is dirty and poisonous, and menstruation was considered a punishment or consequence of sin. Quite contrarily, there may have been times in history when menstruation has been associated with power, sacredness and essential life forces, as well. And to this date, some cultures celebrate a girl's first period, known as menarche, marking her transition into womanhood. In some cases, this milestone comes with responsibilities or the enforcement of traditional gender roles, while in some cultures first periods are acknowledged in a positive and empowering way. Cultural and societal norms around the menses have a profound impact on how menstruation is perceived, discussed and understood.

Addressing misconceptions and challenging harmful norms as well as promoting open conversation and education around the menstrual cycle are needed to this day to foster period positivity.

- **Bleeding dollars—the mythical marketing of menstrual products:** Since the earliest ads for menstrual products emerged in the 1920s, advertising has played its part in perpetuating fears and embarrassment related to periods. Ads have referred to the menstrual cycle as a hygiene nightmare, disguised boxes of pads have been praised for hiding shameful secrets, and mystery blue liquids have been used to show product absorbency (Quint, 2021). In 2024, major menstrual products are still marketed for the "safety" they provide—implying that leaks related to periods are "accidents" and "period dramas" are to be avoided at all costs. It's time to change the narrative.

1.2. THE MENSTRUAL CYCLE: THE EBB AND FLOW OF SEX HORMONES

1.2.1. Sex hormones: Overview

The menstrual cycle is regulated by female sex hormones, the most relevant being estrogen (more specifically estradiol; see section 1.2.2), progesterone, follicle-stimulating hormone (FSH) and luteinizing hormone (LH). The menstrual cycle involves the complex interplay and fine-tuned feedback loops of the hypothalamic-pituitary-gonadal (HPG) axis; in females this is termed the **hypothalamic-pituitary-ovarian (HPO) axis.**

The regulation of the menstrual cycle starts at the level of the hypothalamus. During menses, low levels of estrogen and progesterone trigger the secretion of gondadotropin-releasing hormone (GnRH) from the hypothalamus, which then stimulates the anterior pituitary to release follicle-stimulating hormone (FSH) and luteinizing hormone (LH). These two hormones, which are collectively termed gonadotropins, are released into the bloodstream to the ovaries and in turn stimulate the ovary (more specifically, the follicles) to produce the steroid hormones estrogen and progesterone. In females, estrogen and progesterone are the main sex hormones, both of which act on the reproductive tract and affect many organs throughout the body.

Endocrine basics

Hormones are chemical messengers that are synthesized in endocrine glands and regulate the physiological action of specific target cells. The major **glands of the endocrine system** are the hypothalamus, pituitary, pineal, adrenals, ovaries and pancreas. The **hypothalamus** is located at the base of the forebrain, below the thalamus. It is our "master gland" as it secretes hormones which stimulate other endocrine glands, among them the pituitary gland. The **pituitary gland** (also called the hypophysis) is attached to the hypothalamus at the base of the brain and consists of two organs: the anterior pituitary (a "true" endocrine gland) and the posterior pituitary (an extension of the hypothalamus consisting of neural tissue). The **anterior pituitary** plays an important role in the context of female sex hormones as it releases six hormones: growth hormone, prolactin, thyroid-stimulating hormone (TSH), the gonadotropic or gonad-stimulating hormones, follicle-stimulating hormone (FSH) and luteinizing hormone (LH) (Freeman *et al.*, 2000; Wilkinson and Brown, 2015).

While many hormones are secreted into the bloodstream and travel to target cells, some hormones can activate cells in their immediate neighborhood (**paracrine action**) or even the cell that releases them (**autocrine action**). Hormones are biologically effective in very small quantities. They can be classified as steroid hormones (e.g. estradiol and testosterone) or peptide hormones (e.g. insulin or growth hormone) (Wilkinson and Brown, 2015). An overview of major endocrine glands and hormones related to female health is given in Figure 1.1.

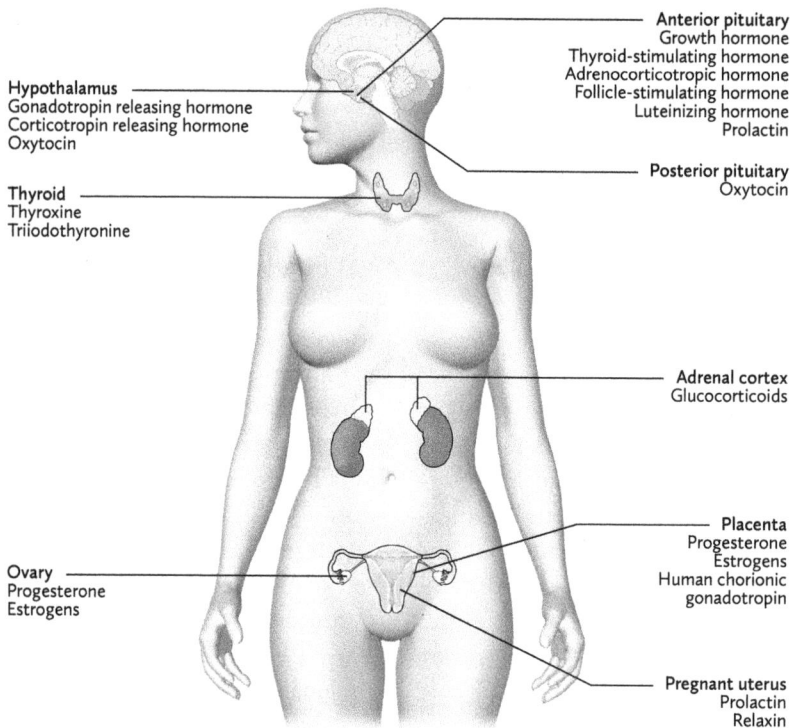

Hypothalamus
Gonadotropin releasing hormone
Corticotropin releasing hormone
Oxytocin

Thyroid
Thyroxine
Triiodothyronine

Ovary
Progesterone
Estrogens

Anterior pituitary
Growth hormone
Thyroid-stimulating hormone
Adrenocorticotropic hormone
Follicle-stimulating hormone
Luteinizing hormone
Prolactin

Posterior pituitary
Oxytocin

Adrenal cortex
Glucocorticoids

Placenta
Progesterone
Estrogens
Human chorionic
gonadotropin

Pregnant uterus
Prolactin
Relaxin

Figure 1.1: Major endocrine glands and representative hormones related to female health (adapted from Wilkinson and Brown, 2015).

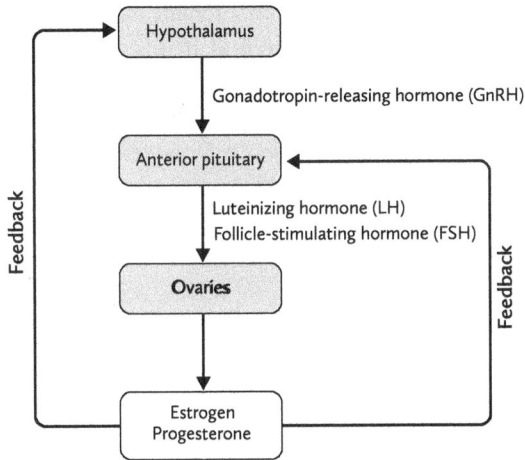

Figure 1.2: Hypothalamic-pituitary-ovarian axis. The reproductive cycle includes complex interactions and feedback loops between the hypothalamus, pituitary and ovaries.

The HPO axis is governed by complex feedback loops: estrogen and progesterone send some feedback to the level of the hypothalamus; however, the more dynamic feedback occurs at the level of the anterior pituitary (Hawkins and Matzuk, 2008). Through a negative feedback loop, increased levels of estrogen and progesterone are recognized by the hypothalamus and pituitary, leading to a reduced release of FSH and LH. In addition, a positive feedback loop is involved in the fine-tuning of the endocrine orchestration of the menstrual cycle: The high estradiol levels produced by the follicle producing the highest amount of estradiol (primary or dominant follicle) alter the sensitivity of the pituitary to the signals from the hypothalamus—the concentration of GnRH needed by the pituitary to produce LH lowers, which leads to the release of significantly more LH from the anterior pituitary. The resulting LH surge triggers ovulation (Messinisi, 2006). Accordingly, estradiol appears to be the main component responsible for this positive feedback loop; the role of progesterone in this positive feedback mechanism is less clear (Messinisi, 2006). Figure 1.2 depicts an overview of the elements and feedback loops of the HPO axis. Section 1.2.2 gives an overview and additional details of the described hormones as well as other female sex hormones. Section 1.2.3 provides a more detailed exploration of the hormonal changes related to each menstrual cycle phase.

1.2.2. Overview of female sex hormones
Gonadotropin-releasing hormone (GnRH)
GnRH belongs to the group of neurohormones, which differ from "true" hormones in that they are produced and released from modified neurons of the hypothalamus (vs. an endocrine gland) (Wilkinson and Brown, 2015).

Follicle-stimulating hormone (FSH)
FSH is produced by the anterior pituitary in response to GnRH and is then released into the peripheral circulation. In females, FSH, as its name suggests, stimulates the growth of the dominant follicle in the ovary, promoting the development of the ovum (Wilkinson and Brown, 2015). The growing egg is surrounded by two layers of cells: the inner granulosa cell layer and the outer theca cell layer. FSH stimulates the growth and function of granulosa cells. In a complex cross-talk with the theca cell layer, FSH also stimulates estradiol production of the granulosa cells (FSH promotes granulosa cells to synthesize aromatase, which converts androgens to estradiol). The resulting high estradiol microenvironment feeds back to the anterior pituitary gland to induce a surge in luteinizing hormone (LH) (Hawkins and Matzuk, 2008).

Luteinizing hormone (LH)
In females, LH stimulates ovulation (ovulation occurs about 8–20 hours after an LH surge) (Kerin, 1982). LH ruptures the follicle, so that the ovum is released into the fallopian tubes. The residual cells of the follicle (the remaining granulosa cells) form the corpus luteum in the ovary, which then secrete progesterone (Wilkinson and Brown, 2015). The name "luteum" means yellow; therefore the corpus luteum is also called yellow body.

Estrogens

Estrogen (or oestrogen) can be synthesized in both reproductive (in premenopausal women these are the ovaries, corpus luteum and placenta) and non-reproductive tissues (such as the adipose tissue, liver, heart, muscle, bone and brain) (Cui, Shen and Li, 2013). Estrogen is produced from cholesterol in a series of reactions; the final step in the process is the conversion of testosterone to estradiol by the enzyme aromatase (Nelson and Bulun, 2001; Chidi-Ogbolu and Baar, 2018). As estrogen receptors are present throughout the body, estrogens exert a broad range of effects in the reproductive, cardiovascular, musculoskeletal, immune and central nervous systems. They also impact metabolism (Heldring *et al.*, 2007; Novella *et al.*, 2019; Rehbein *et al.*, 2021; Bartkowiak-Wieczorek *et al.*, 2024).

There are various types of estrogen, the three main types being:

- estradiol (oestradiol; E2)
- estrone (oestrone; E1)
- estriol (oestriol; E3).

The primary estrogen is estradiol (E2), which is the predominant form in females of reproductive age. During the reproductive years, the ovaries are the main producer of estradiol (the adrenal glands contribute about 4%; during pregnancy, the placenta also contributes some) (Oyelowo, 2007; Cui, Shen and Li, 2013). In postmenopausal women, estrone (E1) is the predominant form of estrogen and production occurs mainly in the adipose tissue, which is high in aromatase activity (Nelson and Bulun, 2001; Chidi-Ogbolu and Baar, 2018). During pregnancy, estriol is produced by the placenta and constitutes the primary form of estrogen.

Estradiol is the most potent form of estrogen as it is 12 times stronger than estrone and 80 times stronger than estriol. Before menopause, blood levels of estradiol are 40–350 pg/ml; after menopause, levels drop to less than 15 pg/ml (Oyelowo, 2007). Estradiol plays an important

role in the onset of puberty, female development in the menstrual cycle and in pregnancy. E2 increases fat in the subcutaneous adipose tissue (particularly in the breasts, thighs and buttocks, making for the characteristic female form). It also has numerous beneficial effects on various tissues and organs. It can protect the heart, support muscle protein synthesis, lower intraocular pressure, prevent and reverse osteoporosis, increase skin collagen production and help with mood swings in postmenopausal women. It may even reduce the incidence of colon cancer (Wilkinson and Brown, 2015).

In oral contraceptive pills, synthetic versions of estrogen such as ethinyl estradiol are used (Wilkinson and Brown, 2015).

In addition to the endogenous estrogens, phytoestrogens—a much less potent form of estrogen—occur in plants, such as in soy, chickpeas and lentils.

Progesterone

Before ovulation, progesterone is synthesized in the follicles and the granulosa cells of the follicle take up a yellow pigment (lutein). In the luteal phase of the menstrual cycle, progesterone is produced in the corpus luteum of the ovary (Mesen and Young, 2015; Nagy *et al.*, 2021). It plays an important role in uterine, vaginal and mammary gland growth. In the context of the menstrual cycle, it prepares the uterus for possible implantation of a fertilized egg by promoting the thickening of the endometrial lining (Wilkinson and Brown, 2015).

Despite its name (i.e. "promoting gestation"), the role of the steroid hormone progesterone is not limited to the menstrual cycle and pregnancy. Progesterone is a precursor of other hormones such as cortisol, estradiol and testosterone. It furthermore affects the central nervous system, cardiovascular system and musculoskeletal system (Taraborrelli, 2015; Nagy *et al.*, 2021). Progesterone can protect neurons and help them recover, as is currently being researched in animal models related to stroke and amyotrophic lateral sclerosis (ALS) (Fréchou *et al.*, 2020, 2021; Ghoumari *et al.*, 2020; De Nicola *et al.*, 2022).

Anti-Müllerian hormone (AMH)
AMH is secreted by follicular cells and regulates the number of growing follicles each month, thereby ensuring that a woman is prevented from ovulating all follicles over only a small number of menstrual cycles during her reproductive years (Durlinger *et al.*, 2002).

Testosterone
Testosterone is produced in the ovary and adrenal glands. In females, it peaks right before ovulation. Testosterone, our principal androgen, plays a key role as anabolic hormone in muscle adaptation following exercise training, in the development of bone, connective and neural tissue, as well as muscle adaptation following exercise training (Sinha-Hikim *et al.*, 2006; Hoffman *et al.*, 2009; Kraemer, Ratamess and Nindl, 2017; Gharahdaghi *et al.*, 2020). Testosterone is binding to androgen receptors (AR).

Prolactin (PRL)
Prolactin is released from the anterior pituitary and plays a key role in initiating milk production in the mammary glands. It also has functions related to growth, fat and carbohydrate metabolism, reproduction and parental behavior. PRL interacts with other hormones such as estradiol, progesterone and oxytocin.

Relaxin
Relaxin is mainly produced by the corpus luteum, decidua (the maternal part of the placenta) and placenta and has mainly been studied in pregnant women (however, it is also found in non-pregnant women) (Parker *et al.*, 2022). Relaxin prepares and maintains the uterine lining during pregnancy (Wilkinson and Brown, 2015). Relaxin has also been reported to weaken collagen in tissues such as the pubic symphysis (Parker *et al.*, 2022).

Oxytocin
Oxytocin has prominently been termed the "love hormone" as it is believed to facilitate feelings of attachment and trust (Wilkinson and Brown, 2015). It is released in large amounts during labor and is a facilitator for childbirth and lactation. Oxytocin has also been linked to behaviors such as social recognition, bonding, and maternal and sexual behaviors (Magon and Kalra, 2011). Like GnRH, oxytocin belongs to the group of neurohormones which differ from true hormones in that they are released from modified nerve cells, rather than an endocrine gland. Oxytocin is mainly produced in the hypothalamus and released into the bloodstream by the posterior pituitary gland, but some is also secreted by the yellow body (corpus luteum) during the luteal phase of the menstrual cycle (Khan-Dawood *et al.*, 1989; Wilkinson and Brown, 2015).

Xenoestrogen
Xenoestrogens are exogenous estrogens and can be found in parabens (preservatives in creams and cosmetics), plastics (e.g. BPA) and environmental pollution. They mimic estrogen, can activate estrogen receptors and interfere with regular estrogenic synthesis and activity. Exposure to xenoestrogens should therefore be limited.

1.2.3. Phases of the menstrual cycle
The menstrual cycle can be divided into three phases (Allen *et al.*, 2016):

1. Follicular/pre-ovulation/proliferative (can be further divided into menses, early, mid and late follicular phase).
2. Ovulation.
3. Luteal/postovulation/secretory (can be further divided into early, mid and late luteal phase).

Note that some classifications count the period or menses as a separate first menstrual cycle phase, making for four menstrual phases. Table 1.1 gives an overview of the menstrual cycle phases. Figure 1.3 provides an overview of female reproductive organs as well as the changes the ovaries undergo with each menstrual cycle (ovarian cycle).

Table 1.1: Menstrual phases based on a 28-day cycle (adapted from Allen *et al.,* 2016)

	Follicular (days 1–10)				Ovulation (days 11–14)	Luteal (days 15–28)		
Change in	Menses	Early	Mid	Late		Early	Mid	Late
Progesterone	Stable	Stable	Stable	Mild increase	Increase	Large increase	Peak	Large decline
Estradiol	Stable	Mild increase	Large increase	Primary peak	Large decline	Mild increase	Secondary peak	Moderate decline
Luteinizing hormone	Stable	Stable	Stable	Stable	Peak	Stable	Stable	Stable

Methodological considerations for menstrual cycle research

Performing research with a focus on the menstrual cycle comes with methodological challenges, such as verifying which cycle phase a subject is in, when and how often to test, and which subjects to include or exclude. Some considerations are shared below:

- **Verification of menstrual cycle phase** of participants at time of testing. Ideally, three methods should be combined: calendar-based counting/menstrual cycle tracking (essential to anticipate measurement schedule), urinary testing of luteinizing hormone surge around estimated time of ovulation (inexpensive method to estimate time of ovulation), and measurement of estrogen and progesterone in the blood serum at time of testing (e.g. to control for or exclude women with anovulatory cycles or luteal deficiency) (Janse De Jonge, Thompson and Han, 2019).

- **Timing of testing.** Most research examining menstrual cycle phases uses a few steady-state time points within the cycle, such as the early follicular phase (testing within days 1–4 of the cycle), late follicular phase (around days 11–14 of the cycle), and mid to late luteal phase (7–9 days after ovulation). It is of note that these time points may represent an oversimplified perspective of the menstrual cycle, as levels of female sex hormones can change drastically within a 24-hour window. These transitions may impact training, performance and wellbeing significantly. Researchers are always challenged to find a balance between comprehensive measurements (e.g. testing every day) and feasibility (regarding funding and logistical practicability). Applying within-subject designs and considering case studies can therefore be valuable tools to understand a woman's menstrual cycle in its entirety (Schmalenberger *et al.,* 2021; Bruinvels, Hackney and Pedlar, 2022).

- Some studies pool together eumenorrheic subjects with oral contraceptive users. This is not to be recommended, since both groups present with different hormonal profiles. Statements about the impact of specific menstrual cycle phases cannot be made in such cases.

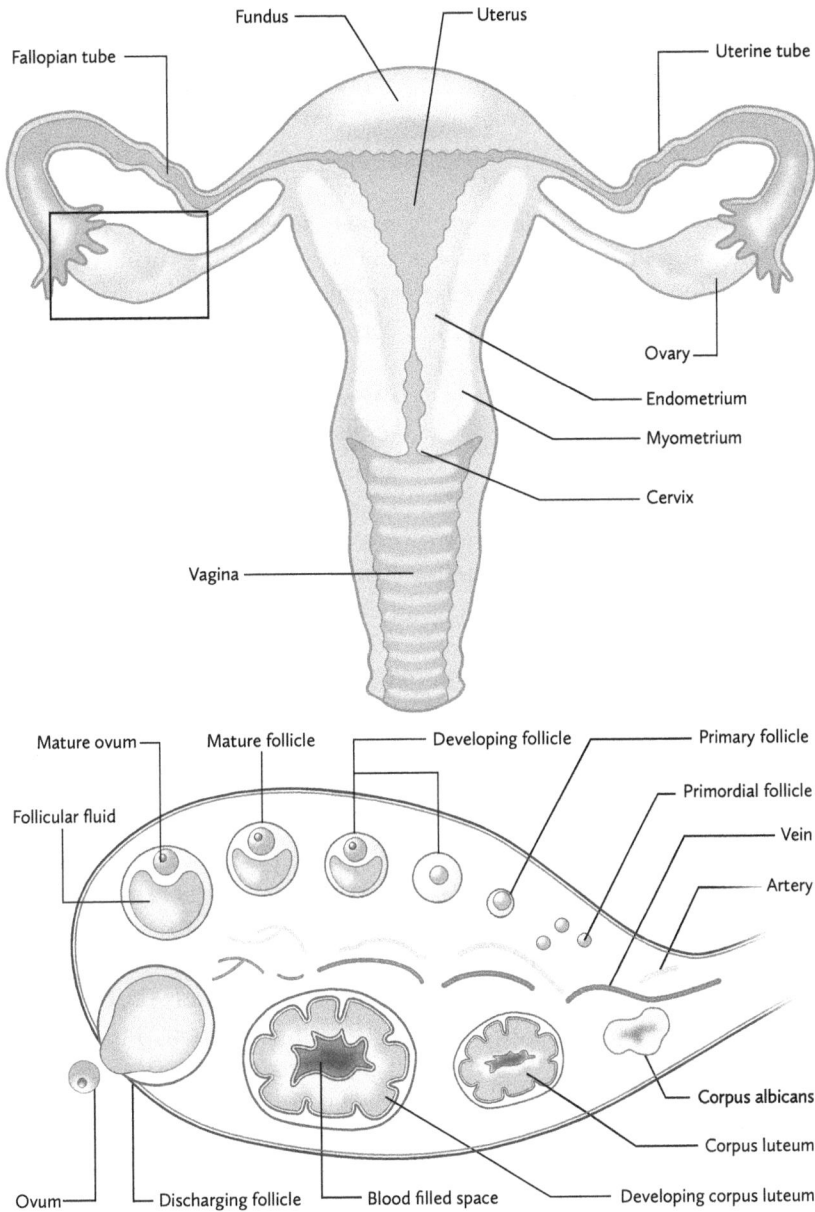

Figure 1.3: Female reproductive organs and ovarian cycle.

Follicular—menses

In 80% of ovulatory women, bleeding occurs over three to six days (range: 2–12 days), with the heaviest flow typically experienced on the second day (Mihm, Gangooly and Muttukrishna, 2011). During the period, levels of estrogen and progesterone are the lowest throughout the cycle, making a woman's hormonal set-up the most similar to their male counterparts throughout menses.

Follicular

Folliculogenesis, the maturation of the ovarian follicle, begins with the recruitment of primordial follicles (the most immature stage of an ovarian follicle's development). The signals that initiate this process are still unknown. After their recruitment, the selected follicles grow and excrete estrogen. The follicle secreting most estrogen becomes the dominant or primary follicle, which also expresses the highest number of FSH receptors, and this enforces the maturation of the follicle (Hawkins and Matzuk, 2008).

Ovulation

The surge of LH triggers ovulation, which occurs about 8–20 hours after the LH peak (see section 1.2.1) (Kerin, 1982). The egg leaves the follicle and passes into the fallopian tube. The remnants of the follicle (the remaining granulosa cells) become the corpus luteum, which is a temporary endocrine structure (Taraborrelli, 2015). Ovulation itself is characterized by high levels of estrogen and low levels of progesterone. When women can potentially conceive, their sexual interests assume greater priority. Though some studies exist that have failed to detect such associations, the evidence suggests that, on average, women experience greater levels of sexual desire and behavior during the late follicular phase and around ovulation (Gangestad and Thornhill, 2008; Gangestad and Dinh, 2022).

Luteal

Progesterone is the dominant hormone in the luteal phase and is produced by the corpus luteum (Mesen and Young, 2015; Nagy et al., 2021). In the days following ovulation, progesterone levels increase to 15–20 nmol/L in the early luteal phase and peak during the mid luteal phase (35–50 nmol/L). In addition to progesterone, the yellow body also secretes relaxin and oxytocin (Khan-Dawood et al., 1989; Nagy et al., 2021). Moreover, a second (smaller) peak in estrogen

occurs in parallel with the progesterone increase. The subsequent steps depend on whether fertilization takes place.

If fertilization occurs and the egg implants into the endometrium, the lining of the uterus changes further (then called decidua), which ultimately develops into the placenta. This lining of the uterus produces human chorionic gonadotropin (hCG), which nourishes and maintains the corpus luteum. The corpus luteum continues to produce progesterone, which in turn maintains the decidua in a self-propagating cycle. Until the ninth week of pregnancy, progesterone is almost entirely produced by the corpus luteum; thereafter the developing structures of the placenta increasingly take over progesterone production. By the twelfth week of the pregnancy, the placenta has formed and is self-sufficient (Csapo, Pulkkinen and Wiest, 1973; Oyelowo, 2007; Taraborrelli, 2015).

If no conception occurs, the rising levels of estrogen and progesterone act via a negative feedback loop on the hypothalamic-pituitary-ovarian axis (see section 1.2.1), which shuts off FSH and LH production (Oyelowo, 2007). The corpus luteum starts to break down around nine to ten days after ovulation and turns into scar tissue (corpus albicans), the mechanisms of which have not been exactly clarified yet (Taraborrelli, 2015; Nagy et al., 2021). Progesterone and estrogen production declines in the late luteal phase (Filicori, Butler and Crowley, 1984; Taraborrelli, 2015). Twenty-four hours before the end of the menstrual cycle (i.e. the end of the late luteal phase), the levels of estrogen and progesterone decrease notably. The blood vessels of the endometrium fail to be nourished, die and are shed off as menstrual bleeding, which results in the start of a new cycle (Oyelowo, 2007; Figueiredo et al., 2021).

Changes in sex hormones, body temperature and endometrial lining during the menstrual cycle are depicted in Figure 1.4.

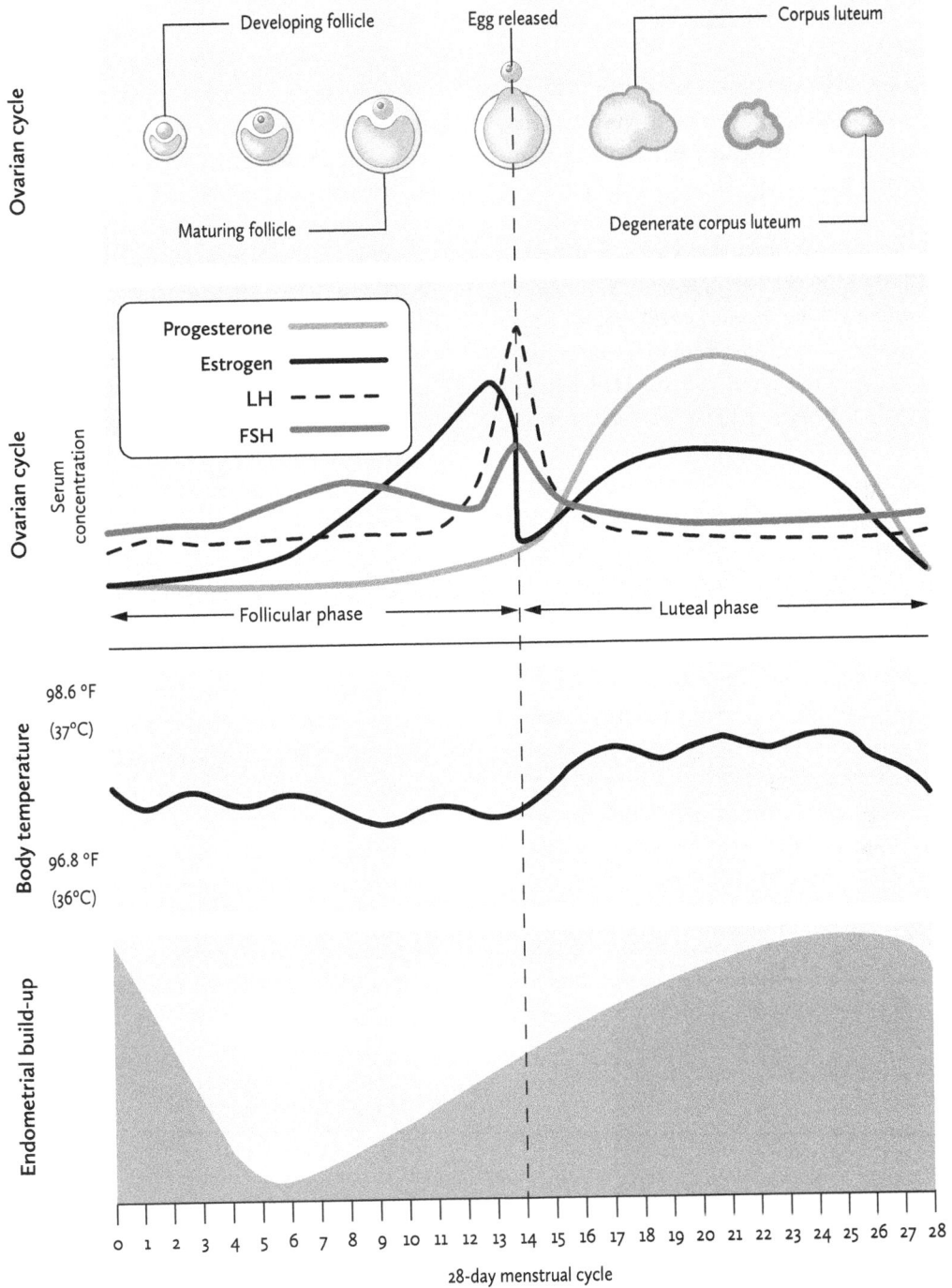

Figure 1.4: Changes throughout the menstrual cycle.

Persistent menstruation in transgender individuals using testosterone

Many trans individuals who identify as male or diverse, but were assigned female at birth, use testosterone gender-affirming hormone treatment (GAHT). Testosterone facilitates the growth of facial and body hair, an increase in muscle mass, and voice lowering in order to align with a person's identified gender (Zwickl *et al.*, 2024). One of the most desired effects of testosterone is the cessation of menstrual bleeding, which is a common cause of gender dysphoria (Schwartz *et al.*, 2022). However, testosterone GAHT does not necessarily result in the end of menses. A 2024 study including 401 trans and gender diverse individuals using testosterone revealed that 22.8% (n = 78) of participants experienced persistent menstruation after at least six months of commencing testosterone GAHT (Zwickl *et al.*, 2024). The odds for persistent bleeding were higher in individuals using testosterone creams or gels compared to injections, and lower in individuals with a body mass index of 30 kg/m^2 or higher. No associations were found between the age at commencement of testosterone treatment or menstrual regularity before starting testosterone. This information is important for people considering testosterone treatment as well as for clinicians advising on the benefits and drawbacks of GAHT.

Menstrual cycle length

The length of the menstrual cycle is 21–35 days, with most females averaging from 26 to 28 days and a "textbook" cycle length (i.e. referred to in most medical and research texts) of 28 days. The duration of the last menstrual cycle phase, the luteal phase, is relatively constant with an average of 14 days. Accordingly, the approximate date of ovulation can be calculated by subtracting 14 days from the length of the menstrual cycle (a woman with a cycle of 35 days will ovulate around day 21 of the cycle; a woman with a cycle of 24 days will ovulate around day 10) (Oyelowo, 2007). However, a regular, normal length cycle is not always a sign of ovulation. One study assessing a group of 3168 women showed that in over a third of normal menstrual cycles, women were anovulatory, meaning that no release of an egg from the ovaries did occur (Prior *et al.*, 2015).

Thus, most of the variability in cycle length is due to a variability in the follicular phase (Wilcox, Dunson and Baird, 2000). Cycle length also changes from menarche (the first occurrence of menstruation) to menopause. The five years following menarche and preceding menopause are marked by high variability in long cycle lengths and bleeding irregularities (Harlow, 2000; Golden and Carlson, 2008).

CHAPTER 2

Symptoms and Disorders of the Menstrual Cycle and Reproductive System

Many women experience symptoms related to the menstrual cycle, often in the late luteal phase or during menstruation (Taim *et al.*, 2023). Over 200 symptoms have been described in the literature for the premenstrual phase alone (Kadian and O'Brien, 2012). However, symptoms can be transient and not all symptoms cause significant impairment (Biggs and Demuth, 2011; O'Brien *et al.*, 2011; Taim *et al.*, 2023). Definitions and classifications of menstrual cycle disorders as well as assessment methods vary across studies (Taim *et al.*, 2023). Menstrual cycle symptoms and disorders can broadly be defined as abnormal uterine bleeding, pain and other symptomatology, which can be related (but are not limited) to premenstrual syndrome (PMS) and premenstrual dysphoric disorder (PMDD) (Taim *et al.*, 2023). Abnormal uterine bleeding includes changes in menstrual cycle pattern (i.e. disturbances in cycle length) and disturbances in bleeding duration/flow (e.g. heavy and/or prolonged bleeding; menorrhagia) (Taim *et al.*, 2023). More detailed efforts to establish formalized classifications of menstrual disorders can be found elsewhere (Practice Bulletin No. 128, 2012; Madhra *et al.*, 2014; Munro *et al.*, 2018, 2022; Taim *et al.*, 2023). Table 2.1 contains a pragmatic overview of menstrual cycle disorders and symptoms.

Table 2.1: Overview of menstrual cycle disorders and symptoms (based on Taim *et al.*, 2023)

Abnormal uterine bleeding	Disruption in: • Cycle pattern (e.g. changes in cycle length such as oligomenorrhea or amenorrhea) • Bleeding duration and/or flow (e.g. heavy menstrual bleeding—menorrhagia)
Pain	Painful periods (dysmenorrhea)
Other symptoms related to the menstrual cycle	• Premenstrual syndrome (PMS) symptoms • Premenstrual dysphoric disorder (PMDD) symptoms • Any affective and physical symptoms related to the menstrual cycle

In addition, polycystic ovary syndrome (PCOS) and endometriosis are among the most common reproductive disorders affecting women. Both disorders arc highly prevalent and can significantly impact a woman's overall wellbeing as well as reproductive health.

2.1. CHANGES IN MENSTRUAL CYCLE PATTERNS

Changes in menstrual cycle patterns present as a continuum, ranging from luteal phase deficiency and occasional failure to ovulate to chronic anovulation/amenorrhea (see Figure 2.1). Optimal menstrual health is characterized by regular ovulatory cycles. Subtle menstrual cycle disturbances, which may or may not occur with noticeable changes in bleeding patterns, include **luteal phase deficiency**, during which a short and therefore insufficient luteal phase (<10 days) results in low progesterone, as well as **anovulation**, where a regular but anovulatory cycle occurs, leading to low progesterone concentrations (Mallinson and De Souza, 2014). Luteal phase deficiency and anovulation can lead to more severe cycle pattern changes. Clinical cycle pattern disturbances include **oligomenorrhea**—long, inconsistent intervals between menstrual cycles—and **amenorrhea**, the most severe irregularity, which is characterized by the absence of bleeding for at least three months (Mallinson and De Souza, 2014).

Ovulation and menstrual bleeding can be understood as a sign of health, as the female hormones associated with the menstrual cycle are governed by intricate feedback mechanisms and are part of a complex body-wide interacting system (see section 1.2.1) (Vigil *et al.*, 2017). In other words, ovulation abnormalities and irregular cycles may point to health issues and could be associated with lifestyle, stress, genetic conditions, drugs, endocrine abnormalities, metabolic conditions and nutrition imbalances, chronic and autoimmune disorders, or tumors. Pregnancy, breastfeeding/pumping and menopause can also be cause of anovulation (Vigil *et al.*, 2017).

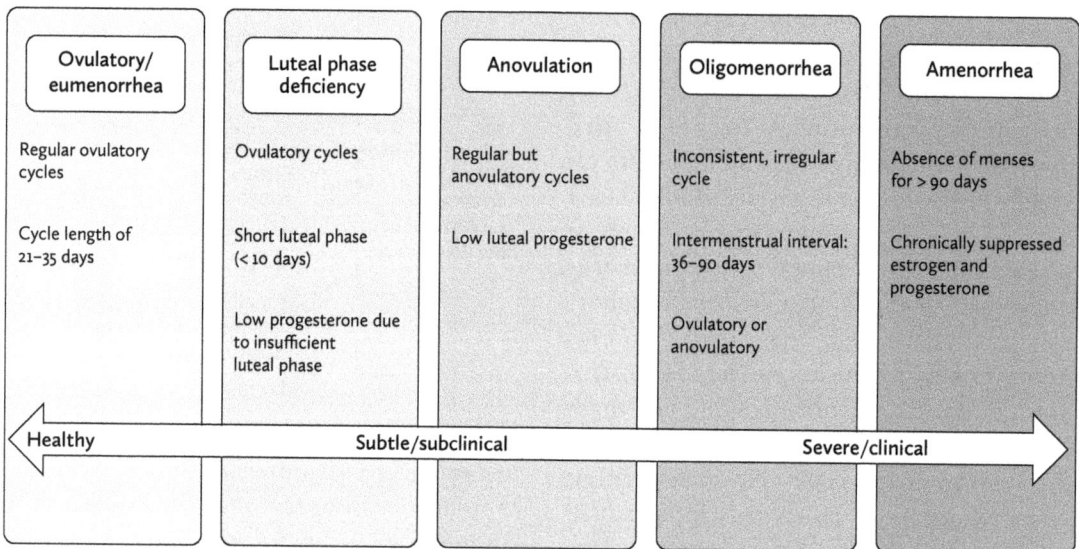

Ovulatory/ eumenorrhea	Luteal phase deficiency	Anovulation	Oligomenorrhea	Amenorrhea
Regular ovulatory cycles	Ovulatory cycles	Regular but anovulatory cycles	Inconsistent, irregular cycle	Absence of menses for > 90 days
Cycle length of 21–35 days	Short luteal phase (< 10 days)	Low luteal progesterone	Intermenstrual interval: 36–90 days	Chronically suppressed estrogen and progesterone
	Low progesterone due to insufficient luteal phase		Ovulatory or anovulatory	

Healthy ← Subtle/subclinical → Severe/clinical

Figure 2.1: Continuum of menstrual cycle pattern changes (adapted from Mallinson and De Souza, 2014). Optimal menstrual health is characterized by regular ovulatory cycles. Subtle/subclinical menstrual irregularities include luteal phase deficiency and anovulation. Inconsistent intervals between menstrual cycles are termed oligomenorrhea, and the absence of menses for at least three months is termed amenorrhea.

The many causes of amenorrhea

Causes for amenorrhea can be manifold. The missing of menses can be physiologic (e.g. during pregnancy, lactation and menopause; when using contraception). Other causes of amenorrhea can be categorized as outflow tract abnormalities (e.g. intrauterine adhesions), hypothalamic or pituitary disorders, other endocrine gland disorders, sequelae of chronic disease, or primary ovarian insufficiency. The following comprises select causes; a comprehensive description can be found elsewhere (Klein, Paradise and Reeder, 2019).

- **Primary and secondary amenorrhea:** Primary amenorrhea is defined as the lifelong absence of menstrual bleeding and requires evaluation if the first menses (menarche) has not occurred by the age of 15, or three years after secondary sexual characteristics start to develop. Secondary amenorrhea is defined by cessation of menstrual bleeding for three months when menses have been regular before, or for six months if menses have previously been irregular (Klein, Paradise and Reeder, 2019).

- **Functional hypothalamic amenorrhea** is characterized by suppression of the hypothalamic-pituitary-ovarian axis. Excessive exercise and stress can alter the rhythmic secretion of GnRH in the hypothalamus. Consequently, FSH and LH are decreased, leading to a decline in estrogen and progesterone, which in turn results in amenorrhea. Extreme weight changes as well as eating disorders can also have an influence on the hypothalamic hormones (Klein, Paradise and Reeder, 2019).

- **Hyperprolactinemia** is related to the pituitary gland and presents with elevated serum concentrations of prolactin (Klein, Paradise and Reeder, 2019). Excessive production of prolactin can create a negative feedback loop, resulting in decreased production of FSH and LH and consequently amenorrhea. Hyperprolactinemia can be caused by benign tumors of the pituitary gland, chronic kidney disease, stress, high levels of activity, nipple stimulation, pregnancy and medications (Freeman *et al.*, 2000; Oyelowo, 2007; Klein, Paradise and Reeder, 2019).

- **Other endocrine causes** comprise polycystic ovary syndrome (PCOS) and thyroid diseases. PCOS manifests with the chronic absence of ovulation, leading to oligomenorrhea or amenorrhea in most patients (Klein, Paradise and Reeder, 2019; Sadeghi, 2022). While hypothyroidism can lead to an increase in prolactin and subsequently impact amenorrhea (see above), hyperthyroidism can interfere with LH (and possibly FSH) production and thereby impact the menstrual cycle (Bahar *et al.*, 2011; Ansari and Almalki, 2016; Ren and Zhu, 2022).

In female athletes, irregularities in menstrual cycle patterns are commonplace, particularly in gymnastics and endurance disciplines (Gimunová *et al.*, 2022; Taim *et al.*, 2023). Information on the prevalence of luteal deficiency and anovulation in female athletes is scarce, which is probably due to the fact that recognition of these irregularities requires daily measurement of LH and ovarian hormones, which is costly and time-consuming. Nonetheless, information about these subtle menstrual cycle changes is valuable for athletes and practitioners as they represent early warning signs of ovarian suppression (Taim *et al.*, 2023). Prevalence of oligomenorrhea and amenorrhea among female athletes appears to be higher than in the general population, supporting the viewpoint that female athletes are more susceptible to severe menstrual cycle pattern changes, particularly as they relate to hypothalamic origin (see text box "The many causes of amenorrhea") (Manore, 2002; Taim *et al.*, 2023). A female athlete's team (coaches, physios etc.) can help monitor menstrual irregularities by creating a safe and welcoming environment where women feel comfortable discussing their reproductive health (Klein, Paradise and Reeder, 2019). Any bleeding pattern irregularity in female athletes requires consideration and priority, as it can lead to lifelong negative health consequences such as poor bone health (Taim *et al.*, 2023). Practitioners should furthermore educate themselves about Relative Energy Deficiency in Sports (RED-S) (see section 4.3), as irregular or missing menses can be part of low energy availability in athletes.

2.2. CHANGES IN BLEEDING DURATION AND/OR FLOW

Heavy or prolonged bleeding (menorrhagia) poses a health problem for many women, affecting up to 30% of women of reproductive age, negatively impacting their quality of life (El-Hemaidi, Gharaibeh and Shehata, 2007; James *et al.*, 2011). Prevalence increases with age and peaks in perimenopause (Duckitt, 2010). Although there is currently no universally accepted definition of menorrhagia, it can broadly be defined as excessive menstrual bleeding and can be characterized by bleeding longer than seven days, blood loss of over 80 mL per menstrual cycle, lowered ferritin levels, passing clots greater than 1.1 in. or 2.8 cm in diameter, and soaking through a pad or tampon within 1 hour (Warner *et al.*, 2004; James *et al.*, 2009, 2011; Davies and Kadir, 2017). There are a number of causes for menorrhagia, including various diseases which should be assessed by medical doctors; in later stages of a woman's life, menorrhagia can be caused by perimenopausal anovulation (James *et al.*, 2011).

In female athletes, prevalence of heavy menstrual bleeding ranges from approximately 3% to 52%. This raises the potential for iron deficiency and anemia, particularly in endurance athletes (Bruinvels *et al.*, 2016; Taim *et al.*, 2023).

2.3. PAINFUL MENSES

Painful menstruations (dysmenorrhea) affect up to 50–90% of women, leading to decreased quality of life, increased risk of depression and anxiety, and absence from school or work (McKenna and Fogleman, 2021). Primary dysmenorrhea is mediated by elevated inflammatory markers (prostaglandin, leukotriene), which cause uterine contractility and cramping pain (ACOG Committee Opinion No. 760: Dysmenorrhea and Endometriosis in the Adolescent, 2018; Oladosu, Tu and Hellman, 2018; McKenna and Fogleman, 2021). Secondary dysmenorrhea accounts for about 10% of cases and is related to pelvic pathology, such as endometriosis, pelvic adhesions or inflammatory conditions (ACOG Committee Opinion No. 760: Dysmenorrhea and Endometriosis in the Adolescent, 2018; McKenna and Fogleman, 2021). Despite its high prevalence, few women seek health care for dysmenorrhea, for example because they assume symptoms are normal/tolerable, feel embarrassed, think providers wouldn't help, and are unaware of treatment options (Chen *et al.*, 2018). Moreover, young women appear to receive little education on dysmenorrhea and experience negative attitudes and stigma regarding menses, resulting in unsupportive environments for young females to learn adequate coping skills (Ní Chéileachair, McGuire and Durand, 2022). Practitioners are therefore called to be part of reforming education and openness related to menses in general, and painful periods in particular.

Dysmenorrhea has been reported to be the most prevalent menstrual cycle disorder among female athletes, with approximately one third commonly experiencing period pain (Taim *et al.*, 2023). Generally, painful periods in athletes are about as common as in the general population; a number of studies, however, report a lower prevalence in female athletes, suggesting that exercise training has beneficial effects on dysmenorrhea (Mukherjee, Mishra and Ray, 2014; Vannuccini *et al.*, 2020; Taim *et al.*, 2023). A 2019 systematic review concluded that exercising for 45–60 minutes, three times per week or more,

regardless of intensity, may reduce menstrual pain intensity significantly. Women may therefore combine exercise with other modalities (such as non-steroidal anti-inflammatory drugs, NSAIDs) (Armour *et al.*, 2019).

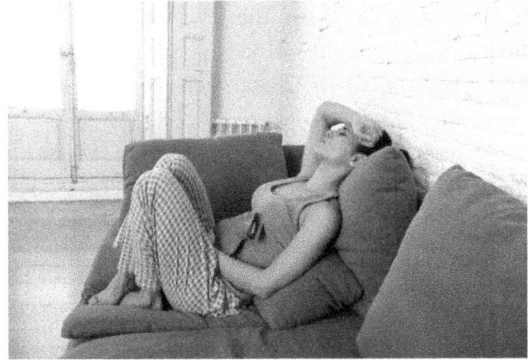

Photo 2.1: Painful periods affect a high percentage of women and are a major cause for absenteeism (McKenna and Fogleman, 2021). Few women seek healthcare for dysmenorrhea, because of stigma and insufficient education related to menstrual cycle pain.

2.4. PREMENSTRUAL SYNDROME (PMS) AND PREMENSTRUAL DYSPHORIC DISORDER (PMDD)

Premenstrual symptoms impair the quality of life of many women (Yonkers and Simoni, 2018; Takeda, 2023). To some degree, most women experience physiological or psychological changes in the late luteal phase of the menstrual cycle (Cary and Simpson, 2024). As diseases with intense symptoms, premenstrual syndrome (PMS) has been classified in the field of gynecology, and premenstrual dysphoric disorder (PMDD) in the field of psychiatry (Takeda, 2023). In recent years, these diseases have collectively been recognized as premenstrual disorders and are thought to exist along a continuum (Takeda, 2023). Premenstrual disorders are characterized by repetitive, cyclical symptoms occurring in the luteal phase of the menstrual cycle. The disorders can present with a wide array of symptoms,

including psychological, physical and behavioral indications (Taim *et al.*, 2023). Criteria for PMS put forth by the International Society for Premenstrual Disorders and the Royal College of Obstetricians and Gynecologists (see Table 2.2) do not stipulate any particular symptom or a minimum number of symptoms (O'Brien *et al.*, 2011; Kadian and O'Brien, 2012; Yonkers and Simoni, 2018). However, women with predominantly physical symptoms or subthreshold levels for PMDD are considered to have PMS (Yonkers and Simoni, 2018), while females suffering from PMDD require at least five predominantly affective symptoms in association with functional impairment to be diagnosed (Yonkers and Simoni, 2018). Thus, PMDD is acknowledged as a severe clinical mood disorder, and criteria for PMDD are more stringent (Yonkers and Simoni, 2018). Examples for affective symptoms include feeling suddenly sad or tearful, increased sensitivity to rejection, marked anxiety, marked depressed mood, feelings of hopelessness, decreased interest in usual activities, sense of being out of control, lethargy, hypersomnia and insomnia. The full list of diagnostic criteria can be found in the *Diagnostic and Statistical Manual of Mental Disorders* (American Psychiatric Association, 2013).

Table 2.2: Criteria for premenstrual syndrome (PMS) (based on O'Brien *et al.*, 2011; Yonkers and Simoni, 2018)

Premenstrual syndrome
Physical or emotional symptoms
Symptoms are present during luteal phase and subside as menstruation begins
A symptom-free week
Symptoms are associated with significant impairment during luteal phase

Prevalence of PMS has been reported to be between 20% and 35%, while PMDD rates range from 1.2% to 6.4% in women of reproductive age (Cohen *et al.*, 2002; Borenstein *et al.*, 2007; Gehlert *et al.*, 2009; Qiao *et al.*, 2012; Yonkers and Simoni, 2018; Prado *et al.*, 2021a). Those approaching menopause may also experience a mix of PMS, heavy bleeding and menopause symptoms (Kadian and O'Brien, 2012). It is of note, though, that estimates of PMS and PMDD are difficult to obtain, because retrospective reports, which are often used in studies, can lead to recall bias (Rubinow and Roy Byrne, 1984). This insight directly translates to the individual work with women suffering premenstrual symptoms; it appears advantageous for females to track data prospectively for at least two menstrual cycles (Kadian and O'Brien, 2012), for example through diaries or apps.

Causes for premenstrual disorders—current theories on allopregnanolone and serotonin

While the precise causes for premenstrual disorders remain to be elucidated, the involvement of hormonal fluctuations appears likely, since premenstrual symptoms occur during a hormonally dynamic phase of the menstrual cycle (Hantsoo and Epperson, 2020; Takeda, 2023). A leading theory suggests that some women may have suboptimal central nervous system sensitivity to neuroactive steroids (Yonkers and Simoni, 2018). Neuroactive steroid hormones interact with neuron receptors such as the γ-amino butyric acid (GABA)-A receptor. One of these hormones, which is thought to play a role in the pathophysiology of PMDD, is allopregnanolone, a progesterone metabolite mirroring the levels of progesterone. The affective symptom expression related to PMDD seems to be associated with an impaired interaction between allopregnanolone and GABA-A receptors (GABA-A receptors respond suboptimally to allopregnanolone fluctuations across the menstrual cycle) (Hantsoo and Epperson, 2020). In addition to the mood symptoms observed in PMDD, women experience greater subjectively perceived stress as well as altered physiologic stress responsivity, such as changes in the hypothalamic-pituitary-adrenal (HPA) axis (see Chapter 5). Alterations in stress response may also be impacted by a poor interaction between allopregnanolone and GABA-A receptors (Hantsoo and Epperson, 2020).

A more classical theory suggests that premenstrual disorders may be rooted in a deficit within the functioning of the serotonin system and serotonin transporters (Eriksson, 2014). Consistent with these theories, evidence supports the efficacy of serotonin reuptake inhibitors in the treatment of premenstrual disorders; they seem to be effective in impacting allopregnanolone levels as well (Gracia *et al.*, 2009).

Periods and menstrual symptoms in transgender and non-binary people

Menses are often distressing for those who are assigned female at birth, but do not identify as female (Schwartz, Bear and Kazak, 2023). Adolescents may experience particular distress in anticipation of menarche (Coleman *et al.*, 2022). Gender diverse people often request menstrual management to alleviate their experienced dysphoria related to menstruation (Schwartz *et al.*, 2022). Menstrual management refers to the use of hormonal treatment to improve menses and related experience, and/or to serve as a bridging method to achieve amenorrhea (Schwartz, Bear and Kazak, 2023). However, little published information on this topic exists. The World Professional Association for Transgender Health Standards of Care suggests the use of progestin for shorter time periods to assist with menstrual cessation before or during the early phases of gender-affirming testosterone therapy; continuous oral contraceptives can also be used as a means to suppress menses, for example for those seeking contraception. In the latter case, individuals should be counseled on the possible side effect of breast development (Coleman *et al.*, 2022).

While evidence remains scarce, some accounts report dysmenorrhea, PCOS and endometriosis in transmasculine individuals. Current treatment options for symptoms vary widely, as there is no data to support one treatment over the other—calling for future research regarding gynecologic conditions in transgender populations (Shim, Laufer and Grimstad, 2020).

Every woman's period is different—changing the narrative

The majority of research on menstrual cycle symptoms reports detrimental conditions, reflecting a negative bias. However, the menstrual cycle—and menstruation in particular—is not experienced similarly by all women. About 5–15% of females experience an increase in wellbeing, energy and excitement during their menses; some also report increased activity and performance as well as heightened sexuality during their period (Logue and Moos, 1988).

Besides biological reasons, such as an individual's response to fluctuating hormone levels, menstruation-related beliefs and expectations could also play a role in these positive experiences (Logue and Moos, 1988).

Both negative and positive effects across the menstrual cycle should be considered by future research as well as from a practical standpoint (Taim *et al.*, 2023). Women should track and understand their menstrual cycle patterns and symptoms and identify potential performance and recovery trends across the cycle. To establish an understanding of the entirety of the menstrual cycle, symptoms as well as performance and recovery patterns should be prospectively charted for at least two menstrual cycles. In creating a welcoming, empathic and informed atmosphere in working with female athletes, practitioners can support their clients through their menstrual cycle to optimize wellbeing and performance.

In female athletes, prevalence of PMS is also high, ranging from 49% to 60% in studies using prospective charting of symptoms; PMDD prevalence in athletes ranges from 1% to 13% across studies (Taim *et al.*, 2023). Treatments supporting positive, mood-stabilizing health habits such as relaxation techniques, yoga, massages and cognitive behavioral therapy have been recommended (Prior *et al.*, 1987; Hunter *et al.*, 2002; Tsai, 2016; Jose *et al.*, 2022). In addition, exercise is a primary intervention and has shown to reduce psychological, physical and behavioral PMS symptoms (Pearce *et al.*, 2020). Various types of exercise have been found to be effective in symptom reduction; however, the most effective type of exercise remains unclear. Individuals are therefore encouraged to choose a type of physical activity to their liking (Liguori, Saraiello and Calella, 2023). Furthermore, exercising regularly over longer periods of time is crucial for favorable outcomes (Maged *et al.*, 2018). For aerobic exercise specifically, a dose of 30 minutes of exercise, three to five times per week, has been found to be effective in reducing physical PMS symptoms (Ravichandran and Janakiraman, 2022). Regarding dietary modifications, some evidence suggests that a carbohydrate-rich diet during the luteal phase can alleviate symptoms, presumably because they increase serotonin availability (Sayegh *et al.*, 1995). An in-depth discussion of available non-pharmacological and pharmacological treatment options exceeds the present work, but can be found elsewhere (Yonkers and Simoni, 2018).

2.5. POLYCYSTIC OVARY SYNDROME

Polycystic ovary syndrome (PCOS) is a lifelong disorder and represents the most common chronic reproductive and metabolic disorder affecting women of reproductive age (Lizneva *et al.*, 2016; Belenkaia *et al.*, 2019). Prevalence amounts to 4–21% worldwide (Rababa'h, Matani and Yehya, 2022). Symptoms comprise:

- **irregularities in menstrual cycle pattern** (infrequent or very light menstruation)

- **hyperandrogenism** (excessive production of androgens such as testosterone, primarily manifesting as acne and hirsutism, i.e. male-patterned hair growth)

- **polycystic ovaries** (20 or more small cysts, measuring 2–9 mm in diameter, present in one ovary) (Azziz *et al.*, 2009; Meier, 2018; Lim *et al.*, 2019; Rababa'h, Matani and Yehya, 2022; Christ and Cedars, 2023; Teede *et al.*, 2023).

Women present with different manifestations of these symptoms depending on age, lifestyle and disease phenotype (Meier, 2018). PCOS is further associated with 80% of anovulatory infertility (failure to conceive) and an increased risk for metabolic disorders such as impaired glucose tolerance and diabetes mellitus (Lim *et al.*, 2019; Rababa'h, Matani and Yehya, 2022). Low health-related quality of life, depression, anxiety and body-image difficulties are common in this population as well (Himelein and Thatcher, 2006; Barnard *et al.*, 2007; Bhattacharya and Jha, 2010; Deeks, Gibson-Helm and Teede, 2010).

To date, PCOS is uncurable, but symptoms can be successfully managed pharmacologically and with lifestyle interventions (Islam *et al.*, 2022). Lifestyle changes primarily target obesity (which accounts for 90% of infertility cases associated with PCOS), insulin signaling and fasting insulin levels (Nandi *et al.*, 2014; Stepto *et al.*, 2020). As overweight constitutes an independent factor of infertility, weight reduction can improve fertility and menstrual cycle irregularities in obese women with PCOS (Bloom *et al.*, 2020). In this context, it is also interesting that morphological and functional changes in adipose tissue are observed in women with PCOS, including increased adipocytes and heightened secretion of proinflammatory cytokines (Dong and Rees, 2023). While an optimal dose-response relationship for exercise in PCOS may not be feasible due to the highly individual manifestation of the syndrome, at least 150 minutes of physical activity per week have been suggested (Woodward, Klonizakis and Broom, 2020). However, women with PCOS report difficulty in losing weight and PCOS patients are found to be more sedentary and don't tend to engage in vigorous exercise (Gu *et al.*, 2022; Dong and Rees, 2023). Barriers to exercise and measures of adherence should therefore be of particular importance when working with PCOS patients. Supervised, structured exercise may help to engage women with PCOS in physical activity (Turan *et al.*, 2015; Vizza *et al.*, 2016). Exercise can furthermore improve psychological wellbeing in women with PCOS (Woodward, Klonizakis and Broom, 2020). For a comprehensive overview of treatment options, especially of a pharmacological nature, reference is made to other sources (Dong and Rees, 2023).

PCOS etiology

The precise mechanism for PCOS-induced anovulation remains to be elucidated (Rababa'h, Matani and Yehya, 2022). A genetic susceptibility appears to be part of the etiology (Diamanti-Kandarakis and Dunaif, 2012). Mechanisms related to hyperandrogenism, insulin resistance and Anti-Müllerian hormone have been discussed in the light of PCOS pathophysiology (Fahs *et al.*, 2023). **Hyperandrogenism** is the biochemical hallmark of PCOS (Kanbour and Dobs, 2022). High levels of androgens can result from an imbalance in the HPO axis (see section 1.2.1): PCOS is characterized by an increased frequency of GnRH pulsatility at the level of the hypothalamus, leading to elevated LH relative to FSH secretion at the pituitary (Saadia, 2020). Heightened LH can result in an enlargement of follicular theca cells in the ovary and consequent increase in testosterone production (Hughesdon, 1982; Haisenleder *et al.*, 1991; Kanbour and Dobs, 2022).

Insulin resistance is considered to be part of the pathophysiology as well; 12–60% of women with PCOS have insulin resistance. While some groups of lean women with PCOS may have normal insulin sensitivity, obese females with PCOS are thought to suffer from insulin resistance for the largest part (Diamanti-Kandarakis and Dunaif, 2012; Kim *et al.*, 2019). Affected women show disruptions in insulin signaling (Diamanti-Kandarakis and Dunaif, 2012). The direct influence of androgens as well as intrauterine androgen exposure have been discussed as contributing factors in insulin resistance related to PCOS (Diamanti-Kandarakis and Dunaif, 2012). Recent studies have suggested the gut microbiota may be also related to insulin resistance in PCOS (Armanini *et al.*, 2022). Insulin resistance and resulting high serum concentration of insulin can impact GnRH secretion at the hypothalamus by increasing its hyperpulsatility, thereby contributing to hyperandrogenism (Fahs *et al.*, 2023). Disturbed regulation of insulin in the central nervous system has also been connected to poor follicular maturation in animal models (Bruning *et al.*, 2000). Thus, PCOS research has brought forward the insight that insulin is an important hormone related to the reproductive system and insulin signaling in the central nervous system is critical for ovulation (Diamanti-Kandarakis and Dunaif, 2012).

Anti-Müllerian hormone (AMH) is secreted by follicular cells and regulates the number of growing follicles and their selection as dominant follicle. Women with PCOS have high concentrations of AMH, produced by numerous small growing follicles. However, no explanation for this overproduction has been identified (Bedenk, Vrtačnik-Bokal and Virant-Klun, 2020; Fahs *et al.*, 2023). Increased AMH production in PCOS may be a factor in LH hypersecretion (Waghmare and Shanoo, 2023).

2.6. ENDOMETRIOSIS

Endometriosis can be defined as the presence of endometrial tissue (tissue similar to the lining of the uterus) in abnormal locations, such as the pelvic peritoneum and ovaries. While it mainly affects the pelvic cavity, endometrial lesions have also been found in other organs such as the lungs and brain (Burney and Giudice, 2012; Marquardt et al., 2019). Endometriosis is the most common reason for pelvic pain in females of reproductive age, affecting 2–10% of this population (Bulun et al., 2019; Zondervan et al., 2022; Tourny et al., 2023). Endometriosis can be asymptomatic; when accompanied by symptoms, disabling pain before and/or during menstruation, painful sexual intercourse, pain when urinating and chronic pelvic pain can be part of the disease pattern (Pugsley and Ballard, 2007; Falcone and Lebovic, 2011; Falcone and Flyckt-Rebecca, 2018). The severe and regular pain can further lead to fatigue, insomnia, depression and stress, and consequently affect the social life and interaction of endometriosis patients (Ramin-Wright et al., 2018; Soliman et al., 2021; Tourny et al., 2023). Endometriosis is also associated with infertility (Bulun et al., 2019).

Symptoms can be differentiated by the localization of the lesions (e.g. lesions in the bladder can lead to pain when urinating) (Maccagnano et al., 2013; Tourny et al., 2023). Due to heterogeneous symptom presentation, diagnosis is complex and it can take many years for affected women to receive a diagnosis (mean latency from onset of symptoms to definitive diagnosis is 6.7 years) (Tourny et al., 2023).

Further hallmarks of endometriosis are inflammation, estrogen dependence/dominance and progesterone resistance (Burney and Giudice, 2012). It has been well established that inflammation and immune dysfunction is a central process in endometriosis (Wang, Nicholes and Shih, 2020). Although being benign in nature, endometrial lesions are considered abnormal tissues by the body due to their anomalous location. Consequently, inflammatory cells may be recruited to the site of endometriosis in an effort to eliminate the lesion. Some lesions might not be cleared by a physiologic inflammatory process and may persist as active inflammatory sites, while other lesions may be replaced with fibrotic tissue (so called white lesions), which can cause adhesions (Wang, Nicholes and Shih, 2020). Several immune cells are prevalent in the microenvironment of endometriosis (e.g. macrophages, B-lymphocytes, T-regulatory cells). The peritoneal fluid is marked by increased levels of immune cells, such as macrophages, and differences in cytokine profiles as well (Burney and Giudice, 2012; Wang, Nicholes and Shih, 2020). This inflammatory environment within the pelvis can contribute to the pain experience of women with endometriosis (Burney and Giudice, 2012). Although it is mostly the ectopic endometrial tissue outside the uterus which is inflammatory, infiltration of macrophages into the endometrial tissue of the uterus in endometriosis patients has also been reported (Berbic et al., 2009; Wang, Nicholes and Shih, 2020).

Another difference observed in women with endometriosis is a disruption in estrogen and progesterone signaling. Patients can exhibit higher activity of estrogen pathways and increased local estrogen production at the endometrial sites, along with lower activity of progesterone pathways and progesterone resistance, which is often linked to reduced progesterone levels. As progesterone has well-described anti-inflammatory properties, low progesterone concentrations and reduced progesterone receptor activity cannot counteract the overactive proinflammatory estrogen pathways in endometriosis (Burney and Giudice, 2012; Wang, Nicholes and Shih, 2020). The hormone imbalance can therefore lead to heightened inflammation and may explain the decreased ability of the uterus to establish pregnancy (Marquardt et al., 2019; Wang, Nicholes and Shih, 2020).

Mechanisms behind endometriosis

Both genetic as well as environmental influences appear to be involved in the etiology of endometriosis, yet the precise mechanisms of endometriosis remain poorly understood (Saha et al., 2015; Rahmioglu et al., 2023). Although various theories shed light on different possible origins of endometriosis, no single theory explains all of the different pathological features and clinical presentations of the disease (Wang, Nicholes and Shih, 2020). Possible mechanisms include the theory of retrograde menstruation (Sampson theory), the coelomic metaplasia theory, the Müllerian remnant theory, the stem cell theory and the vascular and lymphatic metastasis theory (Tourny et al., 2023). Their main assumptions are listed below.

- **Theory of retrograde menstruation (Sampson theory)** purports that menstrual blood containing endometrial cells flows backward through patent fallopian tubes into the peritoneal cavity, where these cells may implant and grow into endometrial lesions. However, a large percentage of women experience retrograde menstruation, but without the development of endometriosis. Risk factors such as longer menstrual flow or uterine outflow obstruction, which increase the quantity of retrogradely flushed cells, might explain why some women develop the disorder. The retrograde menstruation theory is the most widely accepted explanation for the dissemination of endometrial cells. While it can explain ovarian and peritoneal endometriosis, it cannot elucidate lesions outside the peritoneal cavity (Sampson, 1940; Nisolle and Donnez, 1997; D'Hooghe and Debrock, 2002; Burney and Giudice, 2012; Yovich et al., 2020; Lamceva, Uljanovs and Strumfa, 2023).

- **Coelomic metaplasia theory** involves the transformation of cells lining the pelvic cavity (coelomic cells) into endometrial-like tissue outside the uterus due to certain stimuli or conditions. Agents responsible for such transformations remain poorly understood; endocrine disrupting chemicals have been discussed as candidates (Crain et al., 2008; Burney and Giudice, 2012).

- **Müllerian remnant theory** assumes that residual embryonic cells from the Müllerian ducts, which normally develop into the female reproductive system, can persist in the pelvic region. These cells may later develop into endometrial tissue outside the uterus under the influence of estrogen beginning at puberty, or in response to estrogen mimetics (Burney and Giudice, 2012).

- **Stem cell theory** argues that circulating stem cells intended to repair and regenerate the endometrium of the uterus after menstruation become overactive and trapped outside the uterus. These cells then differentiate into endometric tissues, leading to the establishment of endometriotic lesions. Once formed, these tissues become subject to immune surveillance, resulting in chronic inflammation (Wang, Nicholes and Shih, 2020).

- **Lymphatic and vascular (benign) metastasis theory** suggests that endometrial cells can spread from the uterine body to other parts of the body through lymphatic ducts and blood vessels. This theory is supported by histologically proven endometriotic lesions in locations distant from the uterus, such as the lungs, bone and brain (Sampson, 1927; Javert, 1952; Jubanyik and Comite, 1997; Burney and Giudice, 2012; Jerman and Hey-Cunningham, 2015).

Treatment of endometriosis depends on symptomatology and patients' perspectives (Tourny *et al.*, 2023). Complementary medicine, stress relief interventions and physical activity can support women's quality of life and can stabilize symptoms in some cases (Tourny *et al.*, 2023). Various studies have looked at the effects of psychological and mind-body interventions on endometriosis symptoms. A 2019 systematic review found that interventions such as yoga, mindfulness, cognitive behavioral therapy, relaxation training and biofeedback showed promise in alleviating pain, depression, anxiety, fatigue and stress in women with endometriosis. However, the methodological quality of studies was low, making it unfeasible to draw definitive conclusions about the efficacy of the included interventions (Evans *et al.*, 2019). Progressive muscle relaxation techniques have also been found to be effective in improving depression, anxiety and quality of life in women with endometriosis who received GnRH agonist therapy (Zhao *et al.*, 2012). Patients can further benefit from physiotherapy, manual therapy and acupuncture (Mira *et al.*, 2018; Wójcik, Szczepaniak and Placek, 2022).

Evidence regarding the effects of physical activity and exercise on symptom improvement in endometriosis patients is scarce (Tourny *et al.*, 2023). Physical activity and exercise may be beneficial for endometriosis because it has anti-inflammatory effects, may help to lower estrogen levels, and can improve pain (Awad *et al.*, 2017; Ensari *et al.*, 2022; Tourny *et al.*, 2023). However, women with endometriosis have reported to be at risk for physical inactivity. A 2022 study including 1009 women with endometriosis reported a mean weekly frequency of exercise of only 1.43. Walking and yoga were the most frequently reported exercise modalities in the examined sample (Ensari *et al.*, 2022).

In more severe symptomatology, treatment often includes hormone treatment, pain relievers and surgery to remove affected tissue (Bulun *et al.*, 2019). Hormonal therapy aims to block menstruation, for example by inhibiting the HPO axis. GnRH antagonists downregulate the HPO axis and therefore induce a hypoestrogenic state. Combined oral contraceptives are used to inhibit ovarian function; progestin-only preparations are often used for long-term treatment. However, most hormonal therapies are not suitable for women who want to become pregnant; in addition, not all patients respond to progesterone therapy, due to progesterone resistance (Wang, Nicholes and Shih, 2020; Vannuccini *et al.*, 2022; Rzewuska *et al.*, 2023; Tourny *et al.*, 2023).

CHAPTER 3

Move Smartly: How to Align Physical Activity and Training with the Menstrual Cycle

3.1. FEMALE HORMONE EFFECTS ON THE MUSCULOSKELETAL AND OTHER BODY SYSTEMS

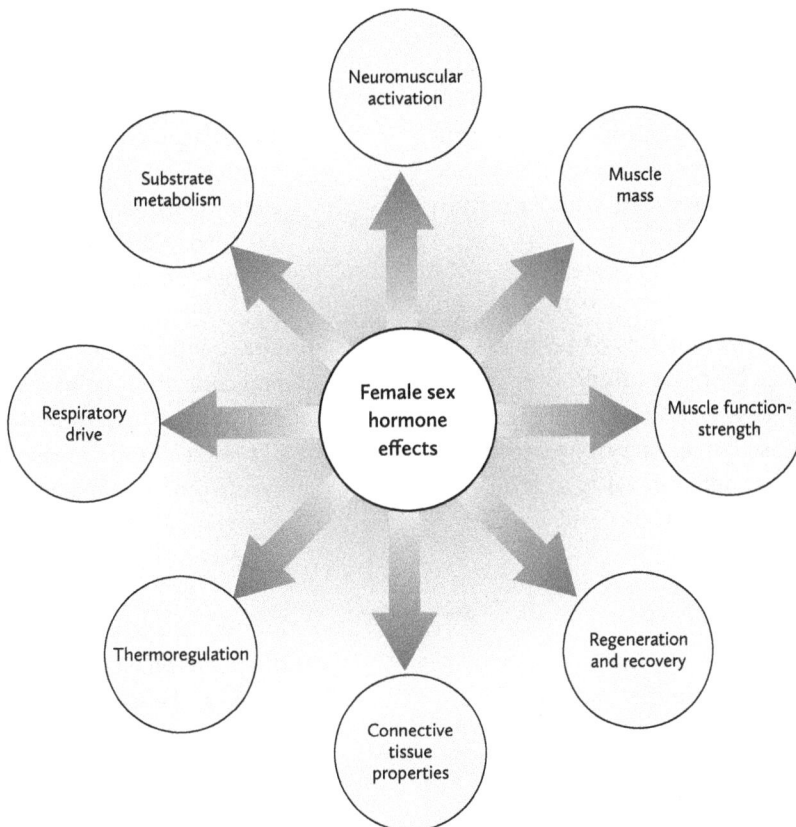

Figure 3.1: Potential direct and indirect mechanisms behind the effects of female sex hormones on the musculoskeletal system.

As far as musculoskeletal system morphology, function and adaptations are concerned, there are no clear answers to the question of whether female hormones are advantageous. Female hormones may concurrently have beneficial as well as non-beneficial effects (Legerlotz and Hansen, 2020). For example, estrogen has been reported to increase muscle mass and strength, while also potentially compromising the mechanical properties of fascial tissues (such as ligaments and tendons). This section discusses potential mechanisms behind the effects of female sex hormones (predominantly estrogen and progesterone) on the musculoskeletal system. Effects on thermoregulation and respiration are also considered.

Proposed mechanisms behind the effects of female sex hormones on the musculoskeletal system—some direct, some more indirect in nature—comprise responses to hormonal alterations related to neuromuscular activation, muscle mass, muscle function (i.e. strength), regeneration, connective tissue properties, thermoregulation, respiratory drive and substrate metabolism.

How are the mechanisms of female sex hormones being studied?

The influence of sex hormones such as estrogen on the musculoskeletal system becomes evident through different types of studies, including (Pellegrino, Tiidus and Vandenboom, 2022):

- Molecular biology

  - For example, studies on the effects of estrogen on satellite cells in cell cultures and analysis of inflammatory markers can provide information about muscle regeneration.

- Animal models

  - In rodents, ovaries are removed to mimic human menopause (i.e. estrogen deficiency); then, hormone replacement is compared with no hormone replacement to study the influence of hormones.

  - Rodents lacking estrogen receptors (e.g. ERα knockout mice) provide a model for evaluating estrogen receptor action (Walker and Korach, 2004).

- Human models/clinical studies

  - Hormone replacement therapy-use in postmenopausal women is compared with non-use to examine the effects of the administered hormones (see section 8.5). In studies using hormonal replacement, combined therapies (estrogen plus progestin) are more commonly used, which may limit the ability to understand the distinct role of single hormones.

  - Oral contraception: Comparison of oral contraception use with non-use can help to understand differences between the downregulated hormonal profile while on the pill with the regular menstrual cycle (see Chapter 6).

  - Menstrual cycle phases: Women in different phases of the menstrual cycle can be examined to draw conclusions about different hormonal profiles. Between-group comparisons as well as within-subject analyses are possible.

- **Neuromuscular activation:** Female sex hormones can be responsible for changes in force production. While estrogen has a neuroexcitatory effect, progesterone can inhibit cortical excitability, which can translate into a positive and negative relationship with force production, respectively (Phillips *et al.*, 1996; Smith *et al.*, 2002; Gordon *et al.*, 2013; Pallavi, Souza and Shivaprakash, 2017; Ansdell *et al.*, 2019). Accordingly, it could be assumed that greater strength and power outputs could be observed during the late follicular phase, when estrogen peaks and progesterone is low (Carmichael *et al.*, 2021).

- **Muscle mass:** Estrogen is known for its anabolic effects on skeletal muscle and may thus regulate the hypertrophic response to resistance training (Lowe, Baltgalvis and Greising, 2010; Kissow *et al.*, 2022). Estrogen deficiency, on the other hand, has shown to decrease muscle cross-sectional area and limit regrowth in animal models (McClung *et al.*, 2006; Kitajima and Ono, 2016). Accordingly, it has been hypothesized that recovery and reconstruction of muscle fibers may be faster when estradiol is high, for example in the mid to late follicular phase (Kissow *et al.*, 2022). It should be noted that much of the work on estrogen and muscle in humans has been done in association with aging, that is, in studies involving postmenopausal women (see text box "How are the mechanisms of female sex hormones being studied?"). Postmenopausal women present with a rapid decline in muscle mass and strength as well as a reduced sensitivity to anabolic stimuli compared to men (Smith *et al.*, 2014; Chidi-Ogbolu and Baar, 2018). Hormone replacement theory has proven to be beneficial for postmenopausal muscle mass and function, particularly in conjunction with exercise, pointing to a possible increase in anabolic response to exercise (Chidi-Ogbolu and Baar, 2018). Progesterone, on the other hand, is thought to have catabolic effects and therefore impact muscle protein synthesis negatively. Healthy women have greater protein degradation during the luteal phase compared to the follicular phase (Lamont, Lemon and Bruot, 1987; Kriengsinyos *et al.*, 2004; Kissow *et al.*, 2022). Moreover, studies with combined oral contraceptives (see Chapter 6) have reported lower levels of myofibrillar protein synthesis associated with oral contraceptive preparations involving particularly high levels of progesterone (Hansen *et al.*, 2011). With progesterone thought to have anti-estrogenic effects, it could be speculated that the beneficial strength performance effects of estrogen are likely to be greater in the late follicular and ovulatory phases when estrogen is high but without the interference of progesterone (compared to mid luteal when both progesterone and estrogen are elevated) (McNulty *et al.*, 2020).

- **Muscle function and strength:** Estrogen is thought to benefit muscle strength (Lowe, Baltgalvis and Greising, 2010). For example, it has been shown that muscle fibers from ovariectomized rats generated less force compared with muscle fibers from ovary-intact rats (Wattanapermpool and Reiser, 1999). Evidence indicates that this is accomplished by improving the intrinsic quality of the muscle, meaning muscle fibers are enabled to generate greater force (Lowe, Baltgalvis and Greising, 2010). As a potential mechanism, it has been proposed that sex hormones affect contractile muscle proteins at the molecular level. In support of this, an animal study showed that ovariectomy in mice led to reductions in strong-binding myosin as well as force generation, while estradiol treatment reversed those reductions (Moran *et al.*, 2007). Thus, myosin appears to be detrimentally affected by the lack of estradiol—not in quantity, but in quality (i.e. how myosin binds to actin) (Lowe, Baltgalvis and Greising, 2010).

Another hypothesis states that fluctuations of bioavailable testosterone throughout the menstrual cycle could lead to changes in strength outcomes. Increases in testosterone can improve performance via improved neural activation, contractile properties and motor system function (Crewther *et al.*, 2011). Testosterone has been shown to peak during ovulation; however, available data stems from basal salivary and serum testing, and it is unknown if bioavailable testosterone rises during ovulation as well (Dougherty *et al.*, 1997; Cook, Kilduff and Crewther, 2018).

- **Muscle regeneration and recovery:** Different key measures—such as satellite cell activity and inflammatory response—can be studied to examine muscle recovery and regeneration. Satellite cells are adult muscle stem cells responsible for repairing and regenerating muscle tissue after exercise, injury or stress. As they express estrogen receptors, satellite cells are directly influenced by estrogen signaling. Beneficial effects of estrogen can have prophylactic effects on muscle satellite cell number and function, which can mitigate injury and enhance the post-damage repair (Pellegrino, Tiidus and Vandenboom, 2022). For example, a positive relationship has been shown between estrogen supplementation and total satellite cell number following exercise in animal models (Tiidus, Deller and Liu, 2005). Estrogen deficiency, in contrast, has been shown to mediate a reduction in satellite numbers and disrupt muscle recovery, and to be associated with a reduced ability to adapt to strength training (Larson *et al.*, 2020; Pellegrino, Tiidus and Vandenboom, 2022). Although cell-cultures and animal models have expanded our understanding of the role of estrogen on satellite function, data from human studies warrants further investigation; studies in humans have mainly been documented in postmenopausal women with or without hormonal replacement therapy (Oxfeldt *et al.*, 2022; Pellegrino, Tiidus and Vandenboom, 2022). A longitudinal study with five women showed that satellite cell numbers reduced by about 15% from perimenopause to early postmenopause (BC Collins, 2019). Estrogen further appears to have antioxidant and membrane stabilizing effects, which might offer protection against exercise-induced muscle damage and reduce inflammatory responses (McNulty *et al.*, 2020; Pellegrino, Tiidus and Vandenboom, 2022). Muscle damage, represented by exercise induced muscle damage (EIMD) and delayed onset muscle soreness (DOMS), both associated with eccentric contractions, is associated with an inflammatory response and negative effects on performance (Fatouros and Jamurtas, 2016). EIMD has been found to be greater in the early follicular phase, when estrogen is low (Romero-Parra *et al.*, 2021).

- **Connective tissue properties:** It has been recognized that female hormones such as estrogen and relaxin can impact connective tissue, for example through altering the extracellular matrix architecture, which contains structural proteins such as collagen and elastin (Fede *et al.*, 2016). Estrogen receptors have been detected in tendons, ligaments and muscular fasciae (Bridgeman *et al.*, 2010; Fede *et al.*, 2016, 2019). Different levels of estrogen can increase fascial elasticity by changing the composition of the extracellular matrix. It has been shown that high levels of estrogen, as observed during ovulation or pregnancy, can reduce the content of collagen type I, and increase the content of collagen type III and fibrillin in muscle fascia. As collagen type III and fibrillin provide a higher degree of compliance for the tissue, this hormonal profile results in more adaptable, less stiff fasciae

(Fede *et al.*, 2019). This increase in elasticity can translate to functional changes around ovulation. A 2015 study reported that plantar fascia became thinner, foot length increased and balance decreased in the periovulatory phase relative to the early follicular phase (Petrofsky and Lee, 2015). Collagen type III expression has also been reported to be significantly higher in female tendon compared to male tissue (Sullivan *et al.*, 2009).

Additionally, it has been suggested that estrogen may enhance connective tissue compliance via reduced cross-linking (Chidi-Ogbolu and Baar, 2018). These findings might have implications for health professionals working with eumenorrheic women when planning their training—for example, they may consider shifting sessions which pose a high challenge to balance into menstrual cycle phases with lower estrogen profiles to avoid falls and injuries. On the other hand, it is possible that women with hormonal dysfunctions present a dysregulated production of extracellular matrix, leading to stiffness, fibrosis and inflammation, which in turn may impact pain generation (Pavan *et al.*, 2014). Changes in tissue properties can impact biomechanical characteristics of connective tissues, such as myofascial force transmission and balance. The stiffness of tendons and ligaments has also been discussed in context of injury, which will further be elucidated in section 3.3.

- **Thermoregulation** can also impact musculoskeletal function. Elevated progesterone levels during the luteal phase alter the thermoregulatory setpoint (Carmichael *et al.*, 2021). As a result, women experience a slight increase in body temperature during the luteal phase. This increase in body temperature could alter subjectively perceived as well as objectively measured physical performance, especially in humid and hot environments (Janse De Jonge *et al.*, 2012; Sims and Heather, 2018). In short duration activity requiring power and speed via better force production and muscle contractility, increased temperature may positively affect performance (Girard, Brocherie and Bishop, 2015). However, research has found that including an active warm-up before physical activity would negate between-phase differences in body temperature, as well as possible performance effects (Somboonwong, Chutimakul and Sanguanrungsirikul, 2015). During prolonged exercise, the body temperature elevation is thought to put greater cardiovascular strain on the body, while cooling mechanisms such as skin temperature and sweat rate do not change throughout the menstrual cycle, thereby potentially limiting endurance performance in the luteal phase (Marshall, 1963; Janse De Jonge, 2003; Giersch *et al.*, 2020; Carmichael *et al.*, 2021).

- **Respiratory drive:** Although in a more indirect way, interactions between respiration and female sex hormones can also impact the musculoskeletal system. Progesterone increases ventilation, resulting in higher rate and depth of breathing in women during the luteal phase as well as during pregnancy when progesterone levels are high (Bayliss and Millhorn, 1992). Progesterone acts on central and peripheral chemoreceptors, thereby increasing sensitivity of the respiratory system to carbon dioxide (Zadek *et al.*, 2022). Whether such changes throughout the menstrual cycle affect ventilatory responses during exercise remains a matter of debate (Rael *et al.*, 2021). A recent study adhering to the highest standards of menstrual cycle phase determination (i.e. verification through ovulation kits as well as measurement of circulating sex hormones) indicated that ventilation during aerobic exercise was 7.6% lower in the late follicular phase compared to the luteal phase (Oxfeldt *et al.*, 2024).

- **Substrate metabolism:** Sex hormones are furthermore thought to alter substrate metabolism, thereby indirectly influencing the musculoskeletal system, which will further be explored in Chapter 4.

3.2. EFFECTS OF THE MENSTRUAL CYCLE ON SPORTS PERFORMANCE

Research on sports performance can be categorized into perceived (subjectively reported) and physical (objectively measured) performance (Vogel *et al.*, 2023).

3.2.1. Perceived performance

With regard to the perceived influence of the menstrual cycle on sports performance, various studies have shown that many athletes believe their performance to fluctuate throughout the menstrual cycle (Jacobson and Lentz, 1998; Armour *et al.*, 2020; Findlay *et al.*, 2020; Solli *et al.*, 2020; Carmichael *et al.*, 2021; McNamara, Harris and Minahan, 2022). Females have reported negative impacts on training, performance and daily life related to their menstrual cycle (Martin *et al.*, 2018; Armour *et al.*, 2020; Findlay *et al.*, 2020; Brown, Knight and Forrest, 2021; Vogel *et al.*, 2023). Performance is perceived to be impaired during late luteal and early follicular phases, which coincides with possible premenstrual and menstrual symptomology. One of the studies referenced above sheds light on how female athletes preparing for Olympic and Paralympic Games experience cycle phases (McNamara, Harris and Minahan, 2022). Two-thirds of the 195 elite female athletes perceived their menstrual cycle to affect their performance; the surveyed women were more likely to be affected in training than during competition. When asked at which time in their menstrual cycle they would choose to ideally compete in their targeted Olympic/Paralympic final, 42% found the window "just after their period" to be most desirable; 4% preferred to compete late in their cycle; and 1% wished to compete during their period (McNamara, Harris and Minahan, 2022).

Another recent study suggests that perception of own physical performance as well as self-reported motivation, pleasure and arousal level are positively correlated with physical performance parameters (Dam *et al.*, 2022). Physical performance impairments (measured via Wingate test and counter-movement jumps) were observed in the late early follicular and late luteal phases compared to the other menstrual cycle phases, which coincided with lower psychological wellbeing and higher pain levels. Fluctuations in sex hormones, however, were not correlated with the performance outcomes. These findings imply that psychological and physical wellbeing are predictors for performance changes. It is further interesting to note that strength-related outcomes (i.e. handgrip strength and isometric elbow flexor strength) did not undergo significant changes throughout the menstrual cycle.

3.2.2. Physical performance

With respect to objective outcomes, research has suggested that female sex hormones, particularly estrogen, might influence physical performance by impacting the cardiovascular, respiratory, neuromuscular and metabolic parameters (Ansdell *et al.*, 2019; Dam *et al.*, 2022) (see section 3.1). Objective physical performance is determined by either testing specific performance characteristics (i.e. strength- and endurance-related measures) or by quantifying sport performance as a collective of performance qualities under match or competitive conditions (Vogel *et al.*, 2023).

Various systematic reviews and meta-analyses have emerged over the last years, examining the effects of menstrual cycle phases and female sex hormones on exercise performance parameters related to strength and endurance outcomes (McNulty *et al.*, 2020; Beníčková, Gimunová and Paludo, 2024; Niering *et al.*, 2024). Narrative and umbrella reviews, as well as individual studies, further elucidate our understanding of the influence of menstrual cycle phases on performance (Carmichael *et al.*, 2021; Colenso-Semple *et al.*, 2023; Vogel *et al.*, 2023). This section primarily draws from research reviews, which provide a synthesis of the current relevant science.

Can we give evidence-based recommendations for menstrual cycle-based training (yet)?

While publications on menstrual cycle effects on performance and training are on the rise and suggested mechanisms make menstrual cycle effects appear plausible, evidence remains inconclusive. Most literature reviews and meta-analyses on the topic note that methodological weaknesses may be responsible for variance in the findings between studies. Here are some possible methodological issues:

- Biphasic comparison (early follicular vs. mid luteal phase), which is frequently used, ignores other phases (e.g. late follicular, ovulatory phases).

- Identification of menstrual cycle phase does not always include hormonal measures, rendering the determination of cycle phases uncertain.

- Numbers of participants in studies are small and a-priori calculations of sample sizes are often lacking.

- Studies show a high variance in sampling, and participant characteristics (e.g. regarding training history) are not always sufficiently considered.

- Variability in methodology between studies is high (e.g. regarding performance measures used).

The current evidence therefore does not warrant general guidance, particularly as findings relate to specific populations such as elite athletes. The conclusion is that we need more robust data to give solid cycle-based training recommendations for different female populations. Does this imply that current scientific findings are useless in practice? By no means. The trends in the research and findings of individual studies can inform practitioners to tailor their approaches to the individual women they work with. Practitioners are encouraged to familiarize themselves with the potential mechanisms of the individual menstrual cycle phases, closely communicate and test strategies with their clients, and not be afraid to look into the depths of research studies to harness information that best represents their use case.

A research-spoiler in advance—the current research reviews on objective performance measures throughout the menstrual cycle do not provide definitive conclusions about if and how performance fluctuates throughout the menstrual cycle. Whenever that's the case in the research, it typically stems from one of the following reasons. Either, the considered measure (here: the influence of the menstrual cycle) does not have a relevant systematic effect in practice, meaning that performance may be uniform across the menstrual cycle, which could be an advantage during competition or training, because if performance doesn't substantially fluctuate throughout the cycle, the timing of a race or exercise bout within the menstrual cycle should not negatively impact performance. Or, the research methods used in current studies do not offer definitive conclusions because they are heterogeneous in nature and may not adhere to the highest methodological standards. A third possibility is that effects of the menstrual cycle on performance may depend heavily on the individual: hormonal profiles of women as well as each female's response to hormonal fluctuations are unique. Even if studies show no systematic effects for their examined study cohorts, effects of the menstrual cycle on performance may be pertinent on an individual level. Which one of these holds most true when it comes to the impact of the menstrual cycle on physical performance remains to be determined. An overview of the research as well as text boxes to shed light on methodological considerations may help the inclined reader to form an opinion of their own.

3.2.3. Strength-based parameters and responses to resistance training

Various reviews conclude that the menstrual cycle may affect strength performance outcomes (Carmichael et al., 2021; Romero-Parra et al., 2021; Niering et al., 2024). In their narrative review, Carmichael and colleagues found that strength performance was most commonly impaired during the late luteal phase (Carmichael et al., 2021). A 2021 systematic review and meta-analysis looking at exercise-induced muscle damage (EIMD) during the menstrual cycle concluded that fluctuations of female sex hormone throughout the menstrual cycle impact delayed onset muscle soreness (DOMS) and strength loss (Romero-Parra et al., 2021). EIMD and strength loss were greater in the early follicular phase, when sex hormones are low, and females are more susceptible to muscle damage. The authors concluded that training loads should be lower and recovery periods longer during this phase. Instead, strength conditioning loads should be enhanced in the mid luteal phase, when estrogen is high. It is of note that peak muscle damage responses in women are observed around 24–72 hours post-exercise,

which should be considered when scheduling load administration.

Another systematic review and meta-analysis from 2024 confirmed that the early follicular phase was unfavorable for all strength classes (Niering et al., 2024). The authors examined the effects of menstrual cycle phases on maximal strength performance, expressed as isometric, isokinetic and dynamic strength, in healthy adults (Niering et al., 2024). Isometric maximal strength describes the force a muscle can produce without significant change in muscle length (maximal voluntary isometric contraction, MVIC), and is tested with the subject exerting force against a stationary object while keeping joint angle and muscle length constant (Maffiuletti et al., 2016). Isokinetic maximal strength is the peak force produced by muscles during a contraction with constant velocity (established through isokinetic dynamometry) (dos Santos Andrade et al., 2012). Dynamic maximum strength measures the force produced during concentric and eccentric phases (e.g. during a 1-repetition maximum lift through full range of motion) (Suchomel et al., 2018). While isometric and dynamic strength were impacted positively in the late follicular phase, isokinetic strength peaked during ovulation.

Further support for menstrual-cycle-based resistance training can be drawn from two individual studies (Sung et al., 2014; Wikström-Frisén, Boraxbekk and Henriksson-Larsén, 2017). Both papers found that women could gain muscle size and strength more efficiently during the follicular phase, compared to training in the second half of the menstrual cycle. However, several methodological shortcomings of both papers have been noted, which may bring the validity of the findings into question (Colenso-Semple et al., 2023): The studies applied biphasic comparison, which does not allow more granular conclusions about the influence of menstrual cycle phases, and determination of cycle phases did not conform to the gold standards (i.e. only body temperature was used in one study; the other did not verify ovulation or menstrual cycle length) (Colenso-Semple *et al.*, 2023) (see text box "Can we give evidence-based recommendations for menstrual cycle-based training (yet)?").

Other reviews, though, find some evidence in favor of no strength differences across menstrual cycle phases, implying that the menstrual cycle does not impact strength performance (Blagrove, Bruinvels and Pedlar, 2020; McNulty *et al.*, 2020; Meignié *et al.*, 2021; Colenso-Semple *et al.*, 2023). In their systematic review and meta-analysis, Blagrove and colleagues found strength-related measures to only be minimally altered by the fluctuations in sex hormones during the menstrual cycle. The authors concluded that women participating in sports or activities relying on maximum or explosive strength are not disadvantaged by their menstrual cycle at any time of the cycle. McNulty and colleagues' systematic review and meta-analysis likewise revealed only trivial performance alterations throughout the menstrual cycle (strength as well as endurance measures were included in the study). The researchers reported a slight reduction of performance during the early follicular phase compared to other menstrual cycle phases, but concluded that this finding was likely to be meaningless to the general population; however, the observed menstrual cycle effects might be of greater relevance to elite athletes, where marginal performance differences can decide between winning and losing (McNulty *et al.*, 2020). Accordingly, the review infers that professionals working with elite athletes should consider performance fluctuations across the menstrual cycle, but should tailor their approach to the individual athlete. Meigniè and colleagues specifically looked at elite athletes' performance in the context of the menstrual cycle and remarked that no solid conclusions regarding the impact of the menstrual cycle on elite athletes could be drawn: The research on this population is limited and where available

is not easily transposable to all of the elite field. The umbrella review by Colenso and colleagues considered some of the sources described in this chapter and determined it would be premature to conclude that fluctuations of sex hormones throughout the menstrual cycle would impact acute exercise performance, strength and hypertrophic adaptations to resistance training. This work, too, favored an individualized approach to exercise planning.

Summing up, various studies and reviews find no impact of the menstrual cycle on strength performance. Those studies reporting impacts of the menstrual cycle phase on strength parameters found the early follicular and late luteal phase to be associated with decreased strength-related performance. The late follicular and ovulatory phase seem to be favorable when it comes to strength performance; however, type of strength may have to be considered.

3.2.4. Endurance-based parameters and response to endurance training

Determining endurance performance includes measures representing anaerobic performance (e.g. short duration tests, jump tests) and aerobic performance (more continuous or longer testing protocols). With respect to anaerobic performance, it is thought that performances of less than three minutes are not impacted by the menstrual cycle phase (Eston and Burke, 1984; Carmichael *et al.*, 2021). Consistent with this, a range of studies showed no difference in sprinting and jump task performance between menstrual cycle phases (Sunderland and Nevill, 2003; Kishali *et al.*, 2010; Tsampoukos *et al.*, 2010; Somboonwong, Chutimakul and Sanguanrungsirikul, 2015; Julian *et al.*, 2017; Tounsi *et al.*, 2018). In those studies finding differences in anaerobic performance across the menstrual cycle, anaerobic performance was mostly reduced in the late follicular phase, but improved in the ovulatory phase (Carmichael *et al.*, 2021).

Regarding aerobic performance, most of the studies report that menstrual cycle phase has no or only marginal effects on aerobic endurance performance (De Souza *et al.*, 1990; Lebrun *et al.*, 1995; Sunderland and Nevill, 2003; Burrows and Bird, 2005; Smekal *et al.*, 2007; Tsampoukos *et al.*, 2010; Vaiksaar *et al.*, 2011; Tounsi *et al.*, 2018; Carmichael *et al.*, 2021; Oxfeldt *et al.*, 2024). In those studies reporting an impact of menstrual cycle phases on endurance, performance appears to be most commonly impaired during the (late) luteal phase, and enhanced in the early follicular phase (Carmichael *et al.*, 2021). However, some studies contradict these findings: one study noted that the percentage of competitive, non-professional runners achieving their best marathon time was higher during luteal phase (57.3%) when compared to follicular phase (Greenhall *et al.*, 2021).

Taken together, many studies conclude that menstrual cycle phase does not affect endurance performance; those that do find effects indicate that anaerobic performance is reduced early in the cycle and improves around ovulation. With respect to aerobic measures, performance mostly appeared to be enhanced in the early follicular phase, but was reduced in the late luteal phase.

Summing up, research results on the effects of the menstrual cycle on performance remain inconclusive to date. Multiple studies and reviews find that the menstrual cycle has no or only minor impact on athletic performance. Where research suggests that the menstrual cycle phases affect performance, the reported effects or trends seem plausible, as they largely align with mechanistic assumptions drawn from basic research (see section 3.1).

With research results being inconclusive and depending on performance measure and specific testing protocols, the type of performance parameter to be targeted should be carefully considered when modifying training according to the menstrual cycle phases (Carmichael *et al.*, 2021). It is also of note that the majority of the current research focuses on sports *performance* markers (i.e. performance at a specific timepoint); few studies have employed longitudinal designs (measuring menstrual-cycle-related adaptations to longer training programs). Therefore, more research is needed to determine how the menstrual cycle affects *adaptations to training*. It is hoped that future studies will yield a clearer picture as to why the research to date is inconclusive: be it that performance in fact stays stable throughout the cycle, methodological issues, or the insight that working with female physiology is largely dependent on each woman's individualized experience.

The matter with "individuality"

Several studies have recognized that individuality—a training approach tailored to the individual woman—appears to be favorable when it comes to considering the menstrual cycle in scheduling of training regimens and load administration. However, the degree to which differences in performance between menstrual cycle phases are individual in nature remains to be quantified (Blagrove, Bruinvels and Pedlar, 2020). It has further recently been noted that the typical phase-based conceptualization of the menstrual cycle (into three or more phases), on which most studies are based, represents an oversimplified perspective of the cycle (Bruinvels, Hackney and Pedlar, 2022): Day-to-day hormonal variations can be significant, which further underlines the importance of tracking each female's menstrual cycle and working with their individual patterns of symptomology, performance and recovery.

3.3. INJURY RISK THROUGHOUT THE CYCLE

Probably the most studied sex difference regarding injuries of the musculoskeletal system is the increased risk of anterior cruciate ligament (ACL) injuries in women compared to men (see Figure 3.2).

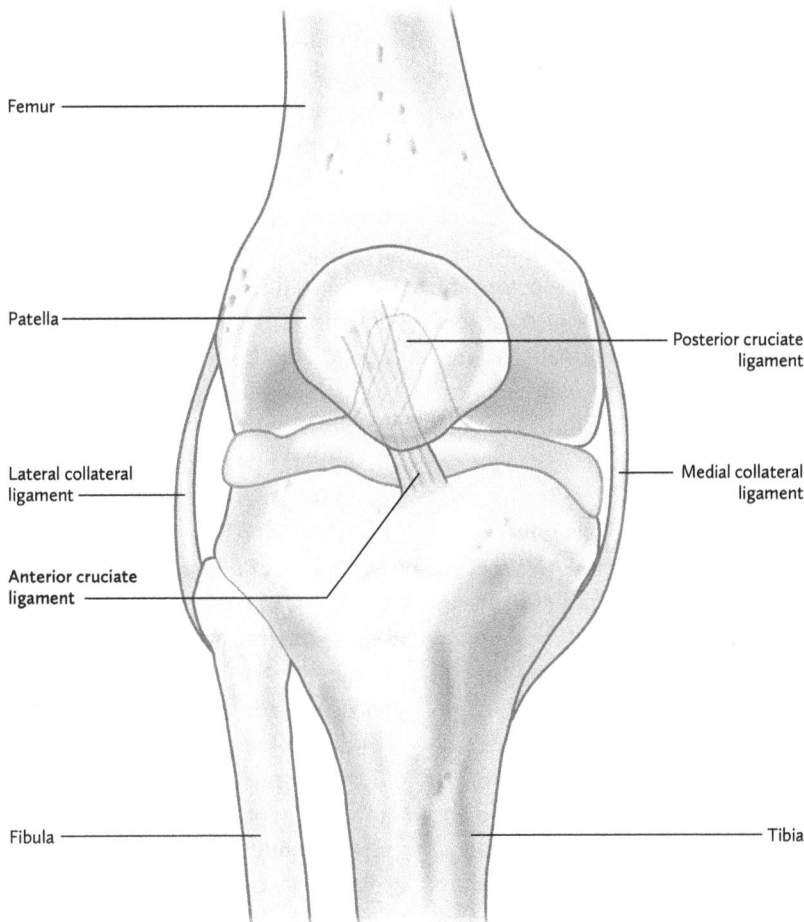

Figure 3.2: Anterior cruciate ligament. Research on differences in ACL injury risk in women and men probably constitutes the most studied sex difference regarding injuries of the musculoskeletal system.

The risk for ACL injuries has been reported to be two to eight times greater in females of reproductive age than males (Majewski, Susanne and Klaus, 2006; Prodromos et al., 2007).

Three main reasons for women's susceptibility to ACL injury have been proposed, the last two of which may be influenced by interventions such as exercise training (Jagadeesh et al., 2021; Seyedahmadi et al., 2022):

• Anatomical/biomechanical differences (e.g. anatomical variations in ACL, alignment of the lower extremity).

- Neuromuscular variation (e.g. different muscle activation patterns).

- Hormonal influences (e.g. influence of menstrual cycle phases on knee laxity).

Greater incidence in ACL injuries in women has previously also been attributed to differences in muscle activation patterns during landing in jump-landing tasks. However, a 2022 systematic review and meta-analysis found no significant differences between muscle activity and contraction timing between men and women. Muscle activation patterns of the lower limb muscles—with the exception of vastus lateralis—before and after foot contact were similar between the two groups. This suggests that other factors (i.e. anatomical/biomechanical and hormonal) can more likely explain the greater susceptibility of ACL injuries in women (Seyedahmadi et al., 2022).

In ligaments, increased stiffness is preferred as it prevents injury and maintains joint stability (note: this is not necessarily true for tendons, where there appears to be a Goldilocks scenario: stiffer tendons can improve force transmission and performance, while too stiff tendons are associated with more injuries) (Chidi-Ogbolu and Baar, 2018). Regarding the ACL and stiffness, a relationship between knee laxity and ACL injuries, as well as between knee laxity and the menstrual cycle, has been established (Shultz et al., 2005; Myer et al., 2008). Moreover, various studies have identified a higher risk of ACL injury shortly before and during the ovulatory phase of the menstrual cycle (Lefevre et al., 2013; Balachandar et al., 2017; Herzberg et al., 2017). Health professionals should be aware of the decrease in joint stability when scheduling training sessions to avoid injury, particularly if training sessions pose a great biomechanical challenge on knee stability. A current meta-analysis suggests that neuromuscular and proprioceptive training may reduce ACL injury (Donnell-Fink et al., 2015). While the meta-analysis considered studies on both male and female subjects, the majority of included studies (15/24) was based on female participants only.

With respect to tendon injury, the picture appears to be more differentiated. Patellar tendinopathy is twice as prevalent in males versus females, which has been hypothesized to be due to reduced force transmission through the patellar tendon in females (Lian, Engebretsen and Bahr, 2005). It has been proposed that reduced power in women may lead to reduced force transmission; it has also been observed that women jump less often than their male counterparts in training sessions of similar length, which may decrease overall force transmission through the patellar tendon (Bahr and Bahr, 2014; Janssen et al., 2015; McMahon and Cook, 2024). However, more research is needed to determine the mechanisms behind this difference in patellar tendinopathy occurrence (McMahon and Cook, 2024). Regarding Achilles tendinopathy, evidence of sex-specific prevalence is conflicting: Some sources find no difference between men and women (Y. Wang et al., 2022), while others report Achilles tendinopathy and tendon rupture to be more common in male individuals than in females (Lantto et al., 2015; McMahon and Cook, 2024). Standardization of research methodology in the future will hopefully clarify the ifs and hows of sex-specific differences in tendon injuries.

3.4. TRADITIONAL CHINESE MEDICINE AND FEMALE HEALTH

While this book offers an overview of western medicine's perspective of female health, broadening one's view to other approaches, such as Traditional Chinese Medicine (TCM), can inform and enrich working with female hormones and the menstrual cycle. Here, Tiffany Cruikshank, founder of Yoga Medicine®, provides an expert's insight into how TCM comprehends and approaches female health.

One of the things I love about TCM is that it so often brilliantly makes sense of what we have yet to figure out in western medicine. This is definitely the case when it comes to female health and an important lens to take to this system as we begin to dig deeper and look at implications for training and lifestyle. It is my belief that we need to take several views to see a full picture of what might be best for the individual, TCM and western medicine being two critical viewpoints for female health. With that said, Chinese medicine has a deep and rich background with a variety of styles, so before we jump in, I'll begin with the caveat that this will in many ways be an oversimplification of a very layered and textured system.

As we shift our perspective to the TCM view, one of the main underlying principles is the idea of balance as a reflection of health. In TCM, balance refers to two main things, appropriate amounts and healthy flow. Appropriate amounts refers to having optimal amounts of the main precious substances (qi, blood, yin and yang) as well as the five elements (earth, wood, fire, metal, water). It's a Goldilocks scenario, meaning we don't want too little or too much. Healthy flow refers to the movement of qi and blood through the body and the meridians and is similar to our circulation but also includes the flow of energy or qi. This flow helps maintain our internal communication and transportation system just as a river would have once provided a necessary route to deliver precious resources. The general idea is that as long as we have all the main resources (qi, blood, yin and yang) and there is a healthy flow to provide those to all the parts then the body can

heal and repair and be resilient to what life throws at us. From this perspective, stagnation in the system can be a major hindrance to health, as can a deficiency or excess of any of these substances. All of this is key to perfectly orchestrate the timing of events and hormone levels throughout this brilliantly constructed four-phase cycle.

As we dig into the details of each phase of the cycle we see that phase 1 begins with menstruation and is where there is the shedding of the uterine lining. In TCM, this quality of release and downward flow is important to clear out and shed all of the endometrium that is crucial to the timing and balance of hormones through the rest of the cycle. It's analogous to clearing a whiteboard before you start to write again—it becomes a much better communication mechanism when we start with a clean slate. Some of the most common issues that show up in this phase are pain, breast tenderness and irritability, which in TCM are generally a reflection of stagnation in this phase of the cycle. Practices here often focus on gentle but tolerable movements, especially locally in the pelvis and generally supporting the downward flow to help encourage the release of the lining. Many females tend to have less energy during this phase, partly due to loss of blood (one of the precious substances), so there can be an inclination toward deficiency in this phase, meaning that we don't necessarily need vigorous practices but we do need to keep the circulation going. This can be done with local massage, gentle circulating and downward flowing yoga, or more vigorous exercise if that feels helpful and not depleting. This can also be a great time to support any type of detoxification that feels helpful to facilitate this release phase.

Phase 2, known as the follicular phase in western medicine, is associated with the growth and development of the follicles and a new endometrial lining. Because of that, in TCM this phase requires more nourishment to provide the building blocks for growth and development that take place here. We know circulation and movement are important in all phases of the cycle, and that's no different in this phase; however, a focus on nourishment through more introspective practices like yin yoga, restorative yoga, recovery practices and meditation is an important adjunct in this phase. For those more susceptible to depletion (especially those who feel more tired during and after their period), this is an important phase to support, and need not replace movement practices or even take large amounts of time but reminds us of the importance of giving back to this precious system. This can also be integrated as short practices added throughout the cycle for additional support, especially helpful when there is exhaustion.

Phase 3 is a short phase but an important one as it correlates with the few days around ovulation. In TCM, this is a quick turnover from the more nourishing (yin) practices of phase 2 to the movement and warmth (yang) practices associated with phase 3. Here we see the spark that triggers a quick shift to ovulation where the egg is released. This phase generally begins a day or two before the expected ovulation and continues for a day or two after; this allows for a primer to the spark and supporting that movement as the egg begins to travel down the fallopian tube. The range also allows for some variability that inevitably can happen in ovulation from one cycle to the next. This phase is associated with more movement, warmth and circulation to help facilitate that turnover from the more nourishing, introspective practices to the release of the egg that happens in ovulation, and the movement associated with it as the egg moves down the fallopian tube. Practices in the phase can be

a bit more strenuous, stirring up more circulation and warmth (especially locally in the pelvis) to support that. I'll add the caveat that for those not trying to get pregnant or unsure of ovulation timing, this phase can seem tedious and if so it may be helpful to focus efforts on the other three phases and skip this one entirely.

Phase 4 is the final phase and the phase in which if the egg is fertilized it will eventually implant in the endometrial lining to receive nourishment and support the growth and development of the egg. During this phase, there are two very different approaches whether one is trying to get pregnant or not. For those trying to conceive, a more balanced practice with both gentle circulating and nourishing components (think calming, stress reduction, restorative yoga, meditation) is important, in addition to more upward lifting qualities (think gentle inversions like legs up the wall) to help support and maintain the pregnancy.

For those not trying to get pregnant and especially for those with premenstrual symptoms like irritability, mood swings, breast tenderness and bloating, which are often related to stagnation in TCM, we take a different approach. If one is not trying to conceive (yet), especially if there are PMS symptoms and/or period pain, this is an important phase to focus on more movement and perhaps more vigorous practices to facilitate and prepare for the shedding of the lining to come in phase 1. Though PMS symptoms may slow us down a bit in this phase, supporting movement and circulation in any form (vigorous or gentle) can be a valuable tool over time.

Keep in mind that all of this can be more detailed and specific and may require a therapeutic specialist to individualize (to find an acupuncturist or yoga teacher trained in female health therapeutics near you, see www.yogamedicine.com). However, we can also draw some simple helpful takeaways. One is that maintaining movement and healthy flow throughout the cycle is key, which could mean finding gentle, palatable ways to do that through the menstrual cycle, or finding an intensity level that is suitable for the individual and their training needs. Another is the importance of nourishment after menstruation through more introspective practices like restorative yoga, yin yoga, meditation, or anything that facilitates recovery. Lastly, consider that if PMS and period pain are an issue, staying active the week or two before the period as well as to some extent during the period can be a valuable approach over time.

There are other models of this system that have equally important applications, so keep experimenting and seeing what works best and stay open to adapting as needed if things shift. Keep in mind we are more than just our cycle, so there may be other things influencing how we feel and perhaps how we may want/need to adapt our training and lifestyle to feel and perform at our best.

Tiffany Cruikshank, L.Ac., MAOM, is a teacher, student, author and educator. Her passion lies in helping people feel their best with a combination of research-based approaches, traditional practices and experience. She has a background in acupuncture, Chinese Medicine, sports medicine and orthopedics, has trained over 15,000 teachers around the world and has worked with thousands of patients and students to optimize their health and performance. www.yogamedicine.com

CHAPTER 4

Fuel Up: Optimizing Nutrition Throughout the Cycle

4.1. SUBSTRATE METABOLISM AND NUTRITIONAL STRATEGIES IN FEMALES

Evidence in the fields of metabolism and nutrition is broad and varied, the totality of which exceeds the scope of this book. This chapter will thus focus on highlighting and summarizing current research reviews and position papers on nutritional concerns for female athletes (Boisseau and Isacco, 2022; Sims *et al.*, 2023; Cabre *et al.*, 2024; Sanchez *et al.*, 2024). Female sex hormones can impact metabolism, energy requirements, fluid balance and recovery (Sims *et al.*, 2023). For example, hormonal fluctuations influence fat, carbohydrate and protein use during physical activity. When comparing the substrate metabolism during exercise of women and men, a key difference is that, generally, females tend to use less muscle glycogen—the stored form of glucose in muscle and liver—than males. This means women favor fat as a fuel source, while men generally rely more on muscle glycogen during exercise. This holds particularly true during moderate-intensity activities. This difference in fuel preference is likely influenced by hormonal variations (i.e. increases in and ratios between estrogen and progesterone as experienced throughout the menstrual cycle) (Sanchez *et al.*, 2024). Through conserving glycogen, women may be able to sustain moderate-intensity exercise for longer periods of activity without depleting their energy stores. This makes females potentially more efficient in longer endurance activities.

While women tend to favor fat as a fuel source during submaximal exercise, they still need readily available carbohydrates for optimal performance. As fat oxidation is a slower process compared to carbohydrate metabolism, carbohydrate utilization is particularly important when the body requires faster, more efficient energy production; for example, when exercise intensity increases (above about 60–65% VO_2 max). Carbohydrate intake is furthermore pivotal to maintain performance levels during physical activity.

In addition to the described general sex differences in substrate metabolism, the menstrual cycle presents with fluctuations in macronutrient utilization patterns. The hormonal profile prevalent in the follicular phase leads to relatively lower fat oxidation and a relatively increased reliance on carbohydrate metabolism. Conversely, the hormonal set-up of the luteal phase results in an uptake in fat utilization (Sims *et al.*, 2023; Cabre *et al.*, 2024). Moreover, progesterone is thought to promote protein catabolism, which can result in reduced stimulus for muscle protein synthesis (Lamont, Lemon and Bruot, 1987; Sims and Heather, 2018). Therefore, the catabolic environment in the luteal phase can negatively impact muscle repair and recovery (Cabre *et al.*, 2024).

How do these findings translate into practice? The International Society of Sports Nutrition

(ISSN) recently released a position paper on nutritional considerations of female athletes, aimed at addressing the unique challenges faced by women in sports (Sims *et al.*, 2023). This outlines a range of strategies to improve overall health, training adaptations and performance by focusing on energy intake and nutrient timing. Adequate overall energy availability is crucial for female athletes, particularly in sports where body composition is of relevance. Section 4.3 will further elucidate the concept of energy availability in sports as well as potential consequences for female athletes if energy requirements are not met.

Regarding carbohydrates, the position paper stresses carbohydrate focus intake during the luteal phase, when sex hormones affect the supression of gluconeogenesis output during exercise to a greater degree. Ensuring carbohydrate intake during this phase can improve performance and recovery. With respect to proteins, females should aim for an intake of around 1.4–2.2 g per kg of body weight, spread throughout the day (every three to four hours). Higher protein intake might be necessary in the luteal phase of the menstrual cycle to counteract the catabolic effects of progesterone.

While these sex-specific mechanisms provide great general insights into the needs of female athletes, it should be noted that each female's hormonal profile is unique. Consequently, menstrual cycle tracking is key to understanding how female sex hormones impact the overall wellbeing, training and recovery of each woman and to tailor individualized training and recovery plans.

Should women exercise in a fasted state?

Sims and colleagues (2023) call into question whether the widely spread practice of exercising in a fasted state is beneficial for women. The authors elaborate that exercising in a fasted state can decrease the efficiency or rate at which fat is used for fuel. While females generally favor fat oxidization when compared to males, fasting may interfere with this process:

- Rises in cortisol during fasting may lead to increased protein breakdown instead of relying on fat stores.

- Females' bodies may be more sensitive to energy deprivation, possibly leading to a greater conservation of fat stores (versus burning them).

- Metabolism may shift to utilize muscle glycogen or muscle proteins, rather than focusing on fat oxidization.

Taken together, fasting may result in poorer exercise performance and recovery in women, rather than an uptake in fat-burning. This implies that proper nutrition before exercise may enhance fat oxidation and energy metabolism, which could potentially improve body composition outcomes.

4.2. CONSIDERATIONS ON FLUID AND ELECTROLYTE BALANCE FOR THE FEMALE ATHLETE

As with nutritional strategies (see section 4.1), female sex hormones interact with fluid regulation processes in a complex manner. Individualized hydration strategies for women, which consider their unique hormonal profile, therefore are important to consider in training and competition. Hormonal fluctuations throughout the menstrual cycle can impact fluid retention and electrolyte handling, which can put females at a higher risk of fluid imbalance, particularly in the luteal phase of the menstrual cycle. Through a complex interplay between progesterone and aldosterone—a hormone which manages sodium (salt) and potassium levels in the blood—sodium retention can be reduced in the luteal phase. This may lead to greater sodium loss during exercise and may leave females at a higher risk of hyponatremia (low sodium concentrations in the blood) (Sims et al., 2007, 2023; Giersch et al., 2020). Excessive water intake during training or competition can further intensify this electrolyte imbalance. Interestingly, thirst regulation may also change across the menstrual cycle. It has been reported that the osmotic threshold for thirst (i.e. the threshold for thirst activation) is lower in the luteal phase, implying that women might perceive thirst earlier in the luteal phase (Vokes et al., 1988). This may further increase the risk for hyponatremia during the luteal phase. Consequently, it is important to monitor hydration status in females during exercise and competition; instead of simply drinking water, adequate electrolyte replenishment (e.g. in the form of sodium tablets during prolonged endurance exercise or competition) needs to be ensured, particularly in the luteal phase of the cycle (Sims et al., 2023).

Moreover, females generally have less total body water compared to males (both in absolute numbers as well as in percentage of body mass; women have 49% water volume, compared to 58% in men) (Ritz et al., 2008). This means that women may lose a higher proportion of their body water when they sweat, which may exacerbate dehydration effects and make the physiological consequences of fluid loss more severe (Wickham et al., 2021). However, the combined impacts of female reproductive impacts and hydration status are not well understood at this time and more research is needed to further elaborate and develop policies and recommendations for fluid balance and hydration in female athletes (Giersch et al., 2020).

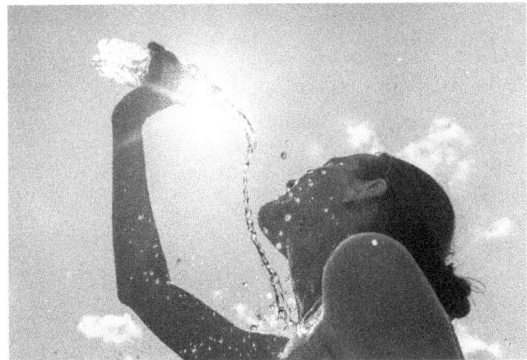

Photo 4.1: Fluid and electrolyte balance in women requires specific considerations. The current state of research suggests that the luteal phase of the menstrual cycle may put female athletes at higher risk for hyponatremia, calling for adequate monitoring of hydration and electrolyte replenishment during exercise and competition. Women may furthermore lose a higher proportion of body water when sweating compared to men, which may exacerbate dehydration effects.

4.3. RELATIVE ENERGY DEFICIENCY IN SPORT (RED-S): WHAT WE KNOW SO FAR

Relative Energy Deficiency in Sport (RED-S) is a syndrome of detrimental effects on health and performance experienced by athletes exposed to low energy availability (LEA) (Mountjoy et al., 2023). Low energy availability describes the imbalance between an athlete's energy intake and energy expenditure. Previously, the term female athlete triad referred to the negative health effects of LEA on reproductive hormonal balance and bone health in women (Mallinson and De Souza, 2014). More recently, it has been acknowledged that male athletes also face the impact of energy deficiency in sports, and the scope of potential health and performance outcomes has been expanded substantially, culminating in the introduction of the term RED-S by the International Olympic Committee in 2014 (Mountjoy *et al.*, 2023).

Risk factors for developing RED-S comprise sports that focus on weight classes or leanness (e.g. ballet, gymnastics, wrestling), aesthetics of the sport (pressure to attain a certain "athletic look"), long-term training at high intensities without proper recovery, psychological factors (e.g. perfectionism, anxiety, depression) and lack of knowledge about adequate nutrition (especially in adolescent athletes) (Mountjoy *et al.*,

2023). RED-S is a multifactorial and complex syndrome and can impact a broad range of body systems, such as the cardiovascular, immune, gastrointestinal, endocrine, psychological and metabolic systems. Figures 4.1 and 4.2 provide an overview of the potential influence of LEA on various health parameters and performance measures. The two graphics are not to be understood separate from each other but rather offer different audiences—one more health-, one more performance-oriented—a perspective of the RED-S consequences most relevant to them (Mountjoy *et al.*, 2023).

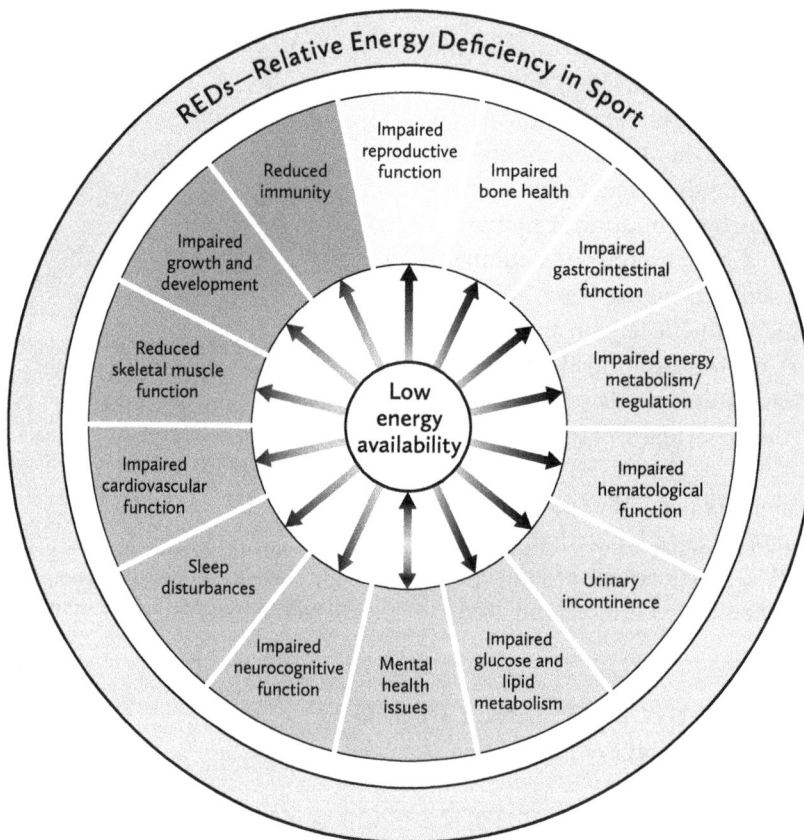

Figure 4.1: RED-S Health Conceptual Model. Potential health effects of low energy availability related to RED-S. Effects exist on a continuum: low energy availability can be mild and transient in nature; problematic low energy availability can result in a variety of adverse outcomes (adapted from Mountjoy *et al.*, 2023).

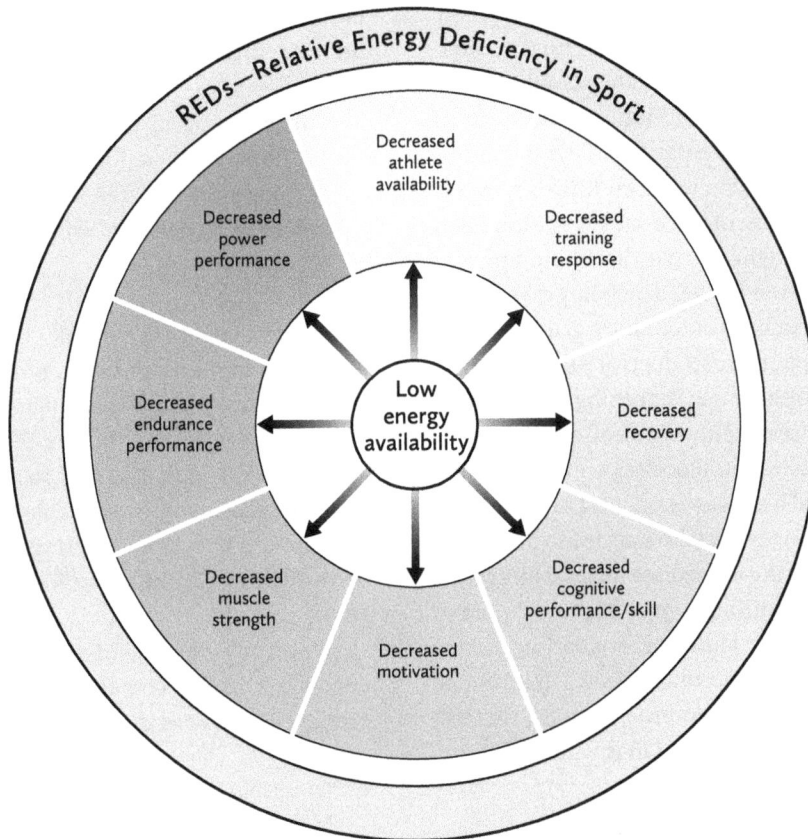

Figure 4.2: RED-S Performance Conceptual Model. Potential performance effects of low energy availability related to RED-S. Effects exist on a continuum: low energy availability can be mild and transient in nature; problematic low energy availability can result in a variety of adverse outcomes (adapted from Mountjoy *et al.*, 2023).

Beyond immediate effects on health and performance, untreated RED-S poses serious long-term health risks. For example, prolonged amenorrhea in females can result in permanent, irreversible loss of bone mineral density and poor bone geometry, which can predispose athletes to bone stress injuries (such as stress fractures) and to osteoporosis at a relatively early age (Soyka *et al.*, 2002; Ackerman *et al.*, 2011, 2019; Gibbs *et al.*, 2014; Tenforde *et al.*, 2017; Taim *et al.*, 2023). Bone density scanning, bone stress injuries, as well as fracture history, may serve as indicators to evaluate the impairment of bone health (Nattiv *et al.*, 2007; Lewiecki *et al.*, 2016; Mountjoy *et al.*, 2023).

LEA is the underlying cause of RED-S and can occur either intentionally (e.g. through dieting or disordered eating behavior), or unintentionally (e.g. when athletes fail to notice how many calories they need to consume to meet their energy needs). Exposure to LEA is graded, meaning it exists on a continuum from adaptable LEA (mild and quickly reversible changes) to problematic LEA (greater and potentially persistent disruption of various body systems) (Mountjoy *et al.*, 2023). Moreover, RED-S may develop subtly over time. Screening for and diagnosing RED-S follows a step-wise graded approach, accordingly. Initial screening may include questionnaires or clinical interviews; if greater than low risk is identified, more sensitive and expensive methods might be used to allow for clear and reliable risk assessment. In cases where risk or severity of RED-S presents as mild to moderate, clinical diagnosis should be combined with clinical history and examination (Mountjoy *et al.*, 2023). The 2023 International Olympic Committee's consensus statement on RED-S provides a current overview of used and recommended methods for studying various health and performance outcomes of RED-S, depending on relevant health or performance outcomes (e.g. measures to determine impaired reproductive function, bone health etc.). For example, screening may include nutritional assessment, physical examination, bone health evaluation, blood tests, menstrual history and mental health assessment. The consensus statement identifies the following list to be serious indicators requiring immediate medical attention, removal from training/competition and potential hospitalization. However, evaluation should always be based on thorough clinical assessment of the athlete by medical professionals; this list should therefore not be used in isolation:

- 75% or less median BMI for sex and age

- Electrolyte disturbances (e.g. hyponatremia, hypokalemia)

- Electrocardiogram (ECG) disturbances (e.g. severe bradycardia)

- Severe hypotension: 90/45 mm Hg or less

- Acute medical problems of malnutrition (e.g. cardiac failure, syncope, pancreatitis)

- Orthostatic intolerance (systolic blood pressure drop of more than 20 mm Hg and diastolic drop of more than 10 mm Hg when coming from supine to standing)

- Any condition that inhibits medical treatment and monitoring while training and competing.

How can energy availability be measured?

> Energy availability is the dietary energy left over and available for optimum function of body systems after accounting for the energy expended from exercise. (Mountjoy *et al.*, 2023)

Energy availability is typically indicated as kcal per kilograms of fat free mass (FFM) per day. Low energy availability describes a situation where the body's total energy needs remain unmet, so the body does not have adequate energy available to support all functions to maintain optimal health and performance (Loucks, 2004; Mountjoy *et al.*, 2018).

Determining an individual's level of energy availability comes with a number of challenges (Burke *et al.*, 2018):

- Determining LEA in a laboratory setting is carried out under scenarios that **do not replicate real-life of an athlete well**; therefore, the data might not be representative of the actual energy availability of an athlete. For example, strict protocols for energy intake (i.e. controlled diet) and energy expenditure (i.e. exercise routine) must be followed in the lab.

- **Gold standard measurements** for energy expenditure such as doubly labeled water are highly accurate, but **expensive and not always available**. More readily available (and potentially less costly) measurement methods, on the other hand, may be less precise.

- Previous, **laboratory-based thresholds** for low energy availability are subject to methodological challenges (for example, the reported threshold of 30 kcal/kg

FFM/day was based on a small sample of sedentary females) and cannot necessarily be extrapolated to a broad athletic population (Burke *et al.*, 2018).

- **Measuring energy intake out of the laboratory** (in free-living athletes) is characterized by a high level of burden and potential inaccuracy. For example, recording dietary intake relies on the meticulous self-report of athletes; such self-reported logs are prone to significant under-reporting and errors in portion size estimation. In addition, athletes might change their eating habits when asked to report their caloric intake compared to their usual diet.

- **Tracking energy expenditure outside the laboratory** is complex, especially in sports which include various activities (e.g. team sports). Tools like accelerometers are helpful, but can produce errors— for example, static exercises as used in strength training involve minimal movement, and are therefore not captured well with accelerometry, even though a large amount of energy is expended.

- Factors such as gender, age and genetics can impact the effect of low energy availability exposure and can vary across individuals.

It has thus been suggested that screening athletes for other risk factors, signs and symptoms of LEA might be more efficient than capturing energy availability (Burke *et al.*, 2018; Mountjoy *et al.*, 2023).

Managing and treating RED-S is a multi-disciplinary endeavor, including coaches, family, as well as sports medicine, nutrition, psychology and sports science personnel (Wells *et al.*, 2020). RED-S practical clinical guidelines include short-term interventions and long-term strategies (Mountjoy *et al.*, 2018, 2023). Here are some examples:

- Short-term measures may include increasing caloric intake and creating a nutrition plan with a sports dietician and/or reducing energy expenditure (i.e. reducing or stopping training).

- Restoring regular menstrual cycles is considered a key goal of treatment. This can involve increasing body weight, reducing training intensities and addressing hormonal imbalances. Treatment can sometimes include temporary hormonal treatment.

- Cognitive-behavioral therapy or counseling may help athletes to develop a healthy relationship with their body, nutrition and exercise, and to manage their psychological stressors.

- Supplementation of calcium and vitamin D, weight-bearing exercises and potentially hormone therapy can be used to support bone health.

- Education, for both coaches and athletes, can increase awareness and mitigate the pressures contributing to energy deficiency.

Raising awareness and knowledge among both athletes and their teams (i.e. coaches, parents, health and performance team) presents a cornerstone in preventing and managing RED-S. Coaches and physiotherapists play a pivotal role in preventing and managing RED-S as they are often the first to perceive shifts in athletes' mental state and physical performance. They should therefore be educated on the signs and symptoms of RED-S, and acquire a sensitive communication approach to create a supportive environment around issues related to body composition, nutrition and female health. Sports organizations should implement policies that promote athletes' health and wellbeing, provide access to nutrition and mental health experts and drive cultural change that values long-term health over short-term performance gains.

More specific examples around prevention-relevant aspects to consider in the daily work with athletes comprise issues around nutrition, body composition, recovery and menstrual health. Athletes should be encouraged to view food as fuel and to understand how to put together a balanced diet, particularly during phases of intense training or competition. Excessive focus on body composition and leanness can result in body-dissatisfaction and long-term negative physiological and psychological outcomes. Body composition assessment should therefore be considered carefully, especially in athletes under 18 years of age, and requires the consensus of athlete and guardians. Practitioners should be aware of how to interpret, manage and communicate topics around body composition to athletes. Athletes should be educated on the importance of rest and recovery to allow for adequate restoration of energy levels. Encouraging female athletes to view their menses as an indicator of health, and normalizing conversation around menstrual health and menstrual cycle tracking, can further shift awareness and create a body-positive culture in sports.

Bringing it all together: A professional triathlete's personal perspective

My name is Anja Ippach and I feel very honored and grateful to share my experiences and personal journey with you, hoping that you can learn a lot from my mistakes and all the extra loops that I went through in my sports career as a professional triathlete. Who am I? First of all, I am a proud mum of two wonderful little kids (three and one years old) and a happy coach for female triathletes. Before becoming a mum, I had the opportunity to live my dream of being a long-distance professional triathlete for more than two decades.

When I started triathlon as a young girl in the 1990s, triathlon training was all about endurance training and the main philosophy was: the longer the better. As I trained with male athletes most of the time, my coaches trained me like a "small" man—just a little less long and less fast than my male counterparts. During that time, this kind of training was the status quo and nobody had thought or heard about gender-specific training methods. Although I grew up in a family where we could talk and ask anything and my mum was very empathetic and took great care of me and my sister, we didn't learn much about our periods and what was going on in our female bodies. This was also typical at the time and nothing out of the ordinary.

Luckily, I never had any big problems with my menstrual cycle—no cramps, no migraine or strong PMS. I just gained weight (and water) in the second phase of the cycle, which wasn't easy in a sport that is very much focused on the physical. Consequently, until nearly the end of my sports career, I thought that my period wasn't affecting my sport performance. Oh my, how wrong I was!

Especially when it came to races or my motivation to perform, I had no clue why I performed well one day, feeling so strong and competitive, and a few days later, felt weak, fat, unsure and just wanted to stay in bed. When I had bad race results and couldn't figure out a reason for it, I suspected that I hadn't trained enough, was physically and mentally not strong enough and my body was too fat. So I trained harder, ate less and consequently my performance sunk and I gained more body fat. I had no idea why this happened and thought it might be related to my genetic predisposition. I never thought about hormones.

Luckily, during my last few years racing as a pro athlete, some evidence-based training methods related to female training theories popped up. I started to read books about the menstrual cycle and training with female physiology and finally found answers as to why I had these massive ups and downs in my physical and mental performance during my whole career: it was my hormones!

I could have saved myself many tears and disappointments and avoided two DNFs (did not finish) at the Ironman World Championships in Kona, Hawaii, where I was in the shape of my life and ended up on the sidewalk with a headache, a swollen body and a big question mark in my mind. Today, I know that I was in the high hormone phase (a few days out from getting my period) and I had borderline hyponatremic issues—I fueled completely wrong. Luckily—or more accurately, incidentally—one year later when I was toeing the start line for the most important race in triathlon in Kona, Hawaii, again, I was in the low hormone phase. I was in second place for most of the race and ended up in fourth place.

In the following paragraphs I share my best practices for achieving high performance—which means training hand in hand with your body and mind; or better yet, training with your hormones and female physiology.

- **Track your cycle:** This advice sounds so simple but most of the women I train don't do it. However, it is so important and the precondition to working with your physiology—and the best thing is, it doesn't take a lot of time. There are plenty of apps and tools on the market that make cycle tracking a quick and easy task. The more you know about your menstrual cycle, the better you can perform. Write comments on your physical sensations, emotional state, thoughts, nutrition, hydration, recovery, sleep, body temperature, heart rate, stress code. The tricky—but at the same time wonderful—point is that every menstrual cycle and every woman is unique and different. Ask the most important question: How do I feel? And don't measure your training progression just by your output (watts, power meter, heart rate). Keep an eye on your input as well: what you eat, how you train, what your daily habits are, and this will improve how you feel and perform.

- **Train with your cycle:** If you are doing an individual sport like I did, you have the big advantage of adapting your training completely based on how you feel on any given day, session or moment. My menstrual cycle was regular: 28 days. So I adapted the usual training rhythm in triathlon 3:1 (three weeks of training followed by one week of recovery) to my cycle. I started my hard training on the day my period started. The following 14 days when my hormones were low (follicular phase), I focused on hard training sessions and lifted maximum weights in my strength workouts. From days 15–20 I reduced the intensity and trained longer and easier. I lifted moderate weights and concentrated on my nutrition and fueling correctly. In my recovery week from days 21–28, I tried to acknowledge that I felt bad because I had trained hard before and my hormones had kicked into high gear. While recognizing PMS symptoms, extra kilos and feelings of wanting to hide, I reminded myself that in a couple of days things would change again.

- **Race with your cycle or your will to perform well:** As a triathlete I could adapt my training regimen to my menstrual cycle but (unfortunately) I couldn't shift the date of the world championship. So, I had to learn to do something differently when the race date fell into the second half of my period, with estrogen and progesterone at their peak levels making high performance more difficult. The good news for endurance sports is that $VO_{2\,max}$ and lactate threshold remain constant throughout your cycle—it is just harder to achieve your personal best and even more important to do some things differently:

  - Consume more carbs and protein during the premenstrual part of your cycle if you race or train more than 90 minutes (10–15 g protein, 40 g carbohydrates before physical activity, 40–60 g carbohydrates combined with protein and fat per hour during physical activity).

  - Drink more before your intense exercise and activate your lymphatic system in that phase (massage, warm water, easy movements) because your plasma volume is low, meaning your blood is thicker, you feel bloated, and less blood is pumped out with every heartbeat, which makes everything feel harder. If you perform in the heat, it is important to preload your body with special hydration products. Even the night before you should preload with high-sodium broth (such as chicken soup or special drinks containing 7.7 g sodium citrate and 4.5 g sodium chloride per liter as well as some carbohydrate).

  - If you have cramps or gastrointestinal issues during that time, which is common, prepare for it! Start one week before your period to take magnesium and omega-3-fatty acids. If you suffer from headaches, increase your hydration and eat more foods high in nitric oxide (beets, watermelon, pomegranate, spinach).

  - If you feel fatigue, foggy in your head or low in mood—which is not very helpful if you want to perform well—find your personal method that makes you happy during that time: more self-care, more family time, more positive talking to yourself, more shopping.

  - If your period starts on race day—celebrate! Before I learned about female physiology, I thought racing during my period was the worst-case scenario; today, I understand you can perform well early in the cycle. In case you have heavy bleeding, keep an eye on your iron level and get your doctor to check it regularly.

I can encourage females or anyone working with female athletes to keep an individual journal to tailor a training regimen for each unique female body. Stop tracking numbers related to performance or sleep and start taking notes of the menstrual cycle and all related sensations during each different phase.

As a retired athlete I—unfortunately—can't prove that these practices led me to my personal best. As I am observing my female triathlon colleagues who get faster year by year (in 2024 the long-distance world record was beaten by Anne Haug, who finished in 8:02 hours), I am sure this is not only because of aerodynamic bikes, carbon shoes or different training and recovery methods, it's also because we have learned to train with female physiology.

It may have taken until I got pregnant with a little miracle growing in my belly for me to fully understand that being a woman and having a menstrual cycle is the most beautiful thing in the world and that there are vast physiological differences between women and men. I hope my experiences are empowering for women as well as anyone working with females, encouraging them to consider each woman's unique physiology.

Female hormones are essential—not only related to high performance, but also when it comes to happiness and freedom in daily life. As a matter of fact, I am writing these words in my first menstrual cycle phase, feeling self-confident, clear-headed and full of positive energy.

Anja Ippach is a former professional triathlete, multiple Ironman winner, winner of the Ironman 70.3 European Championship (2012) and German triathlon long-distance champion (2015). She was placed fourth in the Ironman World Championships in Kona, Hawaii, in 2016. Today, Anja is a proud mom of two kids and shares her knowledge about female hormone-based training with her athletes as a triathlon coach. www.triathlon-maedchen.de

The Mind and the Menstrual Cycle: The Interaction of Psychological Responses with Female Sex Hormones

5.1. MENSTRUAL CYCLE EFFECTS ON PSYCHOLOGICAL RESPONSES

The past decades have produced a substantial body of research suggesting that females and males exhibit different psychological symptomology (Rojiani *et al.*, 2017). It has been suggested that, generally speaking, males are more likely to suffer from conduct disorder and substance use disorder (Lahey *et al.*, 1999; Cotto *et al.*, 2010). When coping with psychological distress, men are thought to "externalize" their distress by distracting themselves or engaging with the environment (e.g. watching TV or playing sports). Women, on the other hand, tend to "internalize" their distress by directing their action and attention inward (e.g. ruminating) (Broderick, 2005; Rojiani *et al.*, 2017). Women are also more likely to experience "internalizing disorders" such as depression and anxiety (Rojiani *et al.*, 2017). In addition to overall gender differences, the menstrual cycle can go along with psychological alterations. Negative psychological changes, such as increased mood disturbances and fatigue, are often observed during the luteal phase (Ossewaarde *et al.*, 2010; Van Wingen *et al.*, 2011; Paludo *et al.*, 2022). In women with PMS (see section 2.4), premenstrual symptom increase in the luteal phase appears to be linked to increased perceived stress and daily rumination (Nayman *et al.*, 2023). Different explanatory models aim to shed light on alterations throughout the menstrual cycle:

- **Prefrontal cortex and amygdala interplay:** Estradiol and progesterone can pass the blood-brain barrier, bind to receptors in the brain and impact the reactivity in the prefrontal cortex and amygdala. In the luteal phase (in comparison to the follicular phase), a decrease in prefrontal cortex function combined with an increased reactivity of the amygdala can be observed. This indicates a reduced ability of the prefrontal cortex to inhibit negative amygdala responses during this phase of the cycle, pointing to a vulnerability window toward negative psychological responses (Bixo *et al.*, 1997; Foy *et al.*, 1999; McEwen, 2001; Van Wingen *et al.*, 2008; Andreano and Cahill, 2010; Pletzer *et al.*, 2019; Prado *et al.*, 2021a).

- **Worst feelings of emotion in the luteal phase:** It has been shown that women report negative emotions when they remember the luteal phase of their cycle (Sabin-Farrell and Slade, 1999). This has been associated with the negative impact of progesterone and cortisol, which increase the excitability of the amygdala and enhance its communication with the medial prefrontal cortex (Herman *et al.*, 2003; Van Wingen *et al.*, 2011; Poromaa and Gingnell, 2014; Prado *et al.*, 2021a).

- **Expression of negative emotions by the action of neuroactive steroids:** Neuroactive steroids such as allopregnanolone can act on the GABA-ergic system and thus be involved in mood regulation. Allopregnanolone fluctuates with the menstrual cycle—because it is a metabolite of progesterone, its levels are higher in the luteal phase. While it generally helps to stabilize mood in the luteal phase and has a calming, anxiety-reducing effect by enhancing GABA activity, some individuals may experience increased anxiety or irritability due to higher allopregnanolone levels. This is thought to be related to altered GABA-A receptor activity in response to fluctuating hormone levels (see text box "Causes for premenstrual disorders—current theories on allopregnanolone and serotonin" in section 2.4) (Andréen *et al.*, 2009; Bäckström *et al.*, 2011; Prado *et al.*, 2021a).

- **Higher stress sensitivity during the luteal phase:** Women may be emotionally more sensitive to stress during the luteal phase. This is primarily due to the complex interplay of hormonal and neurotransmitter fluctuations, as well as a heightened reactivity of the stress response system (Prado *et al.*, 2021a).

Luteal phase and adherence to physical exercise

Physical activity adherence is thought to be related to psychological responses to exercise (Williams, 2008; Prado *et al.*, 2021a). Women are less likely to meet exercise recommendations than men, along with gender differences in physical activity motivators (Van Uffelen, Khan and Burton, 2017; Bennie *et al.*, 2019). Many women appear to be motivated to exercise by pleasant feelings, such as feeling good, as well as social opportunities, such as spending time with others and meeting friends (Sirard, Pfeiffer and Pate, 2006; Beville *et al.*, 2014; Rosenfeld, 2017; Van Uffelen, Khan and Burton, 2017). Physical appearance and weight management have also been shown to motivate women (Egli *et al.*, 2011; Rosenfeld, 2017).

Researchers suggest that the late luteal phase interferes with physical activity levels, probably due to physiological as well as psychological reasons, which can also influence each other: higher core temperature, increased ventilatory rate, as well as levels of progesterone and cortisol can negatively impact the perceived rate of exertion, decrease pleasure while exercising and lower exercise adherence in the luteal phase (compared to the follicular phase) (Pivarnik *et al.*, 1992; Travlos and Marisi, 1996; Hylan, Sundell and Judge, 1999; Schneider *et al.*, 1999; Ekkekakis, Hall and Petruzzello, 2008; Forsyth and Reilly, 2008; Janse De Jonge *et al.*, 2012; Prado *et al.*, 2021b).

Knowing about these physiological and psychological changes can help women to prepare mentally and to adjust their physical activity regimen accordingly; for example, by planning for particularly enjoyable physical activities or working out with friends during the luteal phase.

5.2. THE ABC OF STRESS HORMONES: THE INTERACTION BETWEEN FEMALE SEX HORMONES AND THE STRESS RESPONSE

The HPA axis is the main endocrine axis involved in the stress response, which leads to the production of glucocorticoids, such as the stress hormone cortisol (see Figure 5.1).

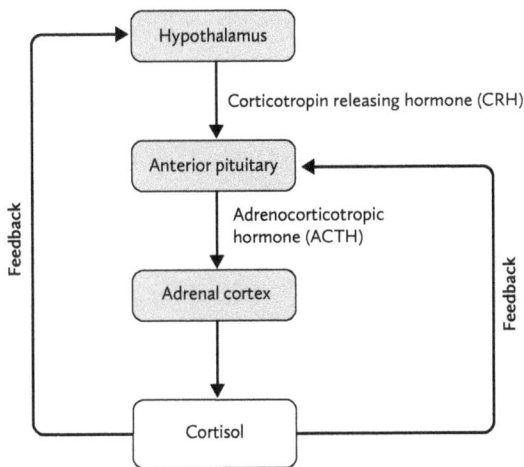

Figure 5.1: Hypothalamic-pituitary-adrenal (HPA) axis.

Cortisol secretion follows a predictable daily rhythm and peaks around 45 minutes after waking (Bartkowiak-Wieczorek et al., 2024). Short-term increases of cortisol are part of the body's natural adaptive response to psychological and physiological stress (including stressors such as exercise) and can stimulate glycogen and glucose synthesis in the liver and increase carbohydrate and fat metabolism, thus helping the body to access energy. Cortisol can also impact immune and inflammatory responses by inhibiting inflammatory and allergic reactions as well as lymphocyte production. This is why synthetic glucocorticoids are used as medication for conditions such as arthritis or as anti-transplant rejection drugs (Wilkinson and Brown, 2015). Prolonged excessive cortisol secretion, however, can have negative effects on a variety of tissues. Possible adverse effects of chronic stress and prolonged cortisol secretion include immunosuppression and increased abdominal fat deposition. Additional adverse effects are depicted in Figure 5.2.

Sex differences in many stress-related psychological disorders such as anxiety, major depressive disorder and post-traumatic stress disorder (PTSD) have been reported (Bangasser and Valentino, 2014; Boyd et al., 2015; Ludwig, Roy and Dwivedi, 2019; Klusmann et al., 2023). As a consequence, an interaction between female sex hormones and stress hormones such as cortisol—and therefore between the HPO (see section 1.2.1) and HPA axes—has been assumed (Heim and Binder, 2012; Wagenmaker and Moenter, 2017; Heck and Handa, 2019; Schumacher et al., 2019). Recent meta-analyses show that the menstrual cycle can affect basal cortisol concentrations (i.e. cortisol levels in an unstressed state), with higher levels in the menstrual compared to the premenstrual (i.e. late luteal) phase, as well as higher concentrations in the follicular compared to the luteal phase (Hamidovic et al., 2020; Klusmann et al., 2022). It has been speculated that lower cortisol concentrations in the luteal phase may be mediated by progesterone metabolites (specifically allopregnanolone) (see also text box "Causes for premenstrual disorders—current theories on allopregnanolone and serotonin" in section 2.4), which are thought to inhibit HPA axis activity.

Another relevant HPA axis marker is HPA reactivity (i.e. the cortisol response to a stressor). A recent systematic review and meta-analysis indicates that HPA axis reactivity is higher in the luteal than in the follicular phase of the menstrual cycle phase (Klusmann et al., 2023). These findings imply that stress reactivity fluctuates throughout the menstrual cycle and that the luteal phase may represent a window of vulnerability for stress-related disorders. Taken together with the above-mentioned meta-analysis on basal cortisol concentrations (Klusmann et al.,

2022), resting cortisol levels may be lower in the luteal phase, but the HPA axis may become more sensitive or reactive to stress in this phase. Accordingly, the luteal phase of the menstrual cycle could be a critical time for interventions aimed at stress reduction. However, the studies included in the meta-analysis were small in sample size and presented with notable variations in methodology (e.g. regarding the determination of menstrual cycle phase or type of stressor—physiological or psychosocial), which emphasizes the need for future studies with larger sample sizes and more standardized and rigorous methodologies to better understand the interaction between ovarian hormones and cortisol.

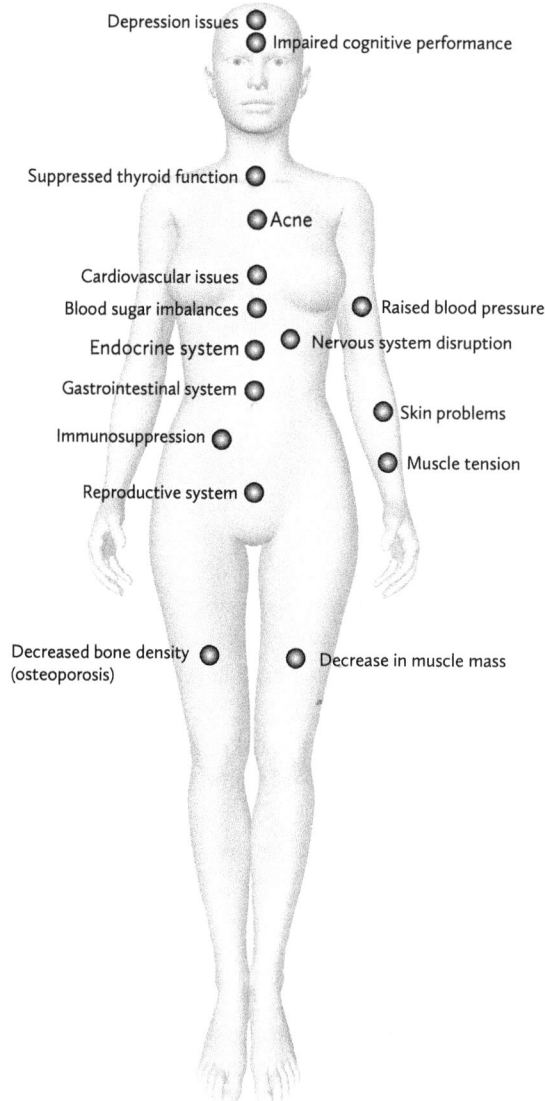

Figure 5.2: Adverse effects of prolonged cortisol secretion. Chronic stress can lead to negative effects on many body systems. In addition, long-term excessive cortisol exposure may lead to an increase in abdominal fat deposition (adapted from Wilkinson and Brown, 2015).

Cortisol levels and stress regulation in transgender people

Research agendas are starting to take a deeper look at stress regulation in transgender individuals. From a biomedical perspective, gender-affirming hormone treatment (GAHT) may impact the stress response. On a psychosocial level, transgender people may be exposed to stigma and other gender minority stressors, which may manifest in neuroendocrinological markers. A 2019 longitudinal study involving ten trans women (female gender identity, assigned male at birth) and 15 trans men (male gender identity, assigned female at birth) tracked their hormonal and stress responses before and after three months of GAHT (Fuss et al., 2019). Trans women showed a 15% increase in cortisol after three months of estradiol and anti-androgen therapy, suggesting enhanced HPA-axis activity. Trans men receiving testosterone treatment, in contrast, exhibited a 58% decrease in cortisol, indicating reduced HPA-axis activity. The study findings demonstrate that GAHT can alter the stress regulation mechanisms and reactivity of the HPA axis in transgender people, with different effects observed between trans women and trans men.

Another 2024 study explored the relationships between gender minority stress and cortisol profiles among 124 transgender and gender diverse individuals (DuBois et al., 2024). Participants who experienced high levels of stigma showed altered cortisol rhythms, characterized by a blunted cortisol awakening response and a smaller decline in cortisol over the course of the day, leading to elevated cortisol concentrations before bedtime compared to those experiencing less stigma. This flattened cortisol pattern represents downregulated HPA-axis functioning, which can also be observed in the context of fatigue, trauma and discrimination. In contrast, community connectedness was positively associated with the cortisol awakening response, pointing to a healthy adaptation to stress experiences. These findings emphasize the importance of addressing stigma and gender minority stress, as well as resilience measures such as social support to improve the stress response and wellbeing of transgender individuals.

Taken together, these studies highlight the influence of biological as well as psychosocial dimensions of transgender health on the stress response.

Changing perspective: Psychological stress and menstrual cycle irregularity

The menstrual cycle can affect the secretion of stress hormones such as cortisol. Conversely, psychological stress also appears to affect the menstrual cycle. A recent review including 41 studies examined the effects of psychological stressors (e.g. academic, occupational or Covid-19-related stress) on menstrual dysfunction (Poitras et al., 2024). The most commonly reported disruptions associated with elevated stress were irregular menstruation and abnormal menstrual flow. These findings support the bidirectional nature of the relationship between the HPO and HPA axes.

5.3. PRACTICES TO ADDRESS THE STRESS RESPONSE

Various interventions have been suggested to address the stress response. Stress-focused interventions include meditation, mindfulness training such as mindfulness-based stress reduction (MBSR), yoga, relaxation techniques, biofeedback and cognitive behavioral therapy (Regehr, Glancy and Pitts, 2013; Agyapong et al., 2023). In addition to improving stress-coping abilities, such interventions may also improve sports performance: for example, mindfulness practices have been recommended as a performance-enhancing complementary training approach, especially in precision sports such as dart throwing (Bühlmayer et al., 2017; Si, Yang and Feng, 2024). However, there is still relatively little research on gender differences for such practices. A few studies have explored whether the use and effects of meditation and mindfulness-based interventions differ across genders. A 2019 study analysed survey data from the 2012 US National Health Interview Survey (including 34,342 US adults) (Upchurch and Johnson, 2019). The authors found that among all meditators, the most common reason for using meditation was to reduce stress (35%). Both women and men found meditation to be helpful (94% and 90%, respectively). Differences emerged in the patterns of using meditation techniques: a higher percentage of females used meditation in combination with yoga, qi gong or tai chi, while male meditators tended to use specific stand-alone meditation techniques (such as mindfulness meditation).

Some experimental studies have looked at the responses of women and men to a meditation/mindfulness intervention. A 2017 study examined the effects of a 12-week meditation course on measures of affect, mindfulness and self-compassion in a group of 77 college students (36 of whom were female) (Rojiani et al., 2017). The study found that women showed greater decreases in negative affect and greater increases in mindfulness and self-compassion compared to men. Women may thus have more favorable responses to meditation. The authors hypothesized that meditation and mindfulness-based interventions may produce better results for women because these techniques decrease ruminative tendencies, which are representative of women's internalized response to distress (Jain et al., 2007; Kingston et al., 2007; Heeren and Philippot, 2011; Rojiani et al., 2017). A 2024 study looked at a relaxation and mindfulness-based intervention in 218 university students (112 females) (Vidic, 2024). It was found that females experienced a greater decrease in maladaptive coping, such as avoidance or detachment from emotions, compared to male participants. Another piece of research looked at sex differences in response to a mindfulness intervention in adolescents (Bluth, Roberson and Girdler, 2017). The researchers noted differences in course engagement and stress after the intervention: females were more engaged in the offered class than males, and practiced mindfulness skills more frequently at home; however, effects on stress per se were inconclusive (which in part was due to the small and unbalanced sample size of ten females and five males). These findings suggest that male and female adolescents may engage with and respond to mindfulness interventions in different ways.

In sports, stress-reducing interventions can be included in the training regimen as part of recovery sessions (to regulate parasympathetic tone to enhance the recovery process), or as part of athletes' mental training (to specifically prepare for situations when pressure during competition or stress and training load are high) (Yu, 2015). Educating athletes about the importance of stress reduction for both physical as well as psychological reasons can help to recognize yoga, meditation and mindfulness approaches as valuable techniques within their toolbox. Female athletes may particularly use phases of their menstrual cycle when perceived performance is reduced to incorporate stress-reducing techniques into their training. Stress-reducing interventions can furthermore be of relevance in the context of "choking under pressure"— freezing and under-performing when it matters most, when a combination of factors increases an athlete's felt pressure and anxiety. Well-known examples in sports include tennis serves, penalty shots in soccer or free throws in basketball. The causes for choking under pressure are multifaceted; one reason for choking can be distraction, when the athlete puts their attention to task-irrelevant cues. Mindfulness-based techniques, meditation and breathing exercises have been found helpful to prevent distraction and promote task-relevant focus (Gröpel and Mesagno, 2019). While the research on sex differences in choking under pressure remains ambiguous (see text box "Coping with stress in sports—sex differences in choking under pressure"), these techniques can generally be used in sports to support athletes when they need to perform the most.

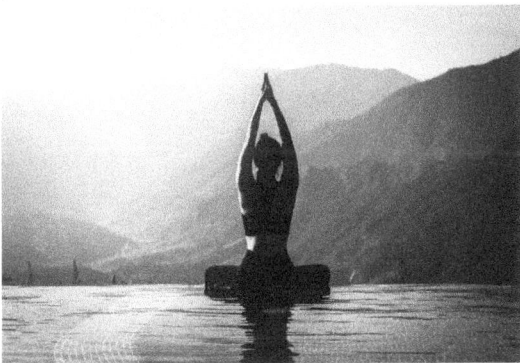

Photo 5.1: Sex differences in response to stress reducing interventions such as yoga, meditation or mindfulness practices remain relatively understudied. The few existing studies suggest that females may engage more in mindfulness trainings and have more favorable responses to meditation than men.

Rolling for relaxation?

Self-myofascial release interventions such as Foam Rolling or techniques using balls have gained popularity among athletes and health professionals. While they are often used to increase range of motion or promote tissue recovery (Wiewelhove et al., 2019; Wilke et al., 2020), self-myofascial release techniques may also impact the stress response by influencing the autonomic nervous system. The fascial system is rich in sensory mechanoreceptors such as Ruffini endings, whose stimulation has been reported to lower sympathetic activity (Schleip, 2003). It has also been shown that fibers of the sympathetic nervous system are present in fascial layers such as the thoracolumbar fascia, and it has been hypothesized that this innervation may be an explanation why low back pain patients report increased pain levels when under stress (Mense, 2019).

While the mechanical load applied through self-myofascial release techniques inevitably impacts all tissue layers, Foam Rolling and other interventions have been used to specifically target the properties of the fascial tissues, including the connection to the (autonomic) nervous system. Myofascial release techniques may thus be a valuable tool to foster relaxation and stress reduction. To date, no studies exist on the influence of gender differences or the menstrual cycle on the effects of self-myofascial release; however, this should not discourage females from trying this technique for themselves and exploring if it can positively impact the autonomic nervous system and stress.

Coping with stress in sports—sex differences in choking under pressure

A few recent studies examined sex differences in choking under pressure: In soccer and basketball, choking appears to happen to the same degree in both women and men, without significant sex differences (Toma, 2015; Santos and Santos, 2024). In alpine slalom skiing, on the other hand, it has recently been reported that women handled pressure better in advantageous situations (i.e. when the course setter was from the same country as the athlete) than men, who were more likely to experience performance declines when expectations were high, particularly in the most decisive moments of competition (Bühren, Gschwend and Krumer, 2024). It is hoped that future studies will further elucidate how differences in choking under pressure are influenced by type of sport, sex and individual characteristics.

Selected breathwork, restorative yoga and self-myofascial release techniques are described in the Appendix. The Appendix covers background and research findings for the different tools, as well as practical tips and suggestions for variations and props.

CHAPTER 6

To Ovulate or Not to Ovulate: Effects of Oral Contraceptives on Hormonal Status, Training and Injury Risk

Contraceptive methods such as withdrawal have been used for millennia, while hormonal methods started to be used in the 1960s (United Nations, 2019). Hormonal contraception comes in various delivery methods, including transdermal patches, injections, implants and vaginal rings. Most commonly, hormonal intrauterine devices (IUDs) or oral contraceptives (OCs; "the pill") are used (Cabre *et al.*, 2024). Hormonal IUDs contain progestin and prevent the sperm from getting into the uterus by thickening the cervical mucus. OCs prevent ovulation and follicular development; they furthermore reduce the endometrial lining and sperm mobility (Elliott-Sale and Hicks, 2018). IUDs are highly prevalent in a handful of countries such as the Democratic People's Republic of Korea (46.9%) and Uzbekistan (36.9%). Oral contraceptives, in contrast, are commonly used worldwide: more than 20% of women of reproductive age in 27 countries are on the pill, with the highest prevalence in European countries (United Nations, 2019). In elite athletes, hormonal contraceptive use is common (approximately 50%), and around one third of female elite athletes (equaling roughly 68% of those using hormonal contraception) have been reported to use the pill (Martin *et al.*, 2018; Clarke *et al.*, 2021). The main reasons for using hormonal contraception include the avoidance of pregnancy as well as the management of menstrual symptoms

(Clarke *et al.*, 2021); in athletes, oral contraceptives are furthermore used strategically to control the cycle, that is, to manipulate the timing of bleeding or to omit it entirely—for example, during competition (Martin *et al.*, 2018; Schaumberg *et al.*, 2018; Elliott-Sale *et al.*, 2020). Since the pill is the most prevalent type of hormonal contraception—both globally as well as among physically active women—this chapter focuses on the types and effects of oral contraceptives.

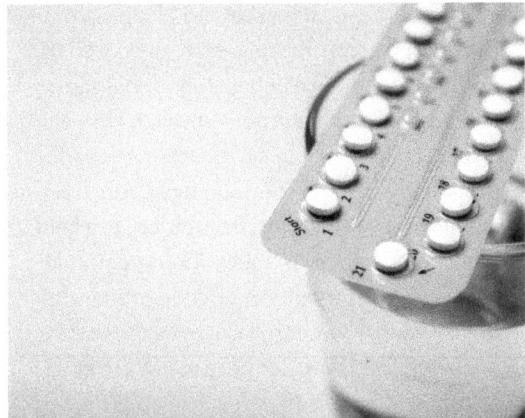

Photo 6.1: Oral contraception ("the pill") is used by many women around the globe. The pill comes in many forms. Most commonly, women use combined monophasic formulations, which contain a fixed amount of synthetic estradiol and progestin to be taken for 21 days (consumption phase), followed by seven pill-free days or placebo pills (withdrawal phase).

Male contraception—*quo vadis*?

This book focuses on female hormones; nevertheless, within a chapter on contraceptives, it seems mandatory to discuss the status of research on male contraception. Novel male contraceptives have been in development for decades and a robust global market has been predicted (Vahdat *et al.*, 2024). Funding, though, has been lacking. Non-profit and governmental agencies are the main advocates for the field; they also provide the limited available funding to develop male contraceptives further. The pharmaceutical industry, however, focuses nearly exclusively on female contraception methods; the industry hasn't been involved much in funding research and development of male contraception and remains a spectator in the current research space (Vahdat *et al.*, 2024).

The lack of involvement of the industry can partly be explained by a lack of guidelines from regulatory agencies (such as the Food and Drug Administration in the US). Open questions remain when it comes to defining biological markers to evaluate efficacy of male contraceptives in clinical trials. For example, sperm count, functional sperm characteristics or hormone levels have been discussed as possible surrogate markers for pregnancy prevention, but have not been agreed on by regulators. In addition, the field faces some obvious methodological challenges: the intervention effect—prevention of pregnancy—is not measured in the patient receiving the treatment (Sitruk-Ware *et al.*, 2024). It is hoped that future research can overcome these funding and regulatory challenges and move this opportunity for shared contraceptive responsibility forward (Vahdat *et al.*, 2024).

Hormonal contraceptives, sexual function and relationship satisfaction

Various studies have looked at the relationship between hormonal contraception and sexual function. It appears that hormonal contraception can have negative sexual side effects in some women. Women using hormonal contraceptives have been reported to have sexual activity less frequently, experience less arousal, pleasure and orgasm, while having more difficulty with lubrication (Smith, Jozkowski and Sanders, 2014). One study reported oral contraceptive users to have poorer sexual function compared with users of copper intrauterine devices (Déa *et al.*, 2024). Within oral contraceptives, for pills with high androgenicity (see section 6.1) these effects might be less pronounced (Handy *et al.*, 2023). Generally, more diversity is needed in research to enhance the understanding of the potential negative sexual side effects of hormonal contraceptives, as current studies are often based on heterosexual college-aged females (Smith, Jozkowski and Sanders, 2014; Handy *et al.*, 2023).

Moreover, potential connections between OC use and the choice of a relationship partner have received much attention. Since hormonal fluctuations throughout the regular menstrual cycle have been associated with temporal variations in the judgement of the attractiveness of men, the use of OCs may alter women's mate preferences (Roberts *et al.*, 2014). More specifically, hormonal contraceptives could influence partner choice when a relationship is formed; relationship satisfaction may then potentially change when the use of hormonal contraceptives is terminated at a later time. This has become known as the **congruency hypothesis** (i.e. relationship satisfaction may be altered if current OC use is not congruent with OC use when the relationship was formed) (Roberts *et al.*, 2014). A 2022 study tested the congruency in four larger samples of couples. The authors only found support for the congruency hypothesis in one of the samples and concluded that the effects of OCs on women's relationships and sexuality show inconsistent patterns (Fiurašková *et al.*, 2022). Fortunately, relationship satisfaction seems to depend on more than exogenous hormones after all.

6.1. TYPES OF ORAL CONTRACEPTIVES

Oral contraception comes in many forms—so many in fact that women can find it difficult to really understand what kind of pill they are taking. For example, a survey among elite football players in Australia revealed that 89% of OC users were not able to identify what type of pill they were using (Clarke *et al.*, 2021).

Since their legal introduction in the 1960s, OCs have been reformulated several times, resulting in four different "generations" of pills. Most females use **combined pill** formulations (Dalgaard *et al.*, 2019). Combined OCs contain synthetic estrogen (ethinyl estradiol) and synthetic progesterone (the type of progestin varies across OC generations). While first-generation pills are no longer available, second-generation OCs are still in use. Newer generations have lower doses of synthetic estrogen and thus produce fewer side effects (such as weight gain, fluid retention, headaches, nausea, breast tenderness). Second-generation OCs are thought to have the lowest risk of blood clots (Elliott-Sale and Hicks, 2018). In addition to combined pills, **progestin-only** OCs (the so called "**mini pills**") are also available for women who do not wish to use exogenous estrogens, for example because they are contraindicated or during lactation (Burrows and Peters, 2007; Thompson *et al.*, 2020). As the mini pill does not contain synthetic estrogen, it tends to have milder adverse effects than the combined pill (Burrows and Peters, 2007). With progesterone-only pills, bleeding can become more irregular or frequent (Elliott-Sale and Hicks, 2018).

Combined pills are available as **mono-, bi- and triphasic** schedules of administration. **Monophasic** OCs contain a fixed amount of estradiol and progestin, typically to be taken every day for 21 days (consumption phase), followed by seven days with placebo pills or free of pills (withdrawal or placebo phase). Most women use combined monophasic OCs (Dalgaard *et al.*, 2019). **Multiphasic** pills use varying doses of synthetic hormones and aim to mimic the rising and falling pattern of estrogen and progesterone of the menstrual cycle (Thompson *et al.*, 2020). Such varying formulas and schedules of administration have been developed to decrease adverse effects of OC consumption (Van Vliet *et al.*, 2006). **Biphasic** products contain the same amount of estrogen throughout the cycle, but the progestin content switches (i.e. increases) once during the consumption phase. **Triphasic** pills contain three different ratios of estrogen and progestin throughout the cycle; estrogen concentration can be constant or variable, while progestin content changes twice during the consumption phase (Burrows and Peters, 2007; Elliott-Sale and Hicks, 2018).

The exogenous estrogens and progestins contained in OCs act on the HPA via a **negative feedback loop** on follicle-stimulating hormone, luteinizing hormone and gonadotropin-releasing hormone (Elliott-Sale and Hicks, 2018). OCs consequently cause the hormonal milieu to be down-regulated at a relatively stable level (Reif *et al.*, 2021). More specifically, use of combined monophasic OCs results in four distinct hormonal environments (Elliott-Sale *et al.*, 2020; Reif *et al.*, 2021) (see Figure 6.1 for a graphic representation):

- A downregulated endogenous estradiol profile.

- A chronically downregulated endogenous progesterone profile (as ovulation is inhibited).

- A daily mild surge of synthetic estrogen and progestin (peak levels are reached within one hour after ingestion).

- Seven OC free days, during which endogenous hormones (estrogen, FSH and LH) may rise slightly (not shown in Figure 6.1).

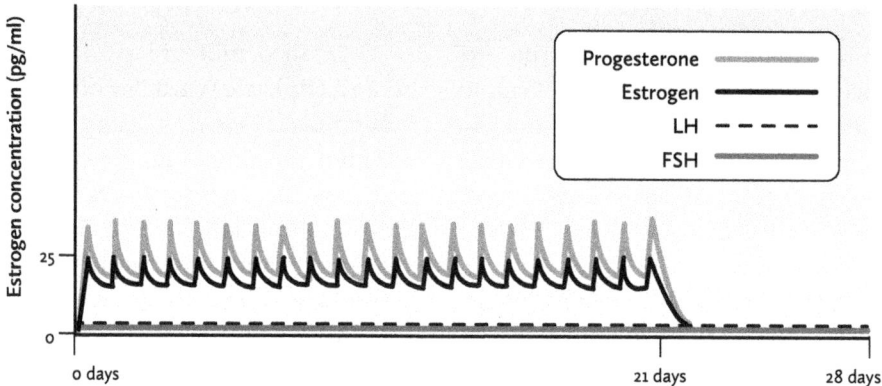

Figure 6.1: Hormonal fluctuations in taking combined monophasic oral contraception containing both estrogen and progestin (adapted from Chidi-Ogbolu and Baar, 2018). Compared to a regular menstrual cycle, the hormonal milieu is downregulated at a relatively stable level, with daily mild surges of synthetic estrogen and progestin during the consumption phase (Elliott-Sale *et al.*, 2020).

Progestins furthermore differ in **androgenicity**, which describes the ability of progestin to produce masculine characteristics such as hair growth or acne (Jones, 1995). The level of androgenicity has been suggested to impact sexual function (see text box above) as well as the responses to resistance training (Thompson *et al.*, 2020). Older progestins (first- and second-generation OCs) have increased androgenic effects because they are synthesized from testosterone and bind to testosterone receptors. Newer progestins (particularly fourth-generation drospirenone, as it is not made out of testosterone) have reduced androgenic or antiandrogenic effects (Dragoman, 2014; Thompson *et al.*, 2021).

Mental health side effects of the pill

In the last couple of years, various documentaries and media reports have stressed the potential mental health side effects of oral contraceptives, including depression, anxiety, low mood and suicidal thoughts. While evidence remains inconsistent, certain subgroups and conditions may be at a higher risk for mental adverse effects, according to the current research (Schaffir, Worly and Gur, 2016; Robakis *et al.*, 2019; Kraft *et al.*, 2024). Adolescents appear to be a particularly vulnerable cohort, and findings indicate a potentially increased mental health risk for adolescent OC users (Skovlund *et al.*, 2016; Kraft *et al.*, 2024). In addition, progestin-only OCs and contraceptives containing more androgenic progestins may lead to higher rates of adverse effects on mood; however, evidence remains inconclusive in this area as well (Schaffir, Worly and Gur, 2016; Kraft *et al.*, 2024). Shockingly, a 2018 study drawing from data of a national cohort including women in Denmark found a positive association between the use of hormonal contraception and subsequent suicide attempt and suicide, with the highest relative risk among adolescent women (Skovlund *et al.*, 2018). Another study from 2022 using data from the Swedish national registries also reported an increased risk for suicidal behavior among young women using oral contraceptives, but found that risk declined with increased duration of use (Edwards *et al.*, 2022). As studies on hormonal contraceptive use and suicidal behavior vary substantially, additional research is needed. The relationship between the pill and mental health side effects should not be taken lightly—even if the overall number of severe mental side effects such as suicides may be small, each individual case should be seen as a devastating consequence and more research efforts are called for to gain important insights for suicide prevention in women using hormonal contraception.

6.2. EFFECTS OF ORAL CONTRACEPTIVE USE ON MUSCLE MASS, STRENGTH AND POWER

The role of synthetic estrogen in OCs use on muscle anabolism is still uncertain. A common measure to evaluate resistance training adaptations is **skeletal muscle hypertrophy**, which is experienced when the average myofibrillar protein synthesis exceeds the average myofibrillar protein breakdown rate over time (Dalgaard *et al.*, 2019). It appears that OCs with high progesterone levels have a negative impact on muscle mass—high-progestin OCs decrease muscle protein synthesis (i.e. myofibrillar protein synthesis) (Hansen *et al.*, 2011; Chidi-Ogbolu and Baar, 2018). This supports the assumption that progesterone has a catabolic effect on muscle mass. However, some have also suggested anabolic effects of progesterone (Smith *et al.*, 2014). Consequently, the anabolic or catabolic effects of OCs remain controversial.

The effects of the pill on strength parameters remain inconclusive. Some work suggests that strength parameters are affected differently when comparing non-OC users with a regular menstrual cycle to OC users: several studies show that OC use produced no changes in strength, while non-users showed changes throughout the menstrual cycle (Wirth and Lohman, 1982; Phillips *et al.*, 1996; Sarwar, Niclos and Rutherford, 1996; Elliott, Cable and Reilly, 2005). Other studies, in turn, contrast with these findings: a 2021 study looked at the effects of a ten-week high-intensity strength and endurance training in hormone contraception users versus non-users. While both groups increased strength parameters, the researchers found no differences between the groups in the observed strength measures (Myllyaho *et al.*, 2021). A 2008 study found similar results in response to a 12-week strength training program in 31 collegiate softball and water polo players (Nichols *et al.*, 2008). More recently, a systematic review and meta-analysis examined the effect of oral contraceptives on muscle hypertrophy, strength and power adaptations in response to resistance training in hormonal contraceptive users and non-users (Nolan *et al.*, 2023). Results indicated that OC use did not significantly affect any of the outcomes. The authors therefore concluded that there is no rationale to advocate for or against OC use when women aim for hypertrophy, strength or power through resistance training. Instead, the decision whether to use OCs should be based on an individualized approach (i.e. reasons for use and an individual's response should be considered).

Regarding strength parameters throughout the OC cycle, numerous studies report no significant changes in strength between the consumption and withdrawal phase (Sarwar, Niclos and Rutherford, 1996; Elliott, Cable and Reilly, 2005; Ekenros et al., 2013), even when considering different combined OCs with various potencies and androgenicity of progestin (Peters and Burrows, 2006). However, the data is not unambiguous: contrasting the findings above, a 2009 study showed that reactive strength measures via a drop jump test were significantly lower in the late withdrawal phase compared to the late consumption phase within a monophasic OC cycle (Rechichi and Dawson, 2009).

Methodological considerations for OC and sports performance research

Some methodological considerations are important to contextualize the findings related to OC effects on sports performance parameters. Generally, studies compare performance:

- in OC use versus non-use with a regular menstrual cycle (e.g. by means of a within-subject design: measurements are taken in eumenorrheic women before introducing OCs, and then after a period of OC consumption in the same women; comparisons between groups—i.e. OC users versus eumenorrheic non-users—are also used in the research)

- between different phases of the OC cycle (e.g. comparing measurements of the consumption and withdrawal phase).

Difficulties in comparing studies arise from the large variance between studies regarding:

- the type of OC pills used (e.g. combined mono- or multiphasic pills, progestin-only OCs, degree of androgenicity, hormone concentrations)

- the phase of OC cycle investigated (e.g. consumption vs. withdrawal phase, early vs. late consumption phase, different phases of multiphasic pills)

- which phase of the menstrual cycle to compare OC data to (e.g. early follicular, late follicular, luteal)

- which performance tests are used (individual performance components such as strength or endurance, sport-specific tests representing complex performance; a multitude of different tests is available for both)

- the characteristics of the cohort researched (e.g. untrained vs. trained subjects, homogeneity within examined sample regarding endogenous hormone concentrations).

With the resulting variability between studies, it's not surprising that the current data on OC effects and sports performance remains inconclusive in several areas. Efforts are being made in the field to clarify and adequately report methodological approaches, so an enhanced execution and reporting of future studies can be ensured (Elliott-Sale et al., 2021). Nonetheless, health practitioners who wish to draw conclusions from the data are encouraged to take a look at the details of studies, to forge an individualized approach for their clients and patients.

6.3. EFFECTS OF ORAL CONTRACEPTIVE USE ENDURANCE MEASURES

The effects of oral contraceptive use on endurance measures—that is, measures of cardiorespiratory fitness such as maximal oxygen consumption ($VO_{2\,max}$)—are less extensively studied than the effects on muscle mass and strength. Some studies suggest that exogenous female sex hormones might reduce endurance performance moderately in active women. A double blind, placebo-controlled study looked at the effects of OC use on maximal aerobic capacity. Women, who initially were on a regular menstrual cycle, were divided into two groups: one received a triphasic OC for a period of two months, the other took a placebo pill. Measures of maximal aerobic capacity were taken twice while women were still on their regular cycle and after two months of the intervention phase. In the OC group, $VO_{2\,max}$ decreased by 4.7%, while a light increase of 1.5% was observed in the placebo group (Lebrun *et al.*, 2003). A 2002 study used a design with two phases to determine the effects of OCs on peak exercise capacity. Women first went through testing while they were on a regular menstrual cycle; they then started taking a triphasic combined pill and were re-tested after four months of OC use. OC consumption led to a significant 11% decrease in peak oxygen consumption compared to the measures taken on the regular menstrual cycle (Casazza *et al.*, 2002). A 2024 study investigated the differences between the consumption and withdrawal phase of combined, monophasic OC use in an incremental running test and found only marginal differences in endurance-related parameters between the two phases. The authors pointed out that while the observed differences may be negligible for most women, even small changes can differentiate winning from losing in elite sports (Mathy *et al.*, 2024).

A systematic review and meta-analysis including cross-sectional observational studies looked at exercise and strength related performance measures (Elliott-Sale *et al.*, 2020). The authors reported only slightly inferior exercise performance in OC users compared to non-users; exercise performance was furthermore consistent across the OC cycle (i.e. no significant differences were observed between the consumption and withdrawal phase). As no significant differences emerged, this study, too, concluded that while OC use may result in small adverse effects on performance in some individuals, the evidence does not warrant general guidance on OC use when it comes to exercise performance. Instead, an individualized approach seems to be more appropriate. The authors also noted that the variance between studies was relatively large, indicating that participant characteristics, research design and measured outcomes might have influenced effects.

6.4. INFLUENCE OF HORMONAL CONTRACEPTIVE USE ON METABOLISM

The exploration of metabolic outcomes in hormonal contraception users is rather limited (Cabre *et al.*, 2024). Only a few studies have investigated the effects of OCs on resting energy expenditure. While one study showed a slight increase in resting energy expenditure with OC use (Kimm *et al.*, 2001), several other studies reported no differences in resting energy expenditure between eumenorrheic women and OC users (Diffey *et al.*, 1997; Eck *et al.*, 1997; Jensen and Levine, 1998). However, the available studies are based on heterogeneous study populations and designs (Cabre *et al.*, 2024). During exercise, OC use may increase lipolytic activity without any effect on substrate utilization (Boisseau and Isacco, 2022).

OCs may further impact metabolic outcomes related to recovery: estrogen is thought to help reduce muscle damage and inflammation after exercise; accordingly, it can be hypothesized that OC users may present with different recovery outcomes due to their downregulated endogenous estrogen level (Cabre *et al.*, 2024). Some studies suggest the notion of pro-inflammatory and stress-amplifying effects of OC use, reporting increased inflammatory markers and cortisol (Meulenberg *et al.*, 1987; Dreon, Slavin and Phinney, 2003; Cauci, Francescato and Curcio, 2017; Bozzini *et al.*, 2021; Cabre *et al.*, 2024).

6.5. ORAL CONTRACEPTIVE USE AND INJURY RISK

The relationship between OC use and injury risk reveals slight differences for various soft tissues (i.e. ligaments, tendons and muscle). Regarding ligaments, research has mainly been conducted related to knee laxity and anterior cruciate ligament (ACL) injury (see section 3.3). Knee laxity has been reported to change with the hormonal fluctuations of the menstrual cycle (specifically, knee laxity increased in relation to estradiol levels), and increased ligament laxity has been associated with a heightened risk for ACL injury (Shultz *et al.*, 2005; Myer *et al.*, 2008). This raises the question of whether eliminating changes in estrogen using OCs has an influence on injury risk (Chidi-Ogbolu and Baar, 2018). In support of this idea, it has been found that young females undergoing surgical ACL repair are 18% less likely to use OCs than matched controls (Gray, Gugala and Baillargeon, 2016). It has furthermore been reported that the relative risk of ACL injury in females who had never used the pill was 20% higher compared to women who were long-term OC users (Rahr-Wagner *et al.*, 2014). Taken together, this suggests that OC use may be protective for ACL rupture (Chidi-Ogbolu and Baar, 2018). While two systematic reviews confirm an association between OC use and decreased knee laxity and ACL injury rates, the strength of the evidence appears to be worth improving. High-quality, long-term observational and intervention studies are needed to verify the relationship between OC use and ACL injury risk and to better understand potential underlying mechanisms (Herzberg *et al.*, 2017; Konopka, Hsue and Dragoo, 2019).

On the other hand, the pill may negatively impact injury risk in **tendon and muscle**: OC use has been associated with increased risk of Achilles tendinopathy (Holmes and Lin, 2006). This may be explained by an altered collagen synthesis in connection with OC use: a group of OC-taking women showed no change in patellar tendon collagen synthesis in response to exercise compared to controls, who were in the follicular phase of their regular menstrual cycle. The latter group increased their collagen synthesis significantly (M. Hansen *et al.*, 2008). OC use has furthermore been related to greater muscle damage and delayed onset muscle soreness, which points to a protective effect of the cyclical rise of estrogen observed during regular menstrual cycles (Savage and Clarkson, 2002; Minahan *et al.*, 2015; Chidi-Ogbolu and Baar, 2018).

Part II

FEMALE FLOW THROUGHOUT THE LIFESPAN

Pregnancy and Beyond: Hormone Changes and their Effects During Childbearing and the Postpartum Period

The period of conceiving, pregnancy and postpartum may very well be the occasion in a woman's life when she consciously becomes aware of her reproductive hormones for the first time, particularly when dealing with infertility issues (Zalewska *et al.*, 2024). In sports research, the existing under-representation of women (see Introduction) is marked during pregnancy and lactation (Zhu, Reed and Van Spall, 2022)—even less data is available for exercising pregnant and breastfeeding/pumping women than for the general female population. This chapter focuses on the physiological adaptations during pregnancy and the postpartum period, preventative aspects of physical activity during this time, and aspects related to musculoskeletal injury. While mentioned briefly in some instances, pathophysiological aspects of pregnancy and the postpartum period (such as pre-eclampsia) are elaborated in detail elsewhere.

7.1. ADAPTATIONS DURING PREGNANCY

7.1.1. Changes in hormone levels

Pregnancy is orchestrated by complex endocrine interactions. The list below provides an overview of some important changes during gestation:

- **Human chorionic gonadotropin (hCG)** produced by the placenta can be detected shortly (approximately 11 days) after conception. It plays an important role in maintaining the corpus luteum (see section 1.2.2), ensuring the production of progesterone to sustain the gestational uterine lining (endometrium).

- **Progesterone** is initially produced by the corpus luteum and later by the placenta. It maintains the endometrium and prevents contractions. Together with cortisol and hCG, it helps to suppress the mother's immune response, protecting the embryo from immunologic rejection.

- **Estrogen (estradiol and estriol)** rises over the course of pregnancy (Robinson and Klein, 2012). Estrogen promotes the growth of the uterus and breasts as well as vascular supply. The increase in vascularization due to estrogen may contribute to vascular varicosities in some pregnant women (Robinson and Klein, 2012; Gavrilov, 2017).

- **Relaxin** softens cervix and connective tissues (Goldsmith and Weiss, 2009).

- **Prolactin** increases to prepare for milk production; in lactating women, prolactin pulses stimulate milk production (Voogt *et al.*, 2001).

- The **thyroid hormones** thyroxine (T4) and triiodothyronine (T3) increase during pregnancy to meet the metabolic demands of pregnancy. Maternal thyroid hormones also play a vital role in fetal neurodevelopment (Feldt-Rasmussen and Mathiesen, 2011).

- **Cortisol** increases due to corticotropin-releasing hormone production in the placenta (which increases over 1000-fold during pregnancy). Cortisol levels peak in late pregnancy and a significant surge is seen in the third trimester and during labor. One proposed reason for cortisol changes may be that cortisol leads to greater glucose levels in the maternal bloodstream, which are then available for fetal consumption (see section 7.1.3) (Gangestad, Caldwell Hooper and Eaton, 2012).

- **Oxytocin** plays a role in labor, lactation and bonding between mother and newborn (Hermesch *et al.*, 2024). A surge in oxytocin levels initiates uterine contractions.

Figure 7.1 depicts hormone changes during pregnancy and postpartum.

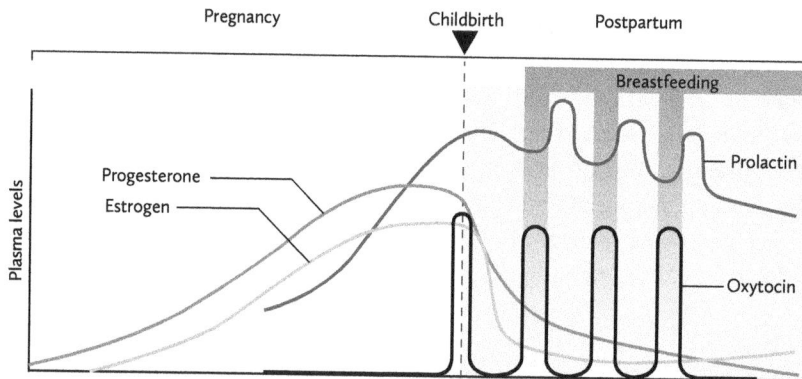

Figure 7.1: Hormone changes during pregnancy and postpartum. Estrogen, progesterone and prolactin rise during pregnancy. A surge in oxytocin levels initiates uterine contractions. After childbirth and removal of the placenta, estrogen and progesterone rapidly drop. In breastfeeding/pumping women, pulses of prolactin concentrations stimulate milk production; oxytocin pulses lead to milk ejection (let-down reflex). In non-lactating women, prolactin levels return to pre-pregnancy values within three weeks postpartum; in breastfeeding/pumping females, prolactin levels remain high in the first weeks postpartum, but eventually decline as well (adapted from Kohl, Autry and Dulac, 2016).

7.1.2. Anatomical and biomechanical changes

Due to the growing uterus and breasts, the center of gravity changes, which results in compensatory postural and movement patterns to avoid falling forward. Postural balance is affected after the first trimester and falling is a common cause of injury later in pregnancy (Vladutiu, Evenson and Marshall, 2010; Cakmak, Ribeiro and Inanir, 2016). Lumbar lordosis and thoracic kyphosis increase in pregnancy (however, not all studies report consistent findings) and back pain is significantly elevated in pregnant women (but this is not significantly correlated with spinal changes such as lordotic or kyphotic angles) (Conder, Zamani and Akrami, 2019). During gait, stride length and velocity decrease, while step width increases, although, again, such patterns are not consistently reported in the literature—each woman appears to adopt unique techniques to optimize balance and distribute load (Conder, Zamani and Akrami, 2019). Changes in hormone receptors may cause changes in skeletal muscle fiber type (from type-I or "slow-twitch" fibers to type-II or "fast-twitch" fibers) (Lontay *et al.*, 2015). Pregnant women appear to rely more on their gluteal muscles instead of their quadriceps muscles for knee extension during gait (Li *et al.*, 2023). Pregnancy is also thought to be accompanied by an increase in tissue compliance (i.e. adaptability of the tissues), which may lead to an increase in injury risk (see section 7.3). Yet, seen from a functional lens, range of motion such as hip flexion and extension has been reported to be reduced in pregnancy (Conder, Zamani and Akrami, 2019).

7.1.3. Cardiorespiratory, metabolic and thermoregulatory adaptations
Cardiovascular changes
Adequate blood supply to mother and fetus needs to be ensured throughout pregnancy. Remodeling of the heart results in increased dimensions of the ventricular cavity—a pregnant woman's heart grows—figuratively, but also literally (Cong *et al.*, 2015)! Maternal cardiac output rises about 50% to ensure sufficient perfusion to the uterus, placenta and maternal organs (Pivarnik, 1996). Maternal resting heart rate rises by 20 beats per minute on average (Sanghavi and Rutherford, 2014) and blood volume may increase up to 50% by late pregnancy (Gilson *et al.*, 1997). Pregnant women are prone to iron deficiency anemia (Zhu, Reed and Van Spall, 2022) due to a mismatch between increased blood plasma and red cell blood count. Blood pressure can change during pregnancy due to increased blood volume, decreased peripheral vascular resistance, and progesterone, which promotes the relaxation of smooth muscles surrounding blood vessels (Ouzounian and Elkayam, 2012). Compression of the inferior vena cava—for example, in supine position—may decrease venous return and cause hypotension; if women experience these symptoms, they should avoid supine position (Avery *et*

al., 1999; Jeffreys *et al.*, 2006; Ibrahim *et al.*, 2015; Bø *et al.*, 2016a).

Pregnancy also affects respiration. Due to the growing uterus, the diaphragm changes shape and elevates; the space for lung expansion thus decreases. In addition, the respiratory system becomes more sensitive to carbon dioxide, resulting in increased respiratory rate and depth (hyperventilation). Hyperventilation decreases carbon dioxide levels in the blood, thus possibly protecting the fetus against acidosis (Wolfe *et al.*, 1998; Heenan and Wolfe, 2000; Bø *et al.*, 2016a). Many women experience respiratory discomfort, especially toward the end of pregnancy (Milne, Howie and Pack, 1978).

Metabolic changes
Maternal blood glucose increases during pregnancy, while liver glycogen storage decreases and liver glucose release elevates; maternal insulin levels also rise. This leads to an increased insulin resistance in muscle tissue and thus decreases the maternal utilization of glucose in peripheral tissues, making more glucose available for the fetus (Buchanan *et al.*, 1990; Catalano *et al.*, 1991; Mottola and Christopher, 1991; Boden, 1996; Bø *et al.*, 2016a). Early during pregnancy, the higher maternal insulin levels result in an increased storage of fat. These adipose stores may provide an energy source later in pregnancy (Boden, 1996). Lipid metabolism is also undergoing alterations with pregnancy. Overall, there is an increase in fatty acids, triglycerides and cholesterol throughout pregnancy. Both the increased insulin resistance as well as estrogens are thought to contribute to the elevation of triglycerides (Feldt-Rasmussen and Mathiesen, 2011).

Thermoregulatory changes
Thermoregulatory changes during pregnancy are important as they help a pregnant woman to regulate her body temperature and protect the fetus from overheating. Hyperthermia should particularly be avoided in the first trimester, as it

can increase the risk for neural tube defects and other developmental abnormalities (Bø et al., 2018). With the progression of the pregnancy, a downward shift in body temperature threshold, at which the body initiates sweating, occurs, resulting in sweating at a lower body temperature (Clapp, 1991). Maternal heat dissipation is essential during pregnancy because fetal metabolism generates additional heat and relies on the maternal body temperature for temperature regulation (Lindqvist et al., 2003; Bø et al., 2016a).

From erasure to opportunity: Transgender men and pregnancy

Transgender men, individuals who identify as men, but were assigned female at birth, may retain their uterus and ovaries as well as the capacity to become pregnant—and some actually do become pregnant. Relatively little research is available about the pregnancy-related needs of transgender individuals, and educational and institutional attention given to this population is sparse, resulting in barriers to receiving adequate healthcare. Taken together, these disadvantageous structural forces are collectively referred to as "institutional erasure" (Makadon et al., 2015). Recently, some consideration has been given to the reproductive needs of transgender men (Hoffkling, Obedin-Maliver and Sevelius, 2017). Below, a few considerations for medical providers are summarized, which are of interest when discussing transition options with transgender men. Hoffkling and colleagues offer a more comprehensive overview.

- Transgender men should avoid getting pregnant while taking testosterone, which is considered a teratogen (i.e. an agent that can cause abnormality in the fetus) (Obedin-Maliver and Makadon, 2015).

- Conception and pregnancy can occur after even long-term testosterone use (Light et al., 2014).

- Chest feeding may be possible after certain forms of chest reconstruction (Obedin-Maliver and Makadon, 2015; MacDonald et al., 2016).

- Genital surgery such as metoidioplasty, scrotoplasty or phalloplasty do not, by themselves, interfere with future pregnancy; they would, however, likely necessitate cesarean section (Hoffkling, Obedin-Maliver and Sevelius, 2017).

- The effects of taking testosterone on the child during lactation are not clearly known. If transgender men initiate or resume taking testosterone during chestfeeding, they should be encouraged to communicate closely with their pediatrician and should be counseled on how to look for signs of androgen exposure in the infant (Hoffkling, Obedin-Maliver and Sevelius, 2017).

7.1.4. Changes in mental health and wellbeing

Poor mental health of pregnant women can have adverse effects on both the mother and the fetus. Mental health issues during pregnancy include mood disorders like depression and anxiety. The prevalence of depressive symptoms in pregnancy has been reported to be much higher than in the general population, at around 23% (versus 7% in the general population). Likewise, anxiety—the expectation of a future threat—is highly prevalent in pregnant women, affecting around 25% of females in the first and second trimesters (compared to 13% of women in the general public). Specific birth-related anxiety has also been reported, including fear of giving birth or anxiety about changing appearance. Specific data on depression and anxiety prevalence in pregnant athletes is not available. Athletes tend to downplay mental health symptoms; in addition, they may have anxiety about being able to return to their athletic career (Bø et al., 2016a).

7.2. EXERCISE DURING PREGNANCY

Inactivity during pregnancy has been associated with weight gain, gestational diabetes and hypertensive disorders, which are risk factors for cardiovascular disease and fetal complications (Beilock, Feltz and Pivarnik, 2001). Nonetheless, only 13% of pregnant women exercise throughout their pregnancy (Rodrigues-Denize, Zolnikov and Furio, 2024). Current recommendations suggest that it is safe for healthy women who were active before pregnancy to engage in exercise, but recommendations regarding the intensity and duration of exercise remain scarce (Sanghavi and Rutherford, 2014; Bø et al., 2016a). Some international guidelines have advised to accumulate 150–300 minutes of exercise per week, with sessions of at least 20–30 minutes on at least three days per week (Ribeiro, Andrade and Nunes, 2021). Most studies of existing guidelines on exercise during pregnancy focus on healthy women who were previously unactive or are recreationally active; information on pregnant competitive and elite female athletes is particularly scant (Bø et al., 2016a; Wieloch et al., 2022). An expert group of the International Olympic Committee (IOC) issued a series of papers summarizing the evidence on exercise in recreational and elite athletes during pregnancy and the postpartum period (Bø et al., 2016a, 2016b, 2017, 2018). This chapter draws from these articles and includes findings from recent reviews and meta-analyses to summarize the research.

7.2.1. Endurance exercise
Aerobic exercise is the most commonly reported type of exercise during pregnancy (Haakstad and Bø, 2011). Most endurance activities, such as walking, swimming and cycling, are considered safe and beneficial during pregnancy. About 85% of pregnant females choose walking as their preferred type of physical activity (White, Pivarnik and Pfeiffer, 2014). Research shows that most recreational and competitive runners voluntarily reduce volume and intensity of training throughout the course of pregnancy (Tenforde et al., 2015). Pregnant athletes who maintain moderate-to-high level of endurance exercise may be able to maintain or even experience slight improvements in $VO_{2\,max}$ (a measure of cardiovascular endurance) (Bø et al., 2016a). Research in elite athletes revealed that exercising at above 90% of maximal heart rate can lead to transient fetal bradycardia (heartbeat lower than 110 beats per minute of the developing baby) in some; whether these heart rate changes affect neonatal outcomes remains unknown. Cautious recommendations therefore suggest to refrain from exercising and performance testing above 90% of $VO_{2\,max}$ (Mottola et al., 2006; Salvesen, Hem and Sundgot-Borgen, 2012; Szymanski and Satin, 2012). Athletes may thus need to adjust their training to avoid overexertion. When it comes to exercising at high altitude, decreased blood flow to the uterus and consequent decrease in fetal oxygen saturation might be of concern (Entin and Coffin, 2004). While concrete research on endurance elite athletes exercising at high altitude is lacking, it appears advisable to refrain from high intensity training at altitudes greater than 1500–2000 m. In addition to physical benefits, walking and running have furthermore been reported to go along with positive mental health effects, such as a decrease in depression and anxiety level (Haakstad and Bø, 2011; Petrovic et al., 2016).

Perceived exertion as a guide for exercise intensity during pregnancy

A rating of perceived exertion (RPE) such as the Borg scale is a practical and affordable tool to guide exercise intensity, as it generally correlates with heart rate (Scherr *et al.*, 2013). In pregnancy, however, RPE does not correlate strongly with heart rate (O'Neill *et al.*, 1992). A pregnant woman using RPE may be exercising at a much higher heart rate than her perceived rating would suggest. Particularly when exercising at more intense ranges (e.g. in elite athletes), additional heart rate measures, such as heart rate monitors, are therefore recommended (Bø *et al.*, 2016a).

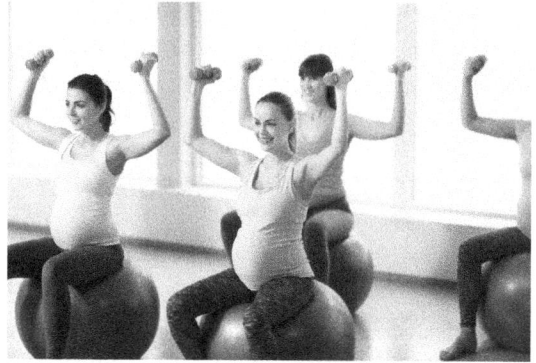

Photo 7.1: Strength training during pregnancy, for example with light weights, is generally considered safe. However, only 10% of pregnant women engage in resistance training.

7.2.2. Strength training

Light-to-moderate strength training (e.g. with free weights or weight machines) is generally considered safe during pregnancy, and substantial strength gains are possible (Clapp, 2000; JF, 2009; O'Connor *et al.*, 2011; Bø *et al.*, 2018). Heavy weightlifting, however, may rapidly increase intra-abdominal pressure and temporarily reduce blood flow to the fetus, the repercussions of which are unknown. Additionally, high intra-abdominal pressure can put a large strain on the pelvic floor, possibly increasing the risk of urinary or anal incontinence or pelvic organ prolapse during or after pregnancy (Bø *et al.*, 2016a). Strength training for the pelvic floor has been shown to prevent and treat urinary incontinence during pregnancy and postpartum (Boyle *et al.*, 2012; Bø *et al.*, 2018). Additional positive effects of resistance training include the reduction of nausea, fatigue and headaches (Fieril *et al.*, 2014). In addition to physical benefits, resistance training during pregnancy has been reported to increase motivation, improve mood swings and decrease stress (Petrov Fieril, Glantz and Fagevik Olsen, 2015; Rodrigues-Denize, Zolnikov and Furio, 2024). However, only 10% of pregnant females engage in resistance training (Rodrigues-Denize, Zolnikov and Furio, 2024).

Female-friendly gyms?

The low rates of pregnant women's engagement in strength training are certainly caused by a variety of reasons. Gym environments may be a contributing factor. Gym spaces have been reported to be gendered, creating barriers for women to access: weight areas are often characterized by gender separation, which can create emotional barriers for women to cross into this "male space." Male exercisers may show performance of their masculinity traits, and the impression may be created to always be "on show" and subject to scrutiny. Moreover, equipment for women's needs may not be provided (Turnock, 2021). It can easily be imagined that pregnant women feel these barriers to access gyms to an even greater extent. Fitness centers specifically tailored to female customers can be a welcomed alternative to make women feel comfortable and enjoy participating in resistance training (Wang, Hsiao and Hsiung, 2022), during pregnancy, or in any other stage of life.

7.2.3. Flexibility training/stretching

As pregnancy, or more specifically estrogen and relaxin, may increase connective tissue compliance and ligament laxity (Dumas and Reid, 1997; Fede *et al.*, 2019), stretching at the end range of motion may not be advisable. However, concrete studies in this area are lacking.

7.2.4. Yoga

Yoga—a mind-body-spirit practice combining physical movement, relaxation and breathing techniques—is a common form of physical activity for pregnant women (Curtis, Weinrib and Katz, 2012; Hall and Jolly, 2014; Babbar *et al.*, 2016; Mooventhan, 2019). Evidence suggests that yoga is safe during pregnancy, particularly when offered with specific adaptations for pregnant women, and is thought to provide the opportunity to foster wellbeing during childbearing (Kwon *et al.*, 2020; Corrigan *et al.*, 2022). A recent systematic review and meta-analysis, including 31 studies, highlighted positive effects of pregnancy yoga on anxiety, depression and perceived stress during pregnancy (Corrigan *et al.*, 2022). However, pregnancy yoga interventions are not standardized in practice and research, which makes it hard to derive recommendations regarding the beneficial characteristics of yoga sessions (i.e. duration, frequency, included elements etc.).

7.2.5. Sports to be avoided

Pregnant women may want to avoid high-risk sports, such as those with a risk of falling, of direct trauma to the abdominal wall, and those with physiologic risks (Bø *et al.*, 2018). Sports with an increased risk of falling or trauma include martial arts and combat sports (e.g. wrestling, boxing, judo, taekwondo), rugby, ice hockey, downhill ski racing, snowboarding, BMX and mountain cycling, ski jumping, bobsleigh, some figure skating events, football, handball, basketball, trampoline and artistic gymnastics. Scuba diving poses physiological risk, as the fetus is not protected from decompression problems and may be at risk of ensuing developmental problems (Bø *et al.*, 2018). However, creating an exhaustive list is not possible and individual risk should be carefully weighed.

"I'm not fine when I'm supine"—exercising in supine position

When exercising in supine position, many pregnant women, particularly after 28 weeks of gestation, experience side effects such as dizziness. This may result from decreased return of venous blood to the heart and reduced blood pressure due to compression of the inferior vena cava by the pregnant uterus (Bø *et al.*, 2016a, 2018). Uterine blood flow can also decrease when exercising supine. Remaining motionless, for example in standing or certain yoga positions, for longer periods of time may lead to the same effects. To reduce potential risk, exercises can be modified—for example, by elevating the torso to 45 degrees or performing exercises in different positions, such as side-lying, sitting or standing. Some studies report that exercising in supine position for two to three minutes at a time leads to no adverse effects (Barakat *et al.*, 2016; Bø *et al.*, 2018).

7.2.6. Contraindications to sports

IOC recommendations have identified a number of absolute (high-risk conditions) and relative (moderate risk conditions) contraindications to exercise during pregnancy (Bø *et al.*, 2018). These conditions are listed in Tables 7.1 and 7.2.

Further issues regarding pregnancy in athletes comprise eating disorders. The frequency of eating disorders is higher among athletes compared to the general public, especially in weight-sensitive sports. Pregnant athletes with eating disorders (as well as their offspring) are at particular risk of pregnancy complications and require close monitoring by a multi-disciplinary team. However, data on the prevalence of eating disorders in pregnant athletes is lacking (Bø *et al.*, 2016a).

Table 7.1: Conditions posing a high risk to the fetus and in which aerobic exercise is absolutely contraindicated (Bø *et al.*, 2018)

Contraindication for aerobic exercise in pregnancy
Hemodynamically significant heart disease
Intrauterine growth restriction in current pregnancy
Poorly controlled hypertension
Restrictive lung disease
Cervical insufficiency/cerclage
Multiple gestation at risk of premature labor
Persistent second or third trimester bleeding
Placenta previa after 26 weeks' gestation
Premature labor during the current pregnancy
Ruptured membranes
Pre-eclampsia/pregnancy-induced hypertension
Severe anemia

Table 7.2: Conditions posing a moderate risk to the fetus and in which aerobic exercise is moderately contraindicated (Bø *et al.*, 2018)

Contraindication for aerobic exercise in pregnancy
History of fetal growth restriction, miscarriage, premature birth or labor
Cervical enlargement
Unevaluated maternal cardiac arrhythmia
Chronic bronchitis or other respiratory disorders
Poorly controlled type 1 diabetes
Extremely underweight
Orthopedic limitations
Poorly controlled seizure disorder

7.3. MUSCULOSKELETAL INJURIES RISK DURING PREGNANCY

Musculoskeletal injuries in pregnancy are relatively common. The center of gravity shifts anteriorly, causing altered biomechanics, which can in turn predispose pregnant women to injuries in falls (Cakmak, Ribeiro and Inanir, 2016). In fact, about one in four pregnant women experiences falls, with multifactorial causes (Cain *et al.*, 2021). Low back pain and pelvic girdle pain are the most common musculoskeletal complaints during pregnancy and may affect up to 71% and 65% of women, respectively (Casagrande *et al.*, 2015; Cain *et al.*, 2021). Biomechanical factors contributing to these pain patterns comprise exaggerated lumbar lordosis, anterior pelvic tilt, increased loading on sacrum and sacroiliac joints, altered gait and neurovascular compression. There is also an increased occurrence of carpal tunnel syndrome symptoms during the third trimester of pregnancy, which is caused by compression of the median nerve. This can result in numbness, tingling and weakness in the hand (Cain *et al.*, 2021).

Moreover, joint and ligamentous laxity have been reported to predispose pregnant women to pain and musculoskeletal injury (Cain *et al.*, 2021). Pregnancy is thought to be accompanied by an increase in tissue compliance (the inverse of tissue stiffness). Recent research on fascial tissues may explain this phenomenon. Fascial tissue samples and fibroblasts exhibit receptors for estrogen and relaxin (Fede *et al.*, 2016). Changes in hormone levels have been shown to modulate extracellular matrix composition: The rise of estrogen as seen during pregnancy resulted in higher amounts of adaptable collagen-III and fibrillin fibers, and a decrease in collagen-I fibers (which have high tensile strength) in vitro (Fede *et al.*, 2019). This altered tissue architecture may come with a loss of stability around the joint and may contribute to back and pelvic pain during pregnancy in vivo (Fede *et al.*, 2019). However, in-vivo data appears inconclusive: Studies report positive associations between estradiol and anterior cruciate ligament laxity (Charlton, Coslett-Charlton and Ciccotti, 2001), while wrist joint laxity did not correlate well with estrogen and progesterone levels in one study (Marnach *et al.*, 2003). Moreover, recent work did not detect any changes in patellar tendon stiffness in pregnant women. However, a progressive increase in tendon rest length has been observed during pregnancy, which may reduce joint stability and thus impact injury risk (Bey *et al.*, 2019; Legerlotz and Hansen, 2020). Hence, the concrete mechanisms connecting changes in female reproductive hormones and biomechanical parameters may be tissue specific or depend on the type of parameter and measurement method used, and need to be further elucidated.

Aquatic training has been suggested as a suitable exercise alternative during pregnancy, as activities in water avoid harsh falls as well as weight load on the musculoskeletal system (Alberton *et al.*, 2019; Rodrigues-Denize, Zolnikov and Furio, 2024).

7.4. TRANSITIONING INTO MOTHERHOOD: CONSIDERATIONS FROM POSTPARTUM DEPRESSION TO BREASTFEEDING

7.4.1. Changes in the postpartum period

With removal of the placenta during the delivery process, estrogen and progesterone concentrations drop sharply within the first 24 hours after birth and reach pre-pregnancy levels by the fifth postpartum day. Cortisol also falls abruptly after birth. In lactating women, pulses of prolactin concentrations stimulate milk production; oxytocin pulses lead to milk ejection (let-down reflex). In non-lactating women, prolactin levels return to pre-pregnancy values within three weeks postpartum; in breastfeeding/pumping females, prolactin levels remain high in the first weeks postpartum, but eventually decline to pre-pregnancy levels over time as well (Hendrick, Altshuler and Suri, 1998; Kohl, Autry and Dulac, 2017). Figure 7.1 depicts hormone changes during pregnancy and the postpartum period.

The respiratory changes related to pregnancy typically resolve within 6–12 weeks postpartum (Bø *et al.*, 2017; Zhu, Reed and Van Spall, 2022). Regarding cardiovascular adaptations during pregnancy, one study with 13 healthy females showed that systemic vascular resistance (which is associated with low blood pressure) remained decreased three months postpartum compared with before conception (Capeless and Clapp, 1991).

One study including a non-athlete female population suggested that it takes at least two months after giving birth for the augmented cardiac response to exercise to subside (Sady *et al.*, 1990). Some study findings indicate that cardiovascular measures such as heart rate and cardiac output gradually return toward baseline over the first postpartum year, but may remain different from pre-pregnancy values a year after birth (Clapp and Capeless, 1997).

Regarding mental health, the most common problem is postpartum depression (depressive symptoms within 12 months after giving birth), which is experienced by approximately 10–20% of new mothers (Gavin *et al.*, 2005; Xu *et al.*, 2023). Despite the high incidence rates, around 90% of patients go untreated (Xu *et al.*, 2023). Symptoms include feelings of hopelessness and helplessness, decreased energy, sleep problems, sad mood, irritability, restlessness, decision-making difficulties— and even suicidal ideation and attempts (Bø *et al.*, 2017). Mild depressive symptoms are encountered by 50–75% of mothers. Very little is known about postnatal depression in athletes. Elite athletes may experience both typical postnatal stressors in addition to stress associated with training for performance at a high level; they may therefore need extra support (Bø *et al.*, 2018).

7.4.2. Exercise in the postpartum period

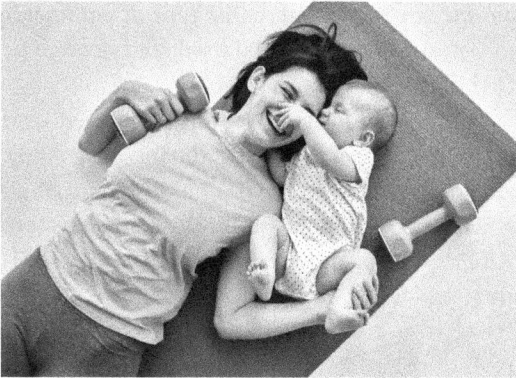

Photo 7.2: Exercise in the postpartum period is considered beneficial—however, a sharp decline in physical exercise occurs in the three years after giving birth. This may be due to physical discomfort, difficulties in prioritizing health over other responsibilities, social isolation and financial constraints.

Despite the positive aspects associated with exercise, there is a sharp decline in physical level reported in the three years postpartum (Brown, Heesch and Miller, 2009). Physical discomfort, difficulties in prioritizing health over other responsibilities, social isolation and possibly financial constraints can contribute to the barriers to sports participation in this period of a woman's life. The concrete effects of sports performance on postpartum physiology and lactation are currently not sufficiently clarified (Zhu, Reed and Van Spall, 2022), making a gradual come-back to physical activity as well as an individual approach essential.

Return to sports

A gradual approach to returning to sports is key—the impact of pregnancy and birth on the maternal musculoskeletal system can be likened to the impact of an acute sports injury, and recovery is multifactorial and complex (Ardern et al., 2016; Bø et al., 2018). Return to sports participation and eventually performance should thus be decided individually in close coordination with healthcare providers. Scientific evidence and guidance on exercises to target some of the most common postpartum complaints (e.g. low back/pelvic girdle pain, diastasis recti) and diseases and how they may impact return to sports remains scarce (Bø et al., 2018). In elite athletes, some accounts find that females may be able to return to training rather quickly: in a retrospective study including 40 Norwegian elite athletes, 38% of participants started jogging within six weeks postpartum (compared to 4.3% in non-athletes) (Bø and Backe-Hansen, 2007). Another study with 34 Norwegian elite athletes and 34 active controls reported that most athletes and every third control returned to sport or exercise within six weeks postpartum (Sundgot-Borgen et al., 2019). Another case study reported that a marathon runner resumed her intense training regimen (training for Olympic qualification) within four weeks of giving birth (Potteiger, Welch and Byrne, 1993). On the other hand, research in physically fit soldiers showed that it took up to 24 months (mean: 11 months) to return to pre-pregnancy performance (Weina, 2006).

Endurance training

Gradual return to physical activity participation typically includes gentle walking when pain allows (often within the first week after birth). Walking distance and speed can be increased step-wise (roughly 10% per postpartum week) (Inge et al., 2022).

Strength training

Pelvic floor training can be started shortly after birth. Strength training should start gradually and care should be given to engage pelvic floor muscles during exercises that increase intra-abdominal pressure (e.g. leg press, squat, bench press, heavy abdominal exercise) (Bø et al., 2018). Regarding strengthening exercises to treat diastasis recti abdominis postpartum, scientific evidence to recommend specific exercises remains scarce. A 2021 systematic review and meta-analysis examined seven trials, including a total of 381 women, to analyse effectiveness of abdominal and pelvic floor muscle training to treat diastasis recti (Gluppe, Engh and Bø, 2021). Very low-level evidence suggested training programs targeting the transverse abdominis were more effective to decrease diastasis recti than minimal intervention. Two studies included curl-up exercises, which have been discouraged in the recent past. Gluppe and colleagues found very low-level evidence that curl-up training was more effective than minimal intervention. Interestingly, pelvic floor muscle training programs were not found to be more effective than minimal intervention; however, again, this finding was based on low- to very low-level evidence.

Exercise and postpartum mental health

A growing body of evidence suggests that physical activity before and during pregnancy as well as during the postpartum period may reduce the risk of postnatal depressive symptoms (McCurdy, Boulé and Sivak, no date; Poyatos-León, García-Hermoso and Sanabria-Martínez, no date; Teychenne and York, 2013; Bø et al., 2018). Cognitive behavioral therapy and interpersonal psychotherapy have been found to provide significant benefits to treat depression, anxiety and trauma-related disorders in the postpartum period. Complementary medicine approaches such as endurance exercise have also been reported to be effective (Nillni et al., 2018). A 2023 meta-analysis found a frequency of three to four bouts of aerobic exercise sessions per week with moderate intensity and a duration of 35–45 minutes to be optimal in the prevention and treatment of postpartum depression (Xu et al., 2023).

Exercise and lactation

Previous concerns that intense physical activity may impair milk production have not been confirmed (Dewey, no date; Dewey et al., 1994). One observational study with 16 participants even showed that women who exercised vigorously for at least 45 minutes daily tended to produce higher milk volume and quality (Lovelady, Lonnerdal and Dewey, 1990). Bone health presents another consideration regarding exercise, and lactation featured in the literature. If calcium levels are insufficient to meet baby's and mother's needs during pregnancy, there may be some bone resorption; this may be exacerbated during the lactation period. However, there is no evidence that this causes fractures or osteoporosis, as mineral content and strength of bones of the maternal skeleton are restored to pre-pregnancy levels after weaning. Nevertheless, excess exercise is considered to be a risk factor for osteoporotic alterations of maternal bone (Kovacs and Ralston, 2015; Bø et al., 2017).

The milkshake study

The components of breast milk differ between individuals with and without obesity. Since exercise has been shown to have beneficial effects on almost all tissues and organs in the body, it has been hypothesized that it may also impact breast milk composition. A current randomized controlled trial aims to determine the effects of an endurance training program, including eight weeks of 25 supervised endurance exercise sessions with moderate or high intensity. Mothers and infants will be followed up after 24 months to track maternal health outcomes, infant growth and infant gut microbiome as well (Moholdt et al., 2023). The results will certainly provide interesting insights into the link between maternal lifestyle during lactation and the ultimate milkshake!

How do research findings on breastfeeding/pumping and exercise translate into practice? A number of regional guidelines mention that exercise does not affect breast milk quantity and composition as long as women ensure adequate food and fluid intake. Beyond that, there are currently no recommendations regarding exercise intensity and breastfeeding/pumping (Bø et al., 2017). Well-fitted sports bras and feeding or pumping before working out may allow postpartum females greater flexibility and comfort during exercise (Wallace and Rabin, 1991; Mottola, 2002; McGhee et al., 2013; Bø et al., 2017).

CHAPTER 8

A New Status Quo: From Perimenopause to Postmenopause

8.1. REPRODUCTIVE AGING—DEFINITIONS

Menopause is experienced by all female humans who live beyond midlife, and yet, it poses an evolutionary mystery: apart from humans, killer whales seem to be the only other mammals going through menopause. While the evolutionary reasoning of menopause may not be fully clarified yet, rigorous scientific efforts have produced precise definitions for the stages of reproductive aging in human females. **Menopause** describes just one day in the life of a woman—the point in time when it's been 12 months since a period last occurred; hence, it can only be determined retrospectively (The North American Menopause Society, 2019).

The transitional stage from a woman's reproductive years to the final menstrual period is termed **menopause transition**, starting with the onset of menstrual cycle irregularities (i.e. persistent difference in cycle length of seven or more days compared to normal cycle) or other menopause-related symptoms (Harlow *et al.*, 2012). **Perimenopause**, which literally means "around menopause," starts with the onset of cycle irregularities (like the menopause transition) and ends with menopause—lasting 12 months longer than the menopause transition accordingly (The North American Menopause Society, 2019). Perimenopause can last five to

fifteen years. Since many women are not naturally menstruating when perimenopause begins (e.g. because of oral contraception or hysterectomy), some authors pragmatically define menopause as the permanent cessation of ovarian function (Davis *et al.*, 2023).

Menopause for "babysitting"?

Only very few species have an extensive lifespan after entering the post-reproductive phase of their lives, making menopause an evolutionary mystery. Why is it that only humans and few other species such as orcas experience menopause? Theories such as the "grandmother hypothesis" or "extended mothering hypothesis" suggest that the support and caregiving of postmenopausal females in a family unit provide evolutionary advantages (Paquin, Kato and Kim, 2020; Watkins, 2021). In studies on killer whales, it has been shown that post-reproductive orcas provide support to their (especially male) offspring: socially inflicted injuries such as tooth rake marks are lower for male offspring in the presence of their post-reproductive mothers (Grimes *et al.*, 2023).

Language matters! Ovarian vs. penile failure

It is interesting to note that there are linguistic differences depending on biological sex when it comes to the topics of aging and reproductive organs. The term "ovarian failure" is used with females in the context of aging, while "penile failure" does not seem to be applied in the same way: a PubMed search in the titles of scientific articles for the term "ovarian failure" produces 1645 results, while a similar search for the term "penile failure" retrieves zero hits (search performed on April 15, 2024). This implies gender-based inequities in the bigger conversation about (reproductive) aging.

menopause is 50–51 years in high-income countries; some countries report an earlier average age of menopause; for example, in India an average age of 46 years (Singh, 2012). Early menopause—happening between ages 40 and 44—occurs in around 8% of females in high-income countries and 12% of females globally. An additional 2–4% experience menopause before the age of 40 (Mishra *et al.*, 2024).

Menopause describes **one particular day** in the life of a woman: the point in time when it has been 12 months since a period last occurred. Pragmatically, menopause can be understood as the cessation of ovarian function. The **menopause transition** refers to the transitional phase starting with the onset of cycle irregularities until the final menstrual period; **perimenopause** includes the time between onset of cycle irregularities to menopause. After menopause has occurred, a woman is in the phase of **postmenopause** for the rest of her life.

While **postmenopause** can pragmatically be described as the stage after menopause, the STRAW +10 framework (the gold standard for characterizing stages of reproductive aging) refers to the time between the final menstrual period and menopause as early postmenopause as well (Harlow *et al.*, 2012). The typical age of

8.2. SLOWING DOWN?! CHANGES DURING REPRODUCTIVE AGING

Reproductive aging comes with changes in hormone levels, and potentially changes in body composition, psychological wellbeing, as well as various other symptoms during perimenopause and postmenopause (The North American Menopause Society, 2019). However, the menopausal transition experienced by women varies greatly—some females go through menopause uneventfully, while for others it is accompanied by severe losses of quality of life due to prolonged symptoms (The Lancet, 2024).

8.2.1. Changes in hormone levels
As a woman experiences the menopause transition, her follicle pool depletes progressively,

driving a series of changes in the hypothalamic-pituitary-ovarian (HPO) axis (K.R. Hansen *et al.*, 2008). While the menstrual cycle becomes more irregular and some symptoms of menopause present themselves more frequently, women do not have consistently low levels of estradiol. Rather, the early stages of perimenopause can be described as **"compensated failure" of the HPO axis**. As the hypothalamus and pituitary gland register the decreasing number of available follicles and amount of estradiol, the body aims to compensate for these changes. It produces **more FSH** to stimulate the ovaries to produce more estrogen and develop follicles, leading to both more extreme FSH levels as well as an overall increase of FSH (Santoro and Randolph, 2011; Hale, Robertson and Burger, 2014). The resulting acceleration in follicle growth can shorten the follicular phase and result in more frequent menstrual periods (The North American Menopause Society, 2019).

Brakes released! The role of inhibin B and anti-Müllerian hormone (AMH)

The decreasing follicle numbers also result in a reduction of anti-Müllerian hormone (AMH) and inhibin B, as both of these hormones are produced by ovarian follicles (Davis *et al.*, 2023). In earlier stages of reproductive life, AMH and inhibin B help to protect the follicle pool by putting a brake on FSH secretion, consequently limiting the number of follicles growing each month. Thereby, a woman is being prevented from ovulating all follicles over only a small number of menstrual cycles (Durlinger *et al.*, 2002; The North American Menopause Society, 2019). With reproductive aging, the reduction of AMH and inhibin B leads to an increase in FSH, which appears to be necessary to maintain follicle growth in this phase (Allshouse, Pavlovic and Santoro, 2018). As a consequence, more follicles are made available for ovulation and to maintain regular menstrual cycles—at the cost of accelerating the diminishing of the follicle cohort (The North American Menopause Society, 2019).

Consistent with the more extreme values of FSH and its impact on follicular growth, perimenopause is characterized by **higher fluctuations of estradiol** than would be observed in a menstrual cycle before perimenopause. Estradiol levels in the follicular phase can be both lower than typically seen during the reproductive years as well as intermittently elevated; estradiol in the luteal phase can sometimes reach levels that are even

double than those normally observed just before ovulation (Shideler *et al.*, 1989; Santoro *et al.*, 1996; Hale *et al.*, 2007; Hale and Burger, 2009; Gordon *et al.*, 2019). One explanation for higher-than-usual estradiol levels during the menopause transition are **luteal out-of-phase (LOOP) events** (Hale *et al.*, 2009). Triggered by elevated FSH levels and related accelerated follicle growth, a second follicle can be recruited in the luteal phase of the menstrual cycle, resulting in a second ovulatory event immediately after or concurrent with the menstrual bleeding of the following cycle. As estradiol from the second ovulatory event is superimposed on the regular estradiol peak in the previous luteal phase, a rise in estradiol can be observed. Cycles with LOOP events are also associated with lower progesterone levels than in typical cycles (Hale *et al.*, 2009; Allshouse, Pavlovic and Santoro, 2018).

In addition, the process of **follicle maturation** may be **altered**: the follicular phase can be shorter and ovulation can occur earlier in the menstrual cycle (Klein *et al.*, 2002), follicle diameter at ovulation can be smaller and corpus luteum formation may fail despite otherwise normal hormone secretion and follicle growth (Santoro *et al.*, 2003). Also, LH may fail to surge as the **HPO axis** may become **less sensitive to estrogen** as women age (Weiss *et al.*, 2004). Taken together, these changes can lead to more frequent and more variable menstrual periods, more variable hormone secretion, and short bouts of amenorrhea.

By the later phases of the menopause transition, the compensatory mechanisms can no longer keep pace. As the follicle cohort shrinks to a critically low level, follicle maturation takes place intermittently, resulting in estrogen deficiency symptoms and amenorrhea of more than 60 days (The North American Menopause Society, 2019). Ovulation consequently occurs less frequently, and when it does, progesterone production is decreased (Santoro *et al.*, 2008). Eventually, the follicle cohort becomes so small that follicle maturation is no longer happening and the production of estradiol and progesterone essentially ceases (The North American Menopause Society, 2019). In the year after the final menstrual period, some estrogen production at variable levels seems to take place; moreover, very little progesterone production can be observed at this point (The North American Menopause Society, 2019). Another change related to the menopausal transition concerns the predominant type of estrogen: while estradiol (E2) prevails during reproductive years (with the exception of pregnancy), estrone is the main type of estrogen produced after menopause (Davis *et al.*, 2023). An overview of hormonal fluctuations before and after menopause is depicted in Figure 8.1.

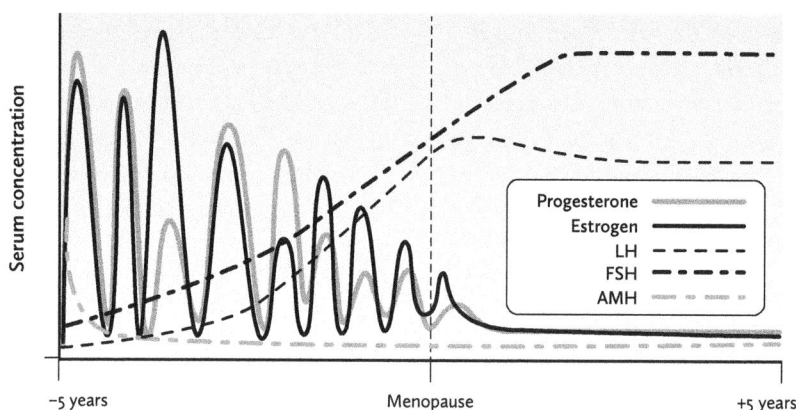

Figure 8.1: Hormonal fluctuations in the years before and after menopause (adapted from Chidi-Ogbolu and Baar, 2018; Nelson *et al.*, 2023).

Can't we just do some blood work? Considerations for menopause stage testing

Laboratory testing to determine which menopause stage a woman is in comes with a number of pitfalls. Considerations for some seemingly obvious candidates for blood work are listed below:

- **FSH:** FSH levels are notoriously variable from day to day within one menstrual cycle as well as from cycle to cycle. Generally, very high FSH levels can predict that a female is likely to go through the menopause transition, but a low or normal FSH value is not informative (Burger *et al.*, 2002).

- **Estradiol:** As estradiol levels fluctuate throughout perimenopause, one-time measurements are not useful to determine menopause stage (Davis *et al.*, 2023).

- **AMH level:** Even though a correlation between AMH and the number of follicles in adulthood has been shown (Kelsey *et al.*, 2011), AMH concentration alone is not useful in predicting the age of imminent menopause in women under 40 years of age. Besides, AMH only captures a quantitative not qualitative view of the ovarian reserve. AMH's predictive value for menopause increases with age as time to menopause shortens, but further clinical studies are needed to correlate AMH with the different menopause stages according to STRAW (The North American Menopause Society, 2019; Nelson *et al.*, 2023).

- **Populations with amenorrhea:** Hormonal changes (and therefore lab values and their interpretation) for women with amenorrhea syndromes may differ from women who have a relatively regular menstrual cycle before perimenopause. For instance, some research has shown that women with PCOS go through menopause later in life and may experience regular menstrual cycles—often for the first time in their lives—during perimenopause: the elevated AMH levels in the menopause transition resolve the chronic suppression of follicle growth associated with PCOS (Brown et al., 2011). Hormonal profiles during the menopause transition in women with PCOS may therefore present differently. Menopausal changes in women with functional hypothalamic amenorrhea remain virtually unstudied (The North American Menopause Society, 2019).

As ovarian hormones fluctuate in perimenopause and plateau at a low level after menopause, women may experience symptoms of:

- relative estrogen excess

- estrogen insufficiency

- a mix of both.

Symptoms related to relative **estrogen excess** include shorter cycle length, shorter follicular phase, breast tenderness, heavy and prolonged menstrual bleeding (menorrhagia), migraine and nausea (Davis et al., 2023). Symptoms associated with estrogen insufficiency comprise vasomotor symptoms such as hot flashes and (night) sweats (see section 8.2.2), changes in body composition (see section 8.2.3) and psychological wellbeing

(see section 8.2.4), urogenital symptoms (vaginal dryness, irritation, urinary frequency, recurrent urinary infections), disturbed sleep (with frequent awakenings) and lessened sexual desire (Davis et al., 2023). Less specific symptoms include headaches and fatigue, as well as impaired concentration and memory (Davis et al., 2023).

How a female perceives and experiences this transitional phase is unique and varies greatly; this depends on the age at which menopause occurs, state of health and wellbeing, environment, culture and ethnicity (Davis et al., 2023).

8.2.2. Hot flashes

Vasomotor symptoms such as hot flashes and night sweats can be described as the hallmark of (peri)menopausal symptoms, with 50-85% of females older than 45 years experiencing them at some point (Mallhi et al., 2018). Impaired sleep often goes along with night sweats and can add to the negative impact of vasomotor symptoms on the quality of life (Utian, 2005; Kingsberg et al., 2023). Various prospective cohort studies have looked at the duration of vasomotor symptoms, a prominent one being the SWAN study (Study of Women's Health Across the Nation) carried out in the US. Frequent vasomotor symptoms may last for approximately 7.4 years in total, thereof about 4.5 years after menopause, with some lasting as long as 20 years (Freedman, 2014; Avis et al., 2015). Moreover, differences in prevalence of vasomotor symptoms have been reported depending on ethnicity. Hot flashes appear to have the highest prevalence in Black women and lowest prevalence in East Asian women, while sleep disturbance seems to be most prevalent in White women (Kingsberg et al., 2023). African American women have been reported to have more persistent vasomotor symptoms, lasting more than ten years for half of the women (Avis et al., 2015). When aiming to predict the duration of vasomotor symptoms, the onset in the earlier phases of perimenopause seems to be the best single predictor (Avis *et al.*, 2015). Additionally, smoking and body composition have been reported as some of the risk factors for the occurrence and higher severity of hot flashes (Whiteman *et al.*, 2003; Gallicchio *et al.*, 2005, 2006).

While frequency, duration and intensity can vary greatly, symptoms seem to be more severe in females with surgical menopause (Mallhi *et al.*, 2018). Some women report hot flashes as often as every hour, while others have only weekly or monthly episodes (Mallhi *et al.*, 2018). Hot flashes typically last between one and five

minutes but can persist for up to 15 minutes. Nausea, agitation, a feeling of pressure in the chest or head as well as an increased heart rate can also accompany hot flashes. Often, shivering or a feeling of cold follows a hot flash (Rossmanith and Ruebberdt, 2009).

Mechanisms

The underlying mechanisms of hot flashes are still under debate (see Figure 8.2). It is likely that vasomotor symptoms comprise multiple interacting processes (The North American Menopause Society, 2019).

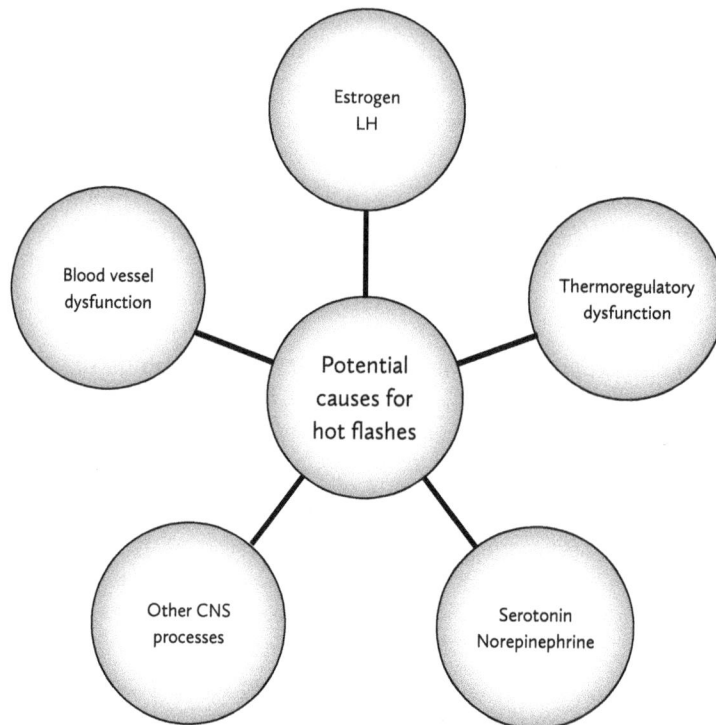

Figure 8.2: Potential mechanisms of hot flashes.

Hormones are an obvious potential contributor, primarily estrogen. Hot flashes occur in the majority of women with surgical menopause, which goes along with an immediate decrease of estradiol; in addition, estrogen supplementation therapy is an efficient therapy to eliminate

hot flashes (Freedman, 2014; Mallhi *et al.*, 2018). Contrary to this, estrogen reduction alone does not explain the occurrence of vasomotor symptoms: estrogen levels (plasma, urinary or vaginal) are not directly related to vasomotor symptoms, and hot flashes usually subside some time after menopause, when estrogen levels have flatlined (Aksel *et al.*, 1976; Freedman, 2014; Mallhi *et al.*, 2018). Therefore, estrogen decreases seem to be an important factor, but are not sufficient to solely explain the occurrence of vasomotor symptoms (Freedman, 2014). Another hormone that has been discussed in the genesis of hot flashes is luteinizing hormone (LH). Some studies showed a temporal relationship between rises in LH and hot flashes. However, hot flashes do also occur independent of LH levels—for instance, in women whose LH levels are suppressed pharmacologically (Freedman, 2014). Accordingly, a straightforward relationship between hormones such as estrogen or LH and hot flashes cannot be assumed.

Another hypothesis for the occurrence of hot flashes relates to changes of the temperature-regulating circuit, a complex system of autonomic and neuroendocrine structures tasked with keeping core body temperature stable, which is crucial for optimal organ function. It is thought that vasomotor symptoms may arise from altered **thermoregulatory functioning** (see Figure 8.3). As long as the body core temperature stays in the thermoneutral zone, no thermoregulatory activities (such as sweating) are induced. If the core body temperature exceeds the upper threshold of this zone, the mechanisms for sweating (such as vasodilation) are activated, so that heat can be released. The upper threshold is therefore termed sweating threshold. If the core body temperature drops below the lower set value (the shivering threshold), the mechanisms for shivering and vasoconstriction are induced to produce heat. Normally, the thermoneutral zone comprises about 0.4 °C; in women who suffer from hot flashes, a narrowing of the thermoneutral zone to practically zero can be assumed (Rossmanith and Ruebberdt, 2009). Accordingly, the body interprets an even minimal temperature change excessively, and reacts to the feeling of overheating with vasodilation and sweating. This is sometimes followed by a compensatory cooling reaction marked by shivering.

What mechanisms may account for the narrowing of the thermoregulatory zone as well as the related reactions? Estrogen makes an appearance once more as it plays an important role in thermoregulation in the central nervous system. During the reproductive years of a woman's life, the brain adapts to the cyclical fluctuation of estrogen; during the menopausal transition the brain may have to undergo adjustments to the changes in hormone levels to regain balance in thermoregulation. When the central nervous system can't adapt quickly or efficiently enough, thermoregulatory dysfunction—and consequently hot flashes—may result (which is referred to as the brain adaptation hypothesis) (Freedman, 2014). Moreover, the hypothalamus—an important central nervous system structure related to thermoregulation—expresses estrogen and progesterone receptors and is therefore sensitive to sex hormones. With changes in these hormones during the menopausal transition, hypothalamic function and thus thermoregulation may be impacted (Boulant, 2000; McEwen, 2001; Witten *et al.*, 2024).

The **neurochemicals serotonin and norepinephrine** (noradrenaline) may also play a role in vasomotor symptoms. Estrogen has been shown to influence serotonin and norepinephrine synthesis, activity, reuptake and degradation. As estrogen levels drop during the menopause transition, the balance of serotonin and norepinephrine is disrupted, which consequently may impact thermoregulation and hot flashes (Witten *et al.*, 2024). Clinically, this has been demonstrated through studies on the efficacy of antidepressants in the treatment of hot flashes: several studies found selective serotonin reuptake inhibitors (SSRIs) and serotonin-norepinephrine reuptake inhibitors (SNRIs) helpful in alleviating hot flashes (Witten *et al.*, 2024). However, efficacy and side effects depend on the type of drug, and not all drugs are approved for reducing hot flashes. Accordingly, treatment decisions should be individualized (Azizi *et al.*, 2022; Witten *et al.*, 2024). Even though SSRIs and SNRIs seem to be an effective relief for hot flashes, their precise involvement in the physiology of vasomotor symptoms is not yet understood (The North American Menopause Society, 2019).

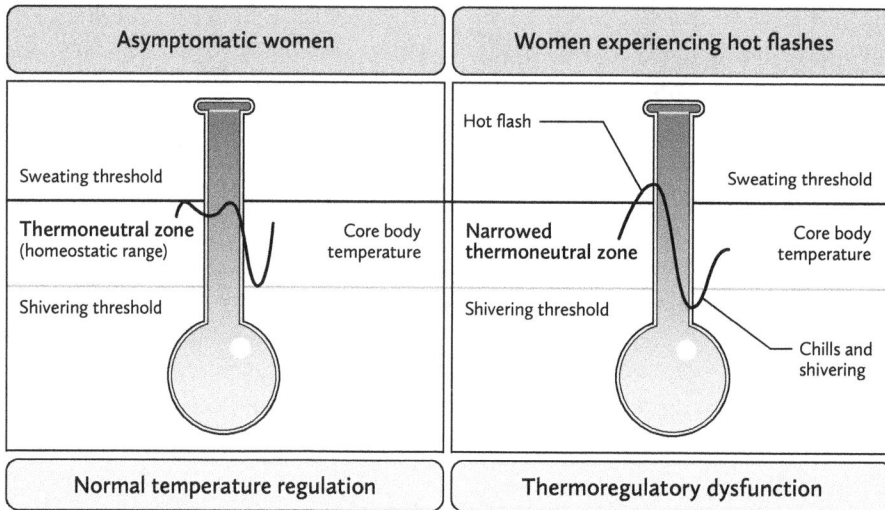

Figure 8.3: Thermoregulation in asymptomatic women and females experiencing hot flashes.

Additionally, **other central nervous system (CNS) structures and processes** have been implicated in hot flashes. Neuroimaging studies have shown that brainstem activity rises before the detectable onset of a hot flash, potentially reflecting the origin of a vasomotor event; this was followed by increased activation of the insula and prefrontal cortex during the hot flash (Freedman *et al.*, 2006; Diwadkar, Murphy and Freedman, 2014).

Blood vessel dysfunction may be another contributing factor to the occurrence of hot flashes. The control of skin circulation through the peripheral vascular system is an important variable in thermoregulation. Some studies indicate that the sensitivity of the blood vessels—particularly in the skin—may change during the menopausal transition and reduce the vasculature's ability to react quickly and appropriately. Such changes in responsiveness have been related to the changes in the threshold for cutaneous vasodilation, which can be influenced by fluctuations in estrogen observed in perimenopause. Furthermore, reduced estradiol levels present in postmenopause can contribute to a reduction of elasticity of the blood vessel walls, which can alter vascular reactivity as well (Joswig *et al.*, 1999; Rossmanith and Ruebberdt, 2009). Conversely, greater blood vessel response in women experiencing hot flashes has been reported in one study (Sassarini *et al.*, 2011). Thus, altered vascular function may accompany hot flashes, but further research is needed (The North American Menopause Society, 2019).

Treatment

Hormone therapy is considered first-line therapy for the relief of hot flashes (see section 8.5). SSRIs and SNRIs have found mention as pharmaceutical treatment earlier in this section as well. Other non-hormonal pharmacological therapies comprise clonidine and gabapentinoids. Note that the approval for hot flashes for these medications (as well as other medications that go beyond the scope of this work) may be regulated differently in different countries.

Beyond prescription therapies, a range of lifestyle changes and mind-body techniques have been researched for the treatment of vasomotor symptoms (The 2023 nonhormone therapy position statement of The North American Menopause Society, 2023).

- **Cooling techniques** include clothing adjustments (e.g. dressing in layers, using breathable clothing materials, avoiding pullover sweaters and scarves), hand or electric fans, cold packs under pillows, lower room temperature. To date, only some small trials have looked at cooling techniques (Baker *et al.*, 2021; Composto *et al.*, 2021) and no strong supporting evidence has emerged as yet.

- **Avoiding triggers** such as alcohol and spicy or hot foods and liquids, which is often recommended to women experiencing hot flashes, has gained little attention in the research. Only one study found a positive association between hot flashes and alcohol intake in a cohort of Chinese women (Zhang *et al.*, 2020), but no clinical trials to date have assessed if avoiding triggers alleviates vasomotor symptoms (The 2023 nonhormone therapy position statement of The North American Menopause Society, 2023).

- **Dietary modification:** A healthy diet is important for overall health; however, there is limited evidence when it comes to improving hot flashes. Some studies associate more vegetable and fruit consumption as well as a Mediterranean-style diet with fewer menopause symptoms, while a high-fat and -sugar diet can increase the risk of hot flashes (Herber-Gast and Mishra, 2013; Beezhold *et al.*, 2018; Soleymani *et al.*, 2019). Another study indicated that females with vasomotor symptoms may benefit from a lower consumption of poultry and skimmed dairy products and a greater consumption of vegetables and soy milk (Herber-Gast and Mishra, 2013).

- **Weight loss:** Adiposity has found to be a risk factor for more frequent and severe hot flashes, and weight loss can decrease vasomotor symptoms. The role of obesity in hot flashes seems to depend on age and menopause stage—weight loss may have greater effects when women are earlier in the menopause transition (i.e. in perimenopause and early postmenopause) (Thurston *et al.*, 2009, 2015; Huang *et al.*, 2010; Thurston, Santoro and Matthews, 2011; Anderson *et al.*, 2020).

- **Cognitive behavioral therapy**—both in group as well as in self-help formats—has shown to be effective in reducing bothersome hot flashes in both breast cancer survivors as well as menopausal women (Mann *et al.*, 2011; Ayers *et al.*, 2012; Hardy *et al.*, 2018; Atema *et al.*, 2019; Green *et al.*, 2019; Fenlon *et al.*, 2020; The 2023 nonhormone therapy position statement of The North American Menopause Society, 2023).

- **Clinical hypnosis**—which involves a deeply relaxed state, mental imagery and suggestion—has been shown to reduce severity and frequency of hot flashes (Elkins *et al.*, 2008, 2013).

- **Mindfulness-based interventions** such as mindfulness-based stress reduction (MBSR) lack data to support their effectiveness in treating hot flashes. Some studies point to positive effects on menopausal symptoms in general, and in some cases vasomotor symptoms in particular. Studies in this group are facing methodological issues such as limited sample sizes or lack of control groups; some are not specifically designed to consider hot flashes (Carmody *et al.*, 2011; Wong *et al.*, 2018; Chen *et al.*, 2021; The 2023 nonhormone therapy position statement of The North American Menopause Society, 2023).

- **Physical activity and exercise** have been looked at in several studies, with a wide array of methods and types of interventions (The 2023 nonhormone therapy position statement of The North American Menopause Society, 2023). Section 8.3 summarizes related findings.

8.2.3. Changes in body composition

On to a topic that causes lots of frustration and suffering among women in the later stages of life. Body composition changes significantly during the menopause transition: 60–70% of midlife women gain weight, on average 1.5 pounds or roughly 700 grams per year, on average between ages 50 and 60 (Karvonen-Gutierrez and Kim, 2016; Baker, Lampio, *et al.*, 2018). Ethnicity has been found to be associated with the risk of weight gain: women of African American and Hispanic descent exhibit higher rates of weight gain than Caucasian women (Persons *et al.*, 2024). The weight gain associated with the menopausal transition can not only be a psychological burden, but also represents a major risk for developing cardiovascular disease (Kodoth, Scaccia and Aggarwal, 2022).

Lean body mass decreases (by about 3–8% yearly after the age of 30, with accelerating numbers after the age of 60), abdominal fat (subcutaneous and particularly visceral fat) increases, and it becomes harder to lose visceral fat, even when women intentionally aim to reduce weight (Park

and Lee, 2003; Volpi, Nazemi and Fujita, 2004; Lovejoy *et al.*, 2008; Franklin, Ploutz-Snyder and Kanaley, 2009). Increased visceral abdominal fat, in particular, can have detrimental effects on cardiovascular health, represented by increases in blood pressure and fasting glucose, as well as changes in cholesterol profiles (i.e. elevated total cholesterol and low-density lipoprotein or LDL levels) (Park *et al.*, 2013).

The specific mechanisms behind the adverse changes in body composition and weight gain have not been clarified yet. Hormonal, age-related and lifestyle changes have been considered as possible influencing factors (Kodoth, Scaccia and Aggarwal, 2022). Within the hormonal realm, changes in estrogen levels have been discussed most prominently: estrogen reduction leads to a change of distribution of adipose tissue (i.e. an accumulation of visceral fat) (Brown and Clegg, 2010). In addition, estradiol has been associated with insulin sensitivity. While premenopausal women exhibit enhanced insulin sensitivity and reduced type 2 diabetes incidence compared to men, estrogen deficiency has shown to be a risk factor for insulin resistance and can contribute to an increase of metabolic syndrome and type 2 diabetes prevalence in postmenopausal women (Yan *et al.*, 2019; De Paoli, Zakharia and Werstuck, 2021). In support of this, it has been shown that women going through surgically induced menopause present with an elevated risk of developing insulin resistance and metabolic syndrome (Pu *et al.*, 2017; Christakis *et al.*, 2020). However, the results on whether body composition changes occur primarily due to hormonal changes are mixed; aging (independent of menopausal status) as well as lifestyle factors have been associated with weight gain as well (Kodoth, Scaccia and Aggarwal, 2022).

Should clinicians focus on weight or health?

Today's culture is focused on dieting and weight loss and many women in midlife are presenting to their healthcare providers with weight gain fears (Persons *et al.*, 2024). Weight-centric interventions with a focus on weight loss or deceleration of weight gain can create frustration—women may perceive their lack of success as a failure, and resume their prior habits (Knight *et al.*, 2021). Clinicians may therefore choose to focus on lifestyle interventions and language that address cardiometabolic risk factors directly, rather than weight loss per se. Additionally, cultural differences in body image perception should inform clinician interactions. It has been shown that obese White women verbalized more internalized weight stigma than Black females, who reported higher body satisfaction and more positive body image. While both groups of women desired empathetic, non-judgmental weight-loss advice, the culturally competent clinician should bear in mind that some women may also need assistance in overcoming stigma and low self-esteem related to weight (Chugh *et al.*, 2013). Clinicians should also recognize that weight management interventions may not be wanted, accessible or affordable for some (Persons *et al.*, 2024). Lifestyle modification attempts in women with economical disadvantages may be aggravated by a sense of powerlessness and resignation to current lifestyle habits. Clinicians should consider barriers to implementing lifestyle changes to ensure that modifications can be realistically implemented; on the level of policy makers, stronger considerations should be given to systemic barriers and upstream health interventions (Audet *et al.*, 2017).

8.2.4. Changes in the musculoskeletal system

Around 70% of midlife women will experience musculoskeletal symptoms, such as loss of muscle mass, loss of bone mineral density, joint pain (arthralgia) and progression of osteoarthritis; 25% will encounter severe symptoms (Lu *et al.*, 2020). Recently, the term **musculoskeletal syndrome of menopause** has been proposed to describe the collective musculoskeletal signs and symptoms, which are largely associated with the fluctuations and loss of estrogen seen in the transition from perimenopause to postmenopause (Wright *et al.*, 2024). In this section, menopause-related changes related to bone, cartilage, muscle and fascia are summarized.

Bone

Estrogen deficiency related to menopause influences bone mineral density and **osteoporosis risk**. Osteoporosis is a multifactorial skeletal disease, marked by reduced bone mineral density and higher susceptibility to fracture (Sandhu and Hampson, 2011). Estrogen deficiency impacts the normal bone turnover cycle, potentially due to the presence of estrogen receptors in osteoclasts. Osteoclastic activity (i.e. bone resorption) increases, while osteoblastic activity (i.e. bone formation) decreases, which results in a net loss of bone mass (Ji and Yu, 2015). Bone loss associated with menopause occurs predominantly in trabecular bone (Rogers *et al.*, 2002) (see Figure 8.4). (A second phase of bone loss, which is marked by a persistent, slower loss of both trabecular and cortical bone, is related to age and starts some years after menopause; this slower form of bone loss also happens to men.) Reduction of bone mineral density during the menopausal transition amounts to about 10% on average (Ji and Yu, 2015). Early menopause may increase the risk for osteoporosis (and cardiovascular disease as well); however, there is a gap in clinical guidance for early menopause (Mishra *et al.*, 2024).

Menopausal hormone replacement therapy has been shown to be effective in the prevention of osteoporotic fractures and to preserve bone mineral density (Wells *et al.*, 2002).

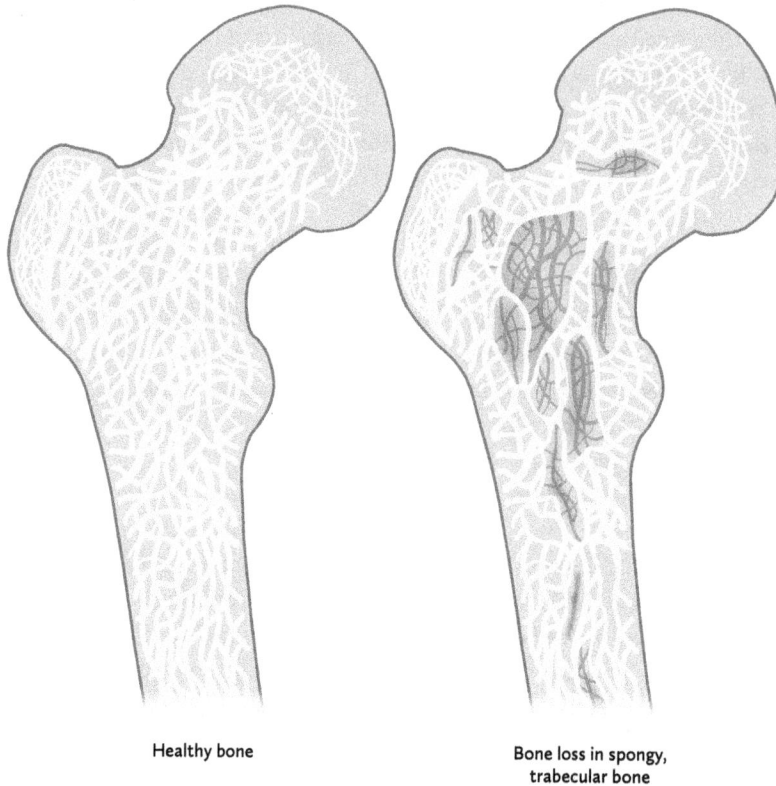

Healthy bone

Bone loss in spongy, trabecular bone

[AQ]Figure 8.4: Decreases in estrogen related to menopause are associated with an accelerated loss in bone mineral density. Bone loss associated with menopause occurs predominantly in spongy, trabecular bone. Bone loss continues with aging, but is characterized by a slower loss of both trabecular as well as cortical bone.

Cartilage

The incidence of osteoarthritis (degeneration of joint cartilage) in women dramatically increases around menopause and females experience more debilitating joint pain than men (Stevens-Lapsley and Kohrt, 2010; Tschon *et al.*, 2021). A possible association between menopausal estrogen deprivation and the frequency of osteoarthritis in knees, hips and fingers as well as the severity of hip osteoarthritis has been suggested (Richette, Corvol and Bardin, 2003). Findings on the effects of menopausal hormone replacement therapy on cartilage health remain inconclusive (Wright *et al.*, 2024).

Muscle

Sarcopenia describes the age-related loss of lean muscle mass (Khadilkar, 2019). While women start losing muscle mass and strength starting in their thirties, the rate of decline accelerates in early menopause (Bondarev *et al.*, 2021). Loss of muscle mass and function can lead to negative impacts on mental health and quality of life and can indirectly contribute to increased risk of disability and reduced independence (Chang *et al.*, 2017; Tricco *et al.*, 2017; Tsekoura *et al.*, 2017; Tan *et al.*, 2023).

Moreover, muscle regeneration may be impaired after menopause: satellite cells, adult muscle stem cells responsible for repairing and regenerating muscle tissue, reduce in numbers by about 15% from perimenopause to postmenopause (BC Collins, 2019). Estrogen deficiency may furthermore impair satellite cell function (Oxfeldt *et al.*, 2022). As estrogen also appears to have antioxidant and membrane-stabilizing effects, these protective mechanisms may decline after menopause, which can negatively impact regenerative processes (McNulty *et al.*, 2020; Pellegrino, Tiidus and Vandenboom, 2022). As sarcopenia and satellite cell activity appear to be driven by estrogen deficiency (also see section 3.1 for effects of estrogen on the musculoskeletal system), hormonal replacement therapy has been found to be a plausible method to counteract losses in muscle mass, strength and regeneration (Dieli-Conwright *et al.*, 2009a, 2009b; Pöllänen *et al.*, 2010; Oxfeldt *et al.*, 2022; Pellegrino, Tiidus and Vandenboom, 2022) (further information on hormonal replacement therapy is given in section 8.5).

Fascial system

In this work, the fascial system is understood as a holistic-functional complex connecting various body components such as muscles, bones, neural tissues and organs. The fascial system includes soft collagenous connective tissue structures such as the intra- and intermuscular connective tissue, superficial fascia, tendons, ligaments, aponeuroses, joint capsules and neurovascular sheaths (Adstrum *et al.*, 2017; Stecco *et al.*, 2018; Schleip, Hedley and Yucesoy, 2019). In this section, special consideration will be given to recent research findings on aging processes related to tendons, deep fascia surrounding muscles and intramuscular connective tissue.

Much of the biomechanical research regarding soft connective tissues has been carried out on tendons. The most consistent finding regarding the effects of aging on tendon structural properties is the accumulation of advanced glycation end product (AGE)-related cross-links, which can increase tissue stiffness and reduce the ability to return elastic energy (Svensson *et al.*, 2016).

Findings regarding other tendon structural properties and aging are less consistent (small increases in cross-sectional areas of tendons and enzymatic cross-links as well as minor reductions in collagen content, fibril diameter and proteoglycan content have been observed) (Svensson *et al.*, 2016). Before menopause, females are at lower risk for Achilles tendon ruptures than men; after menopause, the risk becomes similar in both sexes (Hansen and Kjaer, 2014; Chidi-Ogbolu and Baar, 2018).

Regarding deep fascia, such as the thoracolumbar fascia, it has recently been reported that fascial tissues in the low back are considerably thicker in older versus younger women (Wilke *et al.*, 2019). In the fascia lata (deep fascia of the thigh), however, this pattern was reversed, and younger females were reported to have thicker fascia than their older counterparts. According to the authors, thicker fascial tissues may impact joint flexibility.

With respect to intramuscular connective tissue, recent evidence found that the composition of the extracellular matrix was altered in aging human and mouse samples (Fede *et al.*, 2022). Collagen type I increased, while collagen type III and elastic fibers did not show major changes. Hyaluronan content, critical for maintaining bound water retention and lubrication, was also significantly lower in older subjects. This change in extracellular matrix composition may result in increased tissue stiffness and reduced tissue adaptability.

8.2.5. Changes in psychological wellbeing

Historically, women experiencing depression in midlife were often labeled as "hysterical," reflecting long-held beliefs that females' disturbances in psychological wellbeing were rooted in their reproductive organs (the word hysteria originates from the Greek word for uterus). Affected women were further marginalized as women's mental health issues related to menopause were under-researched and inadequately treated. Until today, the menopausal transition is viewed negatively, and menopausal symptoms of depression are downplayed in many cultures. Lifting off the stigma and normalizing changes in psychological wellbeing related to menopause are long overdue to foster education, lead open conversations and adequately approach and treat symptoms such as menopausal depression.

Women in peri- and postmenopause are at a higher risk for depression, increased stress sensitivity and anxiety (Gordon *et al.*, 2019; Liang *et al.*, 2024). A 2024 systematic review and meta-analysis reported perimenopausal women to be at a significantly higher risk for depressive symptoms and diagnoses compared to premenopausal females (Badawy *et al.*, 2024). Prevalence of postmenopausal depression is also high; however, lack of data to date does not allow direct comparisons between the peri- and postmenopausal phases (Badawy *et al.*, 2024; Li *et al.*, 2024).

However, women are not universally at risk for psychological symptoms during this time of life and a number of protective factors as well as risk factors have been identified (Brown *et al.*, 2024). Among postmenopausal women, those who go through menopause at a later age and therefore have a longer reproductive period are associated with a reduced risk for depression (Georgakis *et al.*, 2016; Li *et al.*, 2024). In fact, each additional year of estradiol exposure decreases the odds of postmenopausal depression by 15% (Marsh *et al.*, 2017). A regular menstrual cycle during premenopause, the number of breastfed infants and physical activity (see section 8.3) appear to be additional protective factors for menopausal depression (Gariépy, Honkaniemi and Quesnel-Vallée, 2016; Li *et al.*, 2024). A primary risk factor for major depressive disorder over the menopause transition is previous depressive episodes—the strongest predictor for depression in women's midlife is a history of mental illness. Further risk factors include severe and prolonged vasomotor symptoms, chronic sleep disturbance, chronic diseases, stressful life events and the number of abortions (Kolte *et al.*, 2015; Soares, 2019; Brown *et al.*, 2024; Li *et al.*, 2024).

Potential mechanisms for depression around menopause include the estrogen withdrawal theory, the domino hypothesis and aspects around the biopsychosocial model (Badawy *et al.*, 2024). According to the **estrogen withdrawal theory**, the reduced level of estrogen and/or dramatic fluctuations of hormones could trigger the onset or worsening of depressive symptoms (Schmidt and Rubinow, 1991). As estrogen has been found to affect neurotransmitter metabolism (e.g. of norepinephrine, dopamine and serotonin), changes in estradiol may influence emotional states (Badawy *et al.*, 2024). Brain-specific changes may provide insights to estrogen-related changes after menopause as well. A 2024 imaging study revealed that in postmenopausal women, a higher density of estrogen receptors was found in brain areas related to mood (Mosconi *et al.*, 2024). Higher receptor density in amygdala, thalamus, frontal areas and posterior cingulate cortex predicted the presence of mood disturbances (low mood, mood fluctuations, tearfulness, irritability) in postmenopausal women. The identified elevations in estrogen receptor density could represent a compensatory neurophysiological response to the loss of estrogen after menopause. The found relationship further provides an explanation for estrogen's modulatory action in emotional processes as well as the relationship between estrogen state and menopausal symptoms (i.e. mood changes). Taken together, peri- and postmenopause can be seen as "window of vulnerability" for mood disturbances and depression according to decreased levels of estrogen (Soares and Zitek, 2008).

The **domino hypothesis** postulates that sleep problems (e.g. related to night sweats) can result in depressed mood (Freeman, 2015). Females with moderate to severe vasomotor symptoms have also been reported to be up to three times more likely to experience moderate to severe depressive symptoms (Worsley *et al.*, 2017). However, findings regarding this hypothesis are conflicting as risk for depressive symptoms has been found to be high in perimenopause in various studies, even after adjusting for vasomotor symptoms (Badawy *et al.*, 2024).

Besides, psychological and social factors as included in the **biopsychosocial model** can impact depression in peri- and postmenopause. Women may be faced with difficult events during perimenopause, such as caring for children as well as aging parents, and cultural attitudes toward menopause and aging have been speculated to increase vulnerability during the menopausal transition (Hunter and Rendall, 2007; Badawy *et al.*, 2024). Additionally, social support has been identified to play a role in postmenopausal depression. Midlife females who receive high social support have a 20% lower risk for depression, and having a spouse can provide social support; accordingly, marital status has been shown to be a protective factor against depression (Gariépy, Honkaniemi and Quesnel-Vallée, 2016; Sassarini, 2016). These associations imply that special psychological care and attention should be attributed to those who are caregivers, single, divorced or widowed (Li *et al.*, 2024).

Taken together, peri- and postmenopausal depression is complex and multifactorial, as it can be impacted by demographic, lifestyle, medical and reproductive health factors. Women in midlife should be educated, encouraged to openly express their experience, and to seek appropriate care.

8.3. PHYSICAL ACTIVITY AND PERFORMANCE IN PERI- AND POSTMENOPAUSE

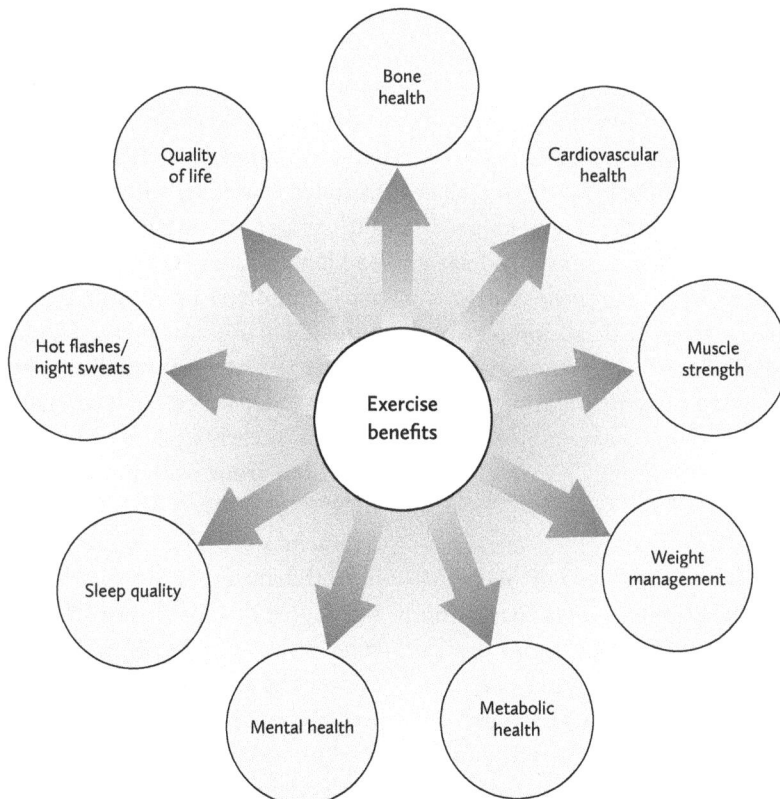

Figure 8.5: Benefits and goals of exercise in peri- and postmenopause.

A word on ideal exercise parameters

While emerging research is helpful to determine the most beneficial forms and dosages of exercise for different aspects of female health in midlife, it can be methodologically challenging to establish ideal exercise recipes. In evidence-based research, meta-analyses are typically used to combine multiple studies available for a given research question, to extrapolate findings to a broader population and to settle controversies from conflicting study findings. To identify optimal exercise protocols, one could carry out a meta-analysis on crucial exercise characteristics for a specified outcome (e.g. the effect of different types of exercise on bone mineral density in postmenopausal women). However, looking at individual factors like type, duration or frequency of exercise necessarily leads to an isolated consideration of single parameters, which doesn't reflect the complexity of exercise interventions and their efficacy. For example, the intensity of an exercise plays a role in bone strengthening, but its relevance also depends on training frequency. Moreover, the progression of a training program is crucial in adaptive processes, particularly when considering longer interventions (Mohebbi *et al.*, 2023). While different methodological approaches can be chosen to capture some of these complexities, one should bear in mind that research findings and related recommendations for single exercise parameters always need to be related to a bigger context.

Physical activity is an effective self-management strategy during midlife, and an increasing amount of research provides insights into how to adapt training for women in the course of reproductive aging. Physical activity and exercise can serve many purposes; for women in peri- and postmenopause, recent research examines the benefits of exercise regarding various outcomes, ranging from bone density and cardiovascular fitness to mental health and sleep quality (see Figure 8.5).

A lot of new research on physical activity, exercise and performance of women in peri- and postmenopause is currently emerging and evidence is becoming more robust as more systematic reviews and meta-analyses are being published. However, in some areas, research remains scarce—for example, studies on interindividual differences in training responses or energy metabolism in perimenopause are very limited (Sanchez *et al.*, 2024). This section therefore summarizes selected benefits and goals of exercise in peri- and postmenopause, mainly drawing from recent reviews and meta-analyses.

8.3.1. Bone health

Exercise is a promising domain for preventing osteoporosis in menopausal women. A 2023 systematic review and meta-analysis provides evidence for a positive effect of exercise on bone mineral density in postmenopausal females (Mohebbi *et al.*, 2023). The meta-analysis included 80 studies with various types of exercise such as aerobic exercise (predominantly walking and jogging), resistance training and combined aerobic and resistance training. A small number of included studies applied tai chi, hopping and jumping. The meta-analysis showed positive effects independent of menopausal status (i.e. women in early as well as late postmenopause benefited from exercise) and supervision (i.e. supervised as well as self-performed exercise regimens were successful). Despite these findings, the authors note that the decision about the degree of supervision should be made with consideration of the specific cohort, aims and budget considerations to provide a safe, efficient and effective training setting. While supervision can enhance adherence, motivation and intensity progression, some exercise formats may need less supervision than others with regard to safety (e.g. jumping training may need less supervision than dynamic resistance exercise). While the meta-analysis did intentionally not identify specific types of exercise to be particularly advantageous (see text box "A word on ideal exercise parameters"), another 2022 systematic review recommended mixed exercise programs (aerobic and resistance training, Pilates) to increase bone mineral density (Kalra *et al.*, 2022).

8.3.2. Cardiovascular health

The menopausal transition is associated with an increased risk of cardiovascular disease, marked by an increase of arterial stiffness (and an associated increase in pulse wave velocity) as well as decreased cardiorespiratory fitness (e.g. expressed by maximum oxygen consumption, $VO_{2\,max}$). A 2024 systematic review reported combined exercise (aerobic and resistance exercise) as well as aerobic exercise alone to improve arterial stiffness and cardiorespiratory fitness (Ferreira *et al.*, 2024). Positive effects were reported for short- (8–12 weeks), medium- (20 weeks) and long-term (51 weeks) interventions. Programs with a frequency of three days per week (on non-consecutive days) and a duration of 90 minutes per session were recommended to improve (i.e. lower) arterial stiffness. Another systematic review and meta-analysis from 2023 found aerobic, resistance as well as combined training effective to increase cardiorespiratory fitness in postmenopausal women (Khalafi *et al.*, 2023). Interesting and important with regard to entry hurdles of exercising is the finding of another study from 2019: even one bout or less than one hour of resistance training per week is associated with reduced risks of cardiovascular disease and all-cause mortality (Liu, Yanghui *et al.*, 2019).

8.3.3. Body composition/ weight management

A specific exercise form that has been increasingly discussed to reduce body weight and adipose tissue is high-intensity interval training (HIIT), which includes repeated bouts of high-intensity efforts (between 80% and 100% of peak heart rate), followed by short phases of recovery or less intense work (Dupuit, Rance, *et al.*, 2020). A 2020 meta-analysis examined the effects of HIIT on body composition in women before and after menopause; 39 articles were included (Dupuit, Maillard, *et al.*, 2020). Overall, HIIT programs decreased body weight and total fat. Regarding the decrease of abdominal fat, HIIT was only effective in females who were overweight. Generally, the effects were more evident in premenopausal women when compared with postmenopausal females. Cycling interventions were found to be more effective than running, particularly among postmenopausal women.

HIIT—varied, hard and satisfactory

Several studies show the beneficial effects of high-intensity exercise—for instance on muscle mass, strength or reduction of body fat. Studies on HIIT are using different modalities such as cardio HIIT, bodyweight HIIT, HIIT with weights, hill runs, or Tabata training. The heterogeneity between studies makes it hard to establish best training regimens. Despite the intensity of HIIT workouts, various studies have shown that HIIT leads to the same or even higher levels of satisfaction and adherence when compared with continuous training (Buckinx and Aubertin-Leheudre, 2019).

8.3.4. Muscle strength

A 2023 systematic review and meta-analysis looked at non-pharmacological interventions to prevent loss of muscle mass and function in menopausal women (Tan *et al.*, 2023). They found that exercise effectively improved muscle mass (i.e. lean body mass) and strength (represented by handgrip strength and knee extension strength).

Resistance training executed three times per week for 20–90 minutes per session proved to be most effective in improving lean body mass, potentially because it increases the secretion of growth hormone, which in turn stimulates muscle protein synthesis (Kraemer and Ratamess, 2005). The findings regarding exercise frequency and duration of this recent meta-analysis support the idea that minimal dose of resistance training can already have beneficial effects: prior research has shown that three times 20–30 minutes of resistance training per week over the course of 16 weeks demonstrated significant improvement in muscle mass and muscle strength (Fisher et al., 2017).

Contrasting with these positive findings, aerobic exercise alone and whole-body vibration interventions resulted in no significant effects on lean body mass (Tan et al., 2023). These findings largely coincide with another systematic review and meta-analysis on muscular strength in postmenopausal women from 2023: upper body strength, lower body strength and handgrip strength all improved in response to resistance training. Combined workouts (aerobic plus resistance training) were also effective for lower body and handgrip strength, while aerobic training alone only improved lower body strength (Khalafi et al., 2023).

8.3.5. Hot flashes, night sweats

Data suggests that moderate exercise can reduce subjectively experienced as well as objectively measured vasomotor symptoms. In women with depression, habitual physical exercise has also shown to decrease hot flash symptoms. However, intensity and type of exercise may make a difference. Some evidence suggests that a very high amount of physical activity may lead to a higher number of reported symptoms—it serves as a trigger for hot flashes (Witkowski et al., 2023). In terms of type of exercise, a 2024 meta-analysis

showed that resistance training can be helpful in reducing hot flashes in postmenopausal women (Choudhry et al., 2024). The effects of aerobic exercise on vasomotor symptoms remain unclear (Money et al., 2024). Current data does not offer findings on different populations, such as perimenopausal versus postmenopausal women and females with different ethnic backgrounds or mental health status. It is also not clear if prescribed exercise is effective (Witkowski et al., 2023).

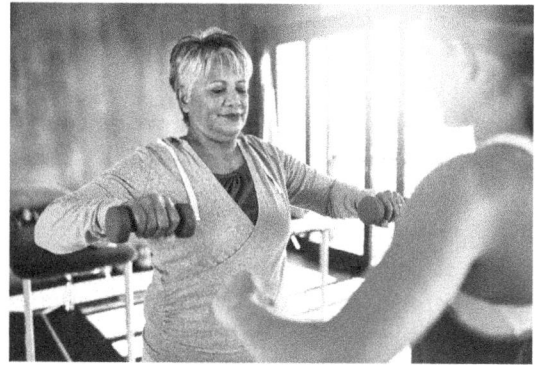

Photo 8.1: Exercise throughout peri- and postmenopause. Physical activity is an effective self-management strategy for peri- and postmenopausal women. Recent research specifically points to resistance and HIIT as helpful interventions.

8.3.6. Mental health

A 2022 systematic review summarized the impact of physical activity on mental health in postmenopausal women (Kalra et al., 2022). Four of the seven included studies used walking as intervention; yoga, Pilates, resistance training and cycling were included in the identified studies as well. Positive effects on measures such as depression, anxiety, sadness, sleep and mental health were found. However, prospective and longitudinal investigations are still scarce, and future research is needed to shed light on the most beneficial forms of exercise, for example for postmenopausal depression (Li et al., 2024).

8.4. LIFESTYLE CONSIDERATIONS FOR PERI- AND POSTMENOPAUSE

Health behavior matters—that holds true for every stage of life and also applies to the menopausal transition. Lifestyle factors, such as physical activity (see section 8.3), sleep, diet, cessation of smoking, limited alcohol consumption as well as actively managing stress, can positively impact the menopausal transition (Kodoth, Scaccia and Aggarwal, 2022; Davis *et al.*, 2023). This section summarizes selected aspects regarding sleep and nutrition, as these are non-pharmacological approaches that can be addressed by health professionals and individuals alike.

8.4.1. Sleep

A substantial number of females experience sleep difficulties during the menopausal transition and beyond—namely difficulties falling asleep, waking up several times throughout the night and waking up early. Clinicians furthermore observe restless legs syndrome, periodic limb movement disorder and obstructive sleep apnea as sleep disturbances in midlife women (The North American Menopause Society, 2019). In 26%, symptoms were found to be so severe that they can impact daytime functioning (Baker, De Zambotti, *et al.*, 2018). Disordered sleep during peri- and postmenopause can have a far-reaching impact on mood, depressive and anxiety symptoms, quality of life, as well as physical health and body composition (Baker, De Zambotti, *et al.*, 2018). For instance, better quality sleep and longer sleep duration have been associated with favorable cardiovascular health, while snoring nearly every night has been shown to negatively impact weight gain in menopausal women (Ayrim, Aktepe Keskin and Özol, 2014; Makarem *et al.*, 2019). Hormonal changes in FSH and estradiol are being discussed as factors contributing to sleep disturbances (Kravitz *et al.*, 2008; Allshouse, Pavlovic

and Santoro, 2018). In addition, nocturnal hot flashes (see section 8.2.2) are associated with an increased number of awakenings and overall wake time, and are therefore a major contributor to sleep complaints in this stage of life. However, the exact mechanisms behind sleep disturbances in midlife are not yet fully understood and further research is needed to better understand what specifically causes sleep problems in midlife (Baker, De Zambotti, *et al.*, 2018).

Sleep and mood

Associations between sleep and mood disturbances are reported for the general population as well as for women during and after the menopausal transition (Grandner *et al.*, 2015). However, the mechanisms behind the interaction between sleep and mood are not well understood. In addition to neurobiological factors (Palagini *et al.*, 2019), circadian rhythm changes as well as psychological mechanisms have been proposed. As an example of the latter, it has been found that unhelpful thoughts and beliefs about sleep mediated the relationship between poor sleep and mood disturbances in perimenopausal women (Kloss, Tweedy and Gilrain, 2004). While it is of advantage that sleep disturbances are a modifiable risk factor and that women can take active measures to protect sleep and prevent insomnia, it should be mentioned that pressuring oneself to create perfect sleep habits can also create further stress and negative thoughts about sleep behavior. This should be considered, particularly when introducing non-pharmacological interventions to improve sleep quality.

Current options for treating sleep disorders include pharmacological treatments (which have been described in detail elsewhere; see, for example, Baker, De Zambotti, *et al.*, 2018) and non-pharmacological interventions, the latter of which have been recommended for people with chronic sleep disorders as they have proven to be effective and have hardly any side effects (MacLeod *et al.*, 2018). Non-pharmacological interventions such as sleep hygiene, cognitive behavioral therapy, exercise, yoga, meditation, acupuncture and aromatherapy have gained popularity in practice over the last years and have also increasingly gained attention in the research. A meta-analysis from 2023 on the effects of such interventions on improving sleep quality and reducing insomnia severity in menopausal women found significant positive effects (Ha *et al.*, 2023). Duration of the intervention had a positive effect on the results, meaning that longer intervention led to bigger effect sizes. This is not surprising, given that behavior changes typically take a certain period of time. Another interesting finding was that effect sizes were larger in studies conducted in Asia than studies carried out in the West, suggesting that acceptance of non-pharmacological interventions for sleep disorders may differ based on culture and society. Additionally, for both older females and males particularly, combined techniques and the inclusion of stress management approaches appear promising non-pharmacological interventions to improve sleep (MacLeod *et al.*, 2018).

Sleep x diet x menopause
Sleeping and eating behavior are not only important factors on their own, but they also interact with each other. Sleep restriction can result in decreased levels of hormones signaling fullness (such as leptin) and increased concentrations of appetite-stimulating hormones (e.g. ghrelin) (Spiegel, Leproult, *et al.*, 2004; Spiegel, Tasali, *et al.*, 2004).

Experimental studies further demonstrate that sleep restriction increases food intake, especially in the evening. However, only a small number of women have been included in sleep restriction studies, and sex-specific analyses are not always performed (St-Onge, 2016). It is not surprising then that research on the interaction between sleep and diet is even more scarce when it comes to menopausal women. A recent explorative study has identified various aspects of eating behavior as potential risk factors for poor quality sleep in menopausal women (Lankila *et al.*, 2024). The following associations were found:

- Snacking-type eating with shorter sleep duration and higher day-time tiredness.
- Externally cued eating with shorter sleep duration.
- Emotional eating with daytime tiredness.

This study is a good reminder that dietary interventions may impact much more than nutritional status!

8.4.2. Diet

The role of nutrition in the development of chronic diseases has been sufficiently proven and is an important determinant for health at every stage in life. As peri- and postmenopause are associated with an increased prevalence of obesity, metabolic syndrome, cardiovascular diseases and osteoporosis, nutrition can help to reduce risk factors and support women in midlife (Erdélyi *et al.*, 2023). It is important to note, however, that investigations involving women in perimenopause and energy metabolism are still extremely limited (Sanchez *et al.*, 2024). Overall, a balanced mixed diet, which can be sustained over a long time, is recommended; however, there is no single, ideal way to achieve a healthy nutritional status (Erdélyi *et al.*, 2023).

As the decrease in estradiol directly impacts

lipid energy metabolism, lipid parameters (i.e. total cholesterol, LDL, triglyceride) worsen rapidly with the onset of the menopausal transition (Anagnostis *et al.*, 2015; Sanchez *et al.*, 2024). Whole-body fat oxidation at rest lowers in post- as opposed to premenopausal women, which contributes to higher levels of circulating lipids (Sanchez *et al.*, 2024). With regard to diet, focus should be put on consuming healthy fatty acids— the composition of ingested **fatty acids** appears to be more important than the total amount. Therefore, dietary intake of omega-3 fatty acids is essential (Erdélyi *et al.*, 2023).

Menopause and the change in estrogen levels also increase the risk of developing **carbohydrate** metabolism disorders (such as type 2 diabetes) due to an impairment of insulin secretion and sensitivity (Paschou *et al.*, 2019). There seems to be a correlation between age of menopause and type 2 diabetes risk: menopause occurring either before the age of 40 or after the age of 49 was associated with an increased risk in a prospective study with over 300,000 women (M. Wang *et al.*, 2022). Dietary considerations should include blood sugar management (i.e. ideally excluding added sugars, eating carbohydrates with low glycemic index and increasing foods rich in fiber, as high fiber contents slow down the absorption of carbohydrates) (Erdélyi *et al.*, 2023). (Gradually) increasing fiber intake also positively changes the intestinal flora, positively impacting isoflavonoids, pre-, pro- and postbiotics (Singh *et al.*, 2023).

Additionally, adequate **protein** intake is needed to maintain or increase skeletal muscle and lean body mass (Thomas, 2007). Adequate intake of protein, as well as vitamin D and calcium, is also among the nutritional recommendations to support bone metabolism (Management of osteoporosis in postmenopausal women: The 2021 position statement of The North American Menopause Society, 2021).

Related to sleep, diet can also affect melatonin levels, for example through foods rich in melatonin and tryptophan (a precursor in melatonin production). Cherries have an exceptionally high melatonin content, making tart cherry juice a popular household remedy to support sleep. Other plant and animal sources with high melatonin content are strawberries, wine grape skin, eggs and fish (Meng *et al.*, 2017; Cortés-Montaña *et al.*, 2023). Tryptophan-rich foods include algae (including spirulina), sesame seeds, soy, sunflower seeds, pumpkin seeds, cheddar cheese, egg whites and sea fish (Zuraikat *et al.*, 2021).

Hormonal changes during reproductive aging can also affect thirst, which may result in a decrease in fluid intake (Stachenfeld, 2014). Women should therefore make sure to take in appropriate amounts of fluid.

Microbiome, estroblome and estrogen recycling in menopause

Estrogen and gut microbiota follow a bi-directional relationship: estrogen levels can affect the microbiome (in part by serving as substrates for microbial metabolism and promoting gut microbe diversity), and gut microbiota can affect estrogen levels as certain microbiota—called the **estroblome**—can produce and metabolize estrogen (Kwa *et al.*, 2016).

Circulating estrogen passes the liver and is metabolized through a process called conjugation, during which estrogen is modified so it becomes more water soluble. Conjugated estrogen can be excreted by bile into the intestinal tract and eventually be removed via feces. Microbiota of the estroblome can **deconjugate** estrogen, allowing estrogen to be reabsorbed into the bloodstream, re-enter circulation and reach other tissues. In fact, a significant proportion of estrogen is being deconjugated by the estroblome, while only a small fraction is found in conjugated form in feces. As postmenopausal women lack ovarian hormone production and have very low levels of estrogen, this form of recycling of hormones by the gut microbiota is important after menopause. Research furthermore suggests that menopause is associated with lower gut microbiome diversity, which may reduce estroblome potential. However, further research is needed to identify and better understand the changes in the gut microbiome in female reproductive aging (Peters *et al.*, 2022).

Safe to soy (milk)?

Perhaps the most common—and at the same time the most controversial—dietary practice during perimenopause is the consumption of soy products and other plant-based estrogens (phytoestrogens). The rationale behind this nutritional strategy is that if you are low in estrogen, there might be benefits in a plant-based diet, containing foods with plant-based estrogens (phytoestrogens), such as soy, chickpeas and lentils. Phytoestrogens activate estrogen receptors, promote mild hormone-like responses, and have been used as an additional hormone supplemental remedy for menopausal symptoms (Patra *et al.*, 2023; Sommer *et al.*, 2023). For example, positive effects on menopause symptoms have been reported for females with asthma and type 2 diabetes (Sommer *et al.*, 2023). Also, it is known that hot flashes are rarer in regions where soy products are more regularly consumed. In terms of quantity, one publication recommended 400 mL of soy drinks per day (corresponding to 20 mg per day of soy supplements or 80 g per day of other soy products such as tofu) for reduction of menopause-related symptoms (Taku *et al.*, 2012).

However, soy consumption has been discussed controversially in the context of breast cancer risk and treatment. While the isoflavone content of soy can have a positive impact on menopausal symptoms, phytoestrogens can have a negative effect on the treatment of hormone-sensitive breast tumors. Regular soy consumption may reduce the efficacy of anti-estrogen therapy, which is used in hormone-sensitive breast cancer (Erdélyi *et al.*, 2023). Meanwhile, other accounts give less cause for concern. One study reported that regular soy consumption did not increase breast cancer risk (Steinberg *et al.*, 2011), and an Asian population-based study reported that among women with breast cancer, soy food consumption (up to 250 mL of soy drink or 10–15 g of soy protein) was considered safe (Shu *et al.*, 2009). It seems safe to say that, to date, there is no consensus among the scientific community on the effect of soy on breast cancer and its treatment. Further research is warranted, especially regarding dosages and molecular subtypes of soy consumption (Shu *et al.*, 2009; Lalioti *et al.*, 2024).

Diet around menopause: How much of what?

A current review on the importance of nutrition in peri- and postmenopause summarizes the recommendations for a balanced diet and fluid intake (Erdélyi *et al.*, 2023). Selected aspects are listed below:

- Protein: 1–1.2 g per kg body weight per day
- Vegetables: 300–400 g per day
- Fruit: 100–200 g per day
- Legumes (beans, peas, lentils, chickpeas, soy): at least once per week
- Nuts and seeds (unsalted): 30 g per day
- Dietary fiber (whole grain, fiber-rich cereals): 30–45 g per day
- Fish (deep-sea fish with fatty meat such as salmon, mackerel, tuna, herring, sardines): 100–120 g per occasion; at least two servings per week

- Adequate intake of vitamin D, C and B
- Adequate intake of omega-3 fatty acids
- If meat is being consumed, no more than 500–700 g of raw (or 350–500 g of boiled/steamed/fried) red meat is recommended (processed meat should only be consumed occasionally)
- Fluids: 33 mL per kg bodyweight per day

With body composition being a main concern of women during reproductive aging, various fasting strategies are being used by women with the intention to positively impact body weight. Generally, there are three fasting strategies, which are also applied in menopausal women: caloric restriction, dietary restriction (decrease of a type of food), and intermittent fasting (Arbour *et al.*, 2021).

- **Caloric restriction:** While it seems plausible that the basal metabolic rate decreases during peri- and postmenopause due to loss of skeletal muscle (Ko and Jung, 2021; Sanchez *et al.*, 2024), focusing heavily on calorie reduction can have negative effects. Diets containing less than 1200 kcal per day are associated with higher risks of micronutrient deficiencies, low-calorie diets lead to a high number of relapses, and diets of 800–1000 kcal/per day do not lead to sustainable weight loss (Yumuk *et al.*, 2015).

- **Dietary restriction:** Low and very low carbohydrate diets are increasingly used to lose weight and treat metabolic disorders. A popular example is the ketogenic diet, which is characterized by less than 20–50 g of carbohydrates per day and elimination of sugar, grains, legumes, as well as some fruits and vegetables. The ketogenic diet includes high-fat and adequate protein intake (Arbour *et al.*, 2021). The goal of the keto diet is to shift the body's metabolism from relying on glucose (derived from carbs) to relying on ketones (derived from fat). Additionally, the lower carbohydrate intake aims to decrease insulin secretion and—as a consequence—reduce fat storage and insulin resistance (Hall, 2017; Arbour *et al.*, 2021). Apart from weight loss, the keto diet is sometimes prescribed in the treatment of cancer and epilepsy (Dozières-Puyravel *et al.*, 2018; Weber, Aminazdeh-Gohari and Kofler, 2018). While the keto diet appears to be effective in reducing body mass and fat mass, it seems to have relatively greater benefits for males (Leaf *et al.*, 2024). Females may even be prone to unfavorable metabolic effects of low-carbohydrate diets (Smolensky *et al.*, 2023). However, more research is needed to determine if these differences may be dampened after menopause due to hormonal changes and if the keto diet may lead to beneficial effects in later life stages of women (Leaf *et al.*, 2024).

- **Intermittent fasting:** This involves varying patterns of feasting and fasting. For example, individuals may choose to fast for 24 hours once or twice a week with normal food intake for the rest of the week. Alternatively, in time-restricted feeding, individuals eat for a set number of hours each day and fast for the rest of the day (e.g. eating for 8 hours, fasting for 16 hours). This is said to force the body to burn more fat, limit the release of insulin, and activate autophagy (a cellular process that cleans up and recycles damaged proteins and cells) (Ahmed *et al.*, 2018; Arbour *et al.*, 2021). Theories suggest that mammalian females evolved to better withstand reduced food supplies due to more severe selection pressures compared to males in times of famine, by becoming more efficient in food metabolism and consequently becoming predisposed to obesity in times of relative feast (Hoyenga and Hoyenga, 1982). In short, a woman's body may fight to preserve energy when she puts herself in a phase of fasting. Supporting the idea that intermittent fasting may not be as beneficial for females, studies have shown that total cholesterol, triglycerides and LDL levels did not change in response to Ramadan fasting in women (HDL, however, increased) (Aksungar *et al.*, 2005). Contradicting these hypotheses and findings, some recent studies have shown better metabolic outcomes in female versus male rodents after intermittent fasting (Emiliano *et al.*, 2022; Bosch de Basea *et al.*, 2024). Initial evidence reports that weight loss and metabolic benefits (such as improved insulin sensitivity) apply to both pre- as well as postmenopausal women with obesity (Cienfuegos *et al.*, 2021; Lin *et al.*, 2021).

Taken together, these findings reflect the state of research in the complex field of nutrition. As in neighboring fields, females have only recently entered the spotlight and our knowledge about sex differences remains controversial for now. Data on energy metabolism is particularly sparse for women in perimenopause (Sanchez *et al.*, 2024). More data is needed for females in later stages of life.

8.5. HORMONE REPLACEMENT THERAPY—WHERE ARE WE NOW?

Estrogen deficiency related to menopause is not a disease, it is a physiological process. However, menopause may have been over-medicalized, for example by commercial companies who are interested in promoting menopausal hormone therapy (The Lancet, 2024). Moreover, females' experience of menopause varies greatly, and while there is no one-size-fits-all approach and some go through the menopausal transition uneventfully, symptoms can range from hot flashes, vaginal dryness and musculoskeletal pain to osteoporosis (The Lancet, 2024). Untreated symptoms may have serious health implications. Hormonal replacement therapy for symptoms is available; it is the most effective treatment for vasomotor symptoms (Langer *et al.*, 2021). Beyond that, research suggests that for women starting treatment before the age of 60, or within ten years of the onset of menopause, all-cause mortality is reduced. Depending on the treatment regimen, hormone replacement therapy can furthermore be protective against dementia and coronary heart disease (Langer *et al.*, 2021). However, it also has potential side effects—some of them serious, such as thromboembolism—which need to be carefully weighed. Ongoing discussion in the research centers around the question of whether hormone replacement therapy increases the risk of serious illnesses such as breast cancer, ovarian cancer and dementia (Beral *et al.*, 2015; Liu, Yang, *et al.*, 2019; Langer *et al.*, 2021). Also, after stopping hormonal treatment, women may experience the return of their vasomotor symptoms, even at higher ages (The Lancet, 2024).

Thus, here is the unsatisfying conclusion to start with: at this time, a definite conclusion on whether the related side effects exceed the risks of untreated symptoms cannot be made. Instead, an individualized assessment and nuanced approach is needed to meet each female's needs (Booyens *et al.*, 2022). Symptom severity, a weighing of risks and benefits including medical history, as well as each female's wishes and expectations, all influence the decision on whether hormone replacement therapy is used (Davis *et al.*, 2023). Enabling women to make empowered and informed choices about hormone replacement therapy requires a basic understanding of the different available options (Hickey *et al.*, 2024). The following overview is intended to outline the overall picture of hormone replacement therapy—it is neither comprehensive, nor is it intended as medical or pharmacological advice.

A breaking point—the Women's Health Initiative (WHI) trial

Before 2002, hormone replacement therapy was the standard of care for menopausal management. This changed abruptly and prescriptions declined steeply when initial results of the WHI trial were published in 2002. What had happened? The WHI trial investigated the effects of hormone therapy on women's health in a cohort of 16,000 women. The study findings published in 2002 suggested that hormone replacement therapy in the form of conjugated equine estrogen (estrogen hormones derived from the urine of pregnant horses) and medroxyprogesterone acetate (a synthetic progestin) increased the risk for breast cancer, stroke, heart attack and thrombosis. The US Food and Drug Administration (FDA) consequently issued a black-box warning on hormone replacement therapy in 2002.

What was not initially taken into account, however, was the average age of the women in the study: WHI evaluated hormone replacement therapy in older women well past their menopause (the average age was 63 years, and mean time since menopause was 12 years; only 30% of the cohort was younger than 60 years at time of enrollment) (Langer *et al.*, 2021). In addition, the majority of women were overweight or obese, which has been recognized as a risk factor for breast cancer (Kuhl, 2005). Early resulting criticism of the study design went unnoticed and the message that hormone replacement therapy was dangerous spread quickly.

Meanwhile, it has been acknowledged that age at starting hormone replacement therapy is critical in determining the risks and benefits of hormone treatment. When initiated before the age of 60—or within ten years of menopause—all-cause mortality is reduced, coronary heart disease risk may be lowered, and breast cancer risk may not be generally increased after all (Manson and Kaunitz, 2016; Langer *et al.*, 2021).

After the reveal of the initial WHI trial results (see text box), women's requests for **compounded bioidentical hormones** accelerated rapidly (Stuenkel, 2021). Such hormones comprise customized formulations, prepared by compounding pharmacies for each patient. In the US, such products are not approved by the FDA. In contrast to hormones used in conventional hormone therapy, women perceive custom-compounded bioidentical hormones as natural (Stanczyk, Matharu and Winer, 2021). The term "bioidentical" has furthermore been used in marketing with the implication that their use is safer and identical to endogenous hormones (Stuenkel, 2021). However, chemical structures used in bioidentical hormone therapy are the same as in conventional hormone therapy (Stanczyk, Matharu and Winer, 2021). Possible reasons why women favor compounded bioidentical hormones are easy to understand: after publication of the WHI results, a strong aversion against conjugated estrogens and an overarching distrust of the pharmaceutical industry with regard to hormone replacement therapy arose. The promise of individualized products added to the attractiveness of these products (Stuenkel, 2021). Current accounts aim to point out that compounded bioidentical hormones are essentially untested and unapproved; also, due to their low aqueous solubility, it is challenging to formulate progesterone and estrogen consistently, which can impact the quality of compounded products. Moreover, the saliva testing used to determine the target level for hormones and thus individualize compounds comes with various problems as data on the correlations between salivary and blood hormone levels remains inconclusive. In the US, the FDA is working toward greater standardization and oversight to assure quality control and safety of compounded products (Stanczyk, Matharu and

Winer, 2021). For women to make empowered decisions, it is important to resolve uncertainties and misconceptions about different types of hormones used in menopausal therapy. Classes of steroid hormones used in hormone replacement therapy are therefore summarized in Table 8.1.

Table 8.1: Types of steroid hormones used in menopausal hormone therapy (adapted from Stanczyk *et al.*, 2021)

Class of steroids	Characteristics	Example/description
A	Found in nature	Conjugated equine estrogens. Can be formulated into a drug without chemical modification.
B	Semisynthetic	Natural starting materials that can be used as precursors for steroid synthesis; found in plants (e.g. in Mexican yam or soybeans). Need to be chemically synthesized (at least 15 chemical reactions necessary).
C	Synthetic	Synthesized from non-steroidal starting material by a "total synthesis" process.
D	Designed/man-made	Steroids not found in humans, animals or plants.

Various steroid hormones can be differentiated. **Class A** steroids are found in nature and can be used in drugs without going through any further chemical modification. The only form of hormone replacement therapy meeting this criterion are **conjugated equine estrogens**, which are extracted from the urine of pregnant mares (Stanczyk, Matharu and Winer, 2021). **Class B** steroids can also be found in nature, for example in **plants** such as the Mexican yam or soybeans, but require further chemical synthesis to be used in drugs. They are therefore **precursors** for the synthesis of steroids such as estradiol. At least 15 chemical reactions in the laboratory are needed to obtain the required substance. Because the starting material for the chemical process is obtained from plant sources, the process is considered "biosynthetic" (Stanczyk, Matharu and Winer, 2021). **Class C** steroids are synthesized from non-steroidal precursors using multiple chemical steps; this process is referred to as **"total synthesis." Class D** steroids are used in drugs such as medroxyprogesterone acetate and include synthetic compounds that are not found in nature. These steroids are **designed or "man-made"** (Stanczyk, Matharu and Winer, 2021).

Types of hormones in hormone replacement therapy—summing up

With the exception of conjugated equine estrogens (which are derived from the urine of pregnant horses and therefore considered truly natural), all hormones used in menopausal hormone therapy are synthesized chemically, whether they are prepared by pharmaceutical companies or custom-compounding pharmacies (Stanczyk, Matharu and Winer, 2021). In the US, bioidentical hormones are available as conventional drugs approved by the FDA, as well as in compounded preparations made by compounding pharmacies (Stuenkel, 2021).

Regarding the routes of administration, oral and transdermal products (such as patches, creams and gels) are available (Booyens *et al.*, 2022). Evidence directly comparing oral and transdermal hormone replacement therapy remains limited and of low quality (Goldštajn *et al.*, 2023). The most relevant difference between the two administration routes appears to be related to the risk for venous thromboembolism. The two routes have different pharmacodynamics: when taken orally, the active ingredients pass the gastrointestinal system first, are absorbed by the gut and then metabolized by the liver (known as the hepatic first-pass mechanism) (Booyens *et al.*, 2022). This process can lead to an increase in procoagulant factors, which consequently may raise the risk for venous thromboembolism. In the application of transdermal products, the increase of procoagulant factors is absent, thus making the transdermal administration the preferred choice in terms of risk for venous thromboembolism (Goldštajn *et al.*, 2023).

The intricacies of different medications are beyond the scope of this book. Medical providers should help to empower women to make informed choices by acknowledging that the females are experts in their own menopause experience and by providing information in a manner that women can become active and equal partners in their own care (Hickey *et al.*, 2024). Furthermore, more diversity in research is needed: the majority of research on menopausal hormone therapy to date is based on western women (Pickar and Baber, 2021).

Framing menopause as a disability and disease can fuel the stigma aging women are already facing. Peri- and postmenopausal women can be happy, healthy and strong. Peri- and postmenopause can be a time to embrace a new phase in life—free of menstruation and potential menstrual pain—and to reassess one's identity. And females deserve nothing less (The Lancet, 2024)!

Trans people and aging: The role of gender-affirming hormone treatment

Many transgender people use gender-affirming hormone treatment (GAHT) to reduce gender incongruence, meaning it allows trans people to achieve physical characteristics more aligned with their gender identity. Trans adults are faced with unique challenges as they age. Only one study so far has looked at trans women's views on menopause (Mohamed and Hunter, 2018). Sixty-seven trans women with an average age of 49 years participated in the study; the majority of them (96%) were taking GAHT. Many of the participants expressed the view that menopause was not relevant to them due to biological differences between them and women going through menopause. Most expected to use GAHT indefinitely. However, several participants expressed concerns and uncertainty regarding prolonged GAHT use.

Picking up on these questions, a 2023 paper addressed possible risks of long-term GAHT use (Cheung, Nolan and Zwickl, 2023). Data on how to manage GAHT with aging remains minimal. For people using feminizing hormone therapy (primarily involving estradiol and anti-androgens), it is unclear if the recommendations from menopausal hormone replacement therapy literature can be applied to trans individuals, who are typically treated with higher doses of estradiol (Cheung, Nolan and Zwickl, 2023). There appears to be an increased risk of venous thromboembolism, stroke and heart attack relative to cisgender individuals (Gooren, Giltay and Bunck, 2008; Wierckx *et al.*, 2013; Gooren, Wierckx and Giltay, 2008; Getahun *et al.*, 2018; Defreyne *et al.*, 2019; Nota *et al.*, 2019). For those with risk factors, the use of ethinyl (oral) estradiol is no longer recommended; transdermal estradiol may be used instead. Regarding bone health, fracture risk has been shown to be higher in older trans women compared to age-matched referenced men, but not to referenced cisgender women (Wiepjes *et al.*, 2020). For transpeople taking masculinizing hormone therapy (primarily involving testosterone), there is even less data available. It appears there is an increased risk of polycythemia (a type of blood cancer), probable higher risk for heart attack and pelvic pain (Cheung, Nolan and Zwickl, 2023).

Individually tailored gender-affirming healthcare is needed for transgender people as they age. Not only shared decision-making approaches between transgender individuals and healthcare professionals, but also more research on the long-term effects and risks of GAHT is needed to balance the risks of continuing GAHT later in life.

Putting it all together: The aging athlete—a personal account
By Alison Slater

Historically, I have been a competitive swimmer at national level, having started training at age five, continuing through to my late teens. I seem to have walked around on an "endorphin high" throughout my youth, enjoying strength, leanness, flexibility, well-above-average lung capacity, and mental and physical endurance. I felt invincible! That changed depressingly quickly following my retirement from swimming, as I gained weight beyond my wildest nightmares, and battled with self-esteem and body image issues, loss of confidence and an evaporation of my personal identity. But once I got my head in gear again, I always felt confident of being able to "channel the warrior," easily able to quickly regain muscle mass, lose weight and retrieve cardiovascular fitness on resumption of any reasonable level of training and competition. This was primarily in the form of triathlon in my early twenties. I took to cycling like (pardon the pun) a fish to water! And while my swimming background stood me in good stead, running was always, and remains, challenging.

Beyond my mid-twenties, life took over and I traveled extensively, working abroad for over 11 years. As an Aussie, the weather in the northern hemisphere wasn't exactly conducive to outdoor activities, and swimming in the winter really did not appeal at all! I moved back to Australia, married, settled down, and then it was back to physical activity and competition. A second iteration of triathlon seemed the perfect fit, allowing variety and flexibility in my training regimen. I even did a number of half marathons, preparing to fulfill the goal of competing in an Ironman 70.3—whatever it took to make 21.1 km seem like not such a long way! Everything was going just fine, and I felt that my body was coping reasonably well with the onset of perimenopause in my late forties. Interestingly, I continued to make gains and improve my times, despite experiencing sleep deprivation and round-the-clock hot flashes at the time. An autoimmune condition affecting my thyroid made maintaining a healthy body weight more challenging, but strict adherence to a ketogenic diet, and discovering intolerances to caffeine, gluten and dairy, helped in preserving a lean and healthy body. The use of prescription bioidentical hormone therapy curbed the flashing, and certainly helped with sleep quality and a general sense of wellbeing.

But then everything seemed to change when I returned to full-time study at the age of 57. Interspersed with running my sole physiotherapy practice, training, commuting interstate (no mean feat in a vast country like Australia) between home and work on a weekly basis, and maintaining a committed marriage, the prolonged sitting was a complete shock to the system. Let's face it, I'd been standing to work for 36 years up until then! I was already eight years into menopause, and all of a sudden, all the symptoms I thought "happened to other people" were actually happening to me! Weight gain, especially belly fat, aches and pains and general body stiffness, loss of strength and endurance, declining muscle mass, swings in energy availability, mood and sleep quality... the list goes on! My recovery, which I'd never really struggled with, became a major issue, taking days to get over heavier training sessions, and even more so, events! At around this time, with a change in prescription legislation here in Australia, getting a hold of my cherished bioidenticals became near impossible.

My keen interest in fascia allowed me to understand the influence that hormones (specifically estrogen and relaxin) have on fascial connective tissue, so the stiffness secondary to relative inactivity shouldn't have come as a surprise. But what about all these other undesirable consequences of a life change that all women of a certain age will face? Why didn't all the tried and trusted strategies to get myself back on track work anymore? The harder I trained, and the more I controlled food intake, the worse it got! None of this yo-yoing helped with mood, my capacity to concentrate or my self-esteem. And that's when the desperation *really* set in! This was not a body I understood anymore! My maintenance regimen, approach to diet and sleep and training as a whole package had to change... Not only did I need to experiment with "biohacking" to work out how to cope, I had to reassess all of the old strategies if I was to be able to keep training to maximize health, functionality and longevity. In other words, I had to "train smarter, not harder!" Worst of all, despite all my years of work regimen, dedicated load-bearing exercise and diligence around eating habits, more recent scanning revealed that my bone mineralization was suffering!

The graduated withdrawal of estrogen with the onset of perimenopause initiates a far-reaching cascade of consequences. With the rapid decline in progesterone production (Delamater and Santoro, 2018) comes relative estrogen dominance, proliferating gut health issues (as microbiome diversity deteriorates), cortisol dominance, a decline in hormone sensitivity and an increase in insulin resistance. These effects combine to disrupt sleep, cause massive fluctuations in energy levels (Sims and Yeager, 2022), and impact thyroid health (a significant problem for someone like me, with already established autoimmune Hashimoto's thyroiditis). This escalates susceptibility to metabolic syndrome, type 2 diabetes, atherosclerotic cardiovascular disease (Seely *et al.*, 1999) and vascular and neurological complications such as stroke (Swarup *et al.*, 2024). And in this modern world, where everyone is seemingly in sympathetic overload, no one is more prone than the peri-/menopausal woman. This "tired and wired" state (Sims and Yeager, 2022) further disrupts the HPA axis, causing cortisol levels to spike, so driving insulin sensitivity. This in combination with reduced sleep quality, when we should be metabolizing our stress hormones... Is it any wonder we struggle with weight gain, especially around the gut? And no conversation about aging is complete without consideration of intramuscular connective tissue (Stecco *et al.*, 2023), and the abundance of estrogen and relaxin receptors therein (Fede *et al.*, 2016). This has a profound influence on the muscles themselves, driving myofascial pain and stiffness and sarcopenia (Geraci *et al.*, 2021).

So, where to start? Seeking the help of experts to counter creeping estrogen imbalance (Sims and Yeager, 2022) seemed the most sensible approach. Eating behaviors, exercise selection and sleep are the crux in this journey of "recovering self." Forearmed is forewarned, but the trick is in finding out what works best for each of us as individuals. I am still negotiating my way through the maze of menopause, honing my regimen to get just the right combination to optimize health, minimize stress and maximize sleep and the benefits of exercise. Perhaps it's time to focus more on heavy resistance training (Carneiro *et al.*, 2022) and reduce the emphasis on my beloved cardio? Any exercise regimen must include a consideration of fascial health and flexibility, but graduated heavy resistance training is critical to promote anabolism (Kerksick and Leutholtz, 2005), so limiting sarcopenia and its consequences of wasting, weakness, balance and confidence issues (Wu *et al.*, 2023). Incorporating through-range movement, skipping, bouncing on a mini-tramp, regular use of gentle rolling incorporating vibration to "cajole" my myofascial mechanoreceptors into a state of relaxation, and jumping exercises to stimulate bone mineralization, have proven helpful. Optimization around sleep hygiene, including restricting food intake two to four hours before bed, regimenting the times for going to bed and getting up, sleeping in a cool to cold dark room to encourage melatonin secretion (Masters *et al.*, 2014) and minimizing screen time after sunset have helped, as have breath practice and meditation.

I'm still hitting PBs (personal bests) from time to time, but the priority is engagement, maintenance, mobility, range of motion and minimizing stiffness and discomfort. Like never before, listening to my body is crucial for being prepared for different things at different times, dependent on energy levels and movement demands. So, in the wise words of Stacy Sims, "reject negative connotations about menopause. It is something every woman experiences. It's a transition we can lean into and push through as we enter a different phase of life that is full of meaning and wisdom" (Sims and Yeager, 2022). And by the way, I achieved my goal and have now completed two Ironman 70.3 events, with two more in the pipeline! Happy training into "old age," ladies.

Alison Slater is a career clinician in manual musculoskeletal physiotherapy. Receiving her undergraduate qualification in 1986 (University of New South Wales and University of Sydney), she went on to complete a Master's in Manual Therapy (University of Western Australia) in 2008, and a Master's in Public Health (University of New South Wales) in 2024.

Since meeting Professor Robert Schleip in 2007, she has maintained an active involvement in the fascia community, attending international workshops, summer and winter schools, congresses and symposia dedicated to the subject. Alison has presented at the Australian Fascia Symposium (2020), Pink Fascia (2021), Fascia Fusion UK (2021) and the Sydney Spine Symposium (2022), as well as maintaining a busy private practice on Sydney's Northern Beaches. Alison has published in Frontiers in Neurology *and* Translational Research in Anatomy *in 2024. She remains an active triathlete and distance cyclist.*

For more information, see www.fasciaaustralia.com.au *and* www.thesourcephysio.com.au.

Appendix: Tools and Practical Tips

PRACTICES TO ADDRESS THE STRESS RESPONSE

Section 5.3 summarizes the research on practices to address the stress response. Here, various techniques are described, some of which have been found to be effective in female health research, and others that have proven their worth in practice. Selected breathwork practices, restorative yoga poses and self-myofascial release techniques are covered. In addition to background information on each technique, practice tips and variations are offered.

BREATHWORK PRACTICES

Breathwork is an umbrella term for techniques employing deliberate control of the breath in order to promote mental, emotional and physical health. Breathwork traditions have their roots in different traditions, such as yoga pranayama from India, practices established in sports and medical communities, and communities looking for consciousness-expanding/psychedelic experiences (e.g. conscious connected breathing, holotropic breathing). Research on the effects of breathwork practices on stress, psychological symptoms and the autonomic nervous system has been growing over the last couple of years. Breath practices have been found to be effective in stress and anxiety reduction (Bentley *et al.*, 2023). Breathing techniques can have an upregulating effect on the nervous system (e.g. techniques using voluntary hyperventilation, such as kapalabhati pranayama) or be downregulating (e.g. slow, diaphragmatic breathing). This section highlights breathing practices with a focus on downregulating the autonomic nervous system that are suitable for everyday use and are universally accessible—they can be practiced anytime, anywhere and in any position (Bentley *et al.*, 2023). The described techniques can be used for just a couple of breath cycles, but can also be part of a full yoga or breathwork practice.

BREATH AWARENESS

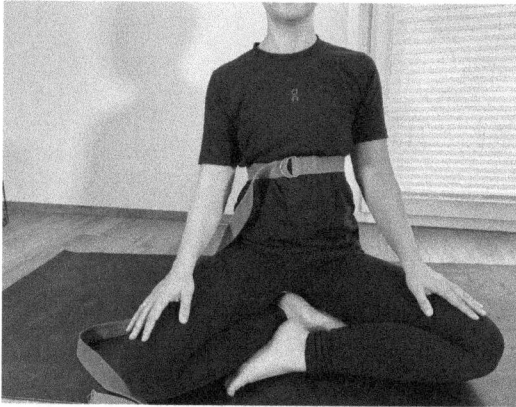

BACKGROUND AND RESEARCH FINDINGS

Simply becoming aware of the breath and observing the breath has been shown to foster a calm state and to positively impact use of attentional resources (Schöne et al., 2018; Sharma et al., 2022). Breath awareness is a great technique to use in everyday situations for just a couple of moments or minutes. It can furthermore serve as a great primer technique should one aim to go through a more extensive session including different breathwork practices.

DO THE PRACTICE

- You can do this practice in any position (seated, supine, in yoga poses such as child's pose, etc.).
- Before beginning, take a couple of rounds of your natural resting breath. If you'd like, slowly close your eyes and let them relax.
- Listen to your breath: the speed of its flow, its sound, its texture and quality.
- Feel the flow and movement of the breath: through the nose or mouth, down into the lungs; become aware of movements in the rib basket/shoulders/belly/elsewhere in the body.
- Observe your reaction to the practice.
- Effortlessness is key—do not force or alter the breath, simply receive the breath and let it flow in its natural rhythm.

VARIATIONS

- With a belt strapped around the chest (in seated or standing position), use the tactile feedback of the belt to notice the three-dimensional aspects of your rib basket as it moves when you are breathing. When using this variation in standing position, try a simple sway from side to side or from front to back to see how it changes your perception of the breath (and the breath itself).
- In child's pose, notice the contact between your belly and your thighs. Notice your gently stretched back body as well. Feel into the three-dimensional aspects of your breath.

SUGGESTIONS FOR PROPS

- Cushion, yoga bolster, chair—something to sit on comfortably if you choose to practice in a seated position.
- Yoga belt.

DIAPHRAGMATIC BREATHING

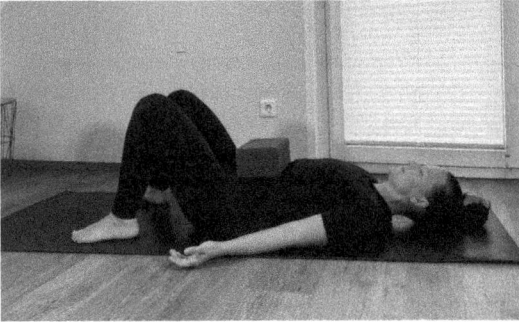

BACKGROUND AND RESEARCH FINDINGS

The goal of this type of breath is to engage the main inhalation muscle—the diaphragm—and rely less on auxiliary inspiratory muscles such as the scalenes, sternocleidomastoid and external intercostals. In practice, diaphragmatic breathing is therefore often referred to as "belly breathing," implying that the movement amplitude of the diaphragm inferiorly is facilitated, which typically presents with more pronounced movement of the abdominal wall. Diaphragmatic breathing has been shown to facilitate slow respiration, increase venous return to the heart and decrease stress (e.g. marked by reduced blood pressure and cortisol levels) (Kolář et al., 2009; Byeon et al., 2012; Dick et al., 2014; Stromberg, Russell and Carlson, 2015; Hopper et al., 2019). Men's lungs display a pyramidal, triangularly shaped lung geometry (i.e. lower lung width is greater than the width at the apices of the lungs), reflecting greater diaphragmatic movement in breathing. Women's diaphragms are shorter and female lung geometry can be described as prismatic (more similar widths at upper and lower lungs), resulting in increased muscle action of intercostals (Bellemare, Jeanneret and Couture, 2003; Mitchell et al., 2018; Torres-Tamayo et al., 2018). In short, male lung anatomy may facilitate diaphragmatic movement better, while women tend to rely more on auxiliary muscle recruitment. Even more reason for females to consciously use this technique to take advantage of its benefits!

DO THE PRACTICE

- You can do this practice in any position (seated, supine, in yoga poses, etc.).
- As a supine position fosters the excursion of the diaphragm inferiorly, facilitated by less activity of abdominal muscles, lying on your back is particularly suitable to start practicing this technique (Romei et al., 2010). If you choose to practice supine, place your feet on the floor, with the knees bent.
- Before beginning, take a couple of rounds of your natural resting breath. If you'd like, slowly close your eyes and let them relax.
- Let your abdominal area be as relaxed as possible and notice the abdominal wall rising with your inhale, and moving back toward your spine as you exhale.

VARIATIONS

- In supine position, place your hands, a yoga block or folded blanket/towel on your abdomen. Use the tactile feedback of the prop to help guide the breath into your belly area.
- Try different positions such as seated, side-lying or standing. Notice how the different mechanical loads change your ability to breathe into the belly and let the diaphragm move through its full excursion.

SUGGESTIONS FOR PROPS

- Cushion, yoga bolster, chair—something to sit on comfortably if you choose to practice in a seated position.
- Yoga block, blanket or towel.

EQUAL RATIO BREATHING (E.G. COHERENT BREATHING, BOX BREATHING)

BACKGROUND AND RESEARCH FINDINGS

Equal ratio breathing comprises similarly long inhalations and exhalations (ratio 1:1), as well as techniques that add breath holds (e.g. holding the breath after inhalation and exhalation). A well-studied version of the former is coherent breathing, establishing a rhythm of slow regular breaths at a pace of six breaths per minute (i.e. counting to five with each inhalation and exhalation). A popular form of the latter rhythm is "box breathing," with a ratio of inhale:breath, hold, exhale:breath, hold of 1:1:1:1 (e.g. counting to four on each inhalation, exhalation and breath hold between). In the yogic pranayama tradition, equal ratio breathing is known as samavritti. In military and law enforcement personnel, box breathing patterns have been studied under the term "tactical breathing."

Long, slow inhalations and exhalations of equal length have been shown to augment parasympathetic activity, thus shifting autonomic nervous system balance toward parasympathetic dominance, decreasing stress on the cardiovascular system and helping with lung function (Bernardi et al., 2001; Russo, Santarelli and O'Rourke, 2017; Zhang et al., 2017; Zaccaro et al., 2018). Box breathing has been reported to reduce physical arousal (e.g. marked by heart rate) (Bouchard et al., 2012; Röttger et al., 2021; Balban et al., 2023).

DO THE PRACTICE

- You can do this practice in any position (seated, supine, in yoga poses such as child's pose, etc.).
- Before beginning, take a couple of rounds of your natural resting breath. If you'd like, slowly close your eyes and let them relax.
- Start with equally long inhalations and exhalations, for example by counting to four or five during each inhale and exhale.
- If you'd like to add breath holds progressively, start adding in breath retentions in a step-wise manner, starting with the breath hold after inhalation; add the breath hold after exhalation later on.
- If you are comfortable with adding breath holds, try box breathing with different durations, e.g. start with a four-count breath and work your way up toward longer durations (e.g. six- or eight-count breath) over time.

SUGGESTIONS FOR PROPS

- Cushion, yoga bolster, chair—something to sit on comfortably if you choose to practice in a seated position.

RESTORATIVE YOGA

Restorative yoga is an internal practice, combining passive yoga postures, relaxation and possibly meditation. It focuses on restoration and inner stillness, thereby aiming to positively target the stress response. Restorative yoga has been shown to effectively mitigate stress—for example, among female nurses and medical students (Miyoshi, 2019; Thompson et al., 2023). It has also been reported that restorative yoga can alleviate depressive symptoms, emotional outcomes and fatigue in breast cancer survivors (Danhauer et al., 2009; Taylor et al., 2018). Regarding cardiovascular parameters, restorative yoga has been found to reduce blood pressure and heart rate, suggesting it is a potential complementary therapeutic option for hypertensive patients (Pandey and Huq, 2017).

SUPPORTED RELAXATION POSE (SAVASANA)

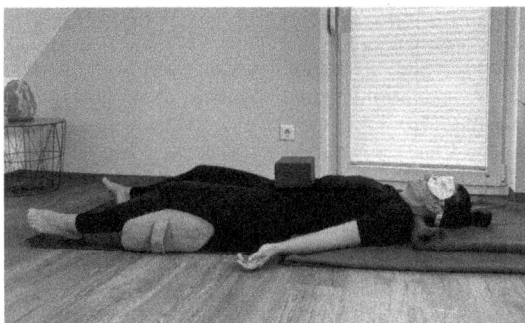

BACKGROUND AND RESEARCH FINDINGS

Research suggests that this pose blunts the sympathetic response and reduces load on the heart; savasana may therefore enhance one's ability to withstand stress (Madanmohan *et al.*, 2002). While you can practice the relaxation pose without any props, adding blankets, bolsters and eye pillows can support relaxation and a sense of groundedness.

DO THE PRACTICE

- Fold up a blanket twice: start with the blanket completely unfolded, then fold the blanket in half lengthwise; then fold it in half widthwise. If using a beach towel, fold the blanket once widthwise, creating a similar shape. Place the blanket or towel on your mat. Have the rounded edge to start at your waist; the rest of the blanket or towel can extend upward toward your head.

- Place a bolster, cushion or rolled up blanket/beach towel under your knees.

- Let your hands rest next to your body, with the palms facing toward the ceiling or sky.

- Duration: you can remain as long as you like; five to ten minutes is recommended.

VARIATIONS

- If your neck tends to overextend in supine position, fold a blanket or towel to an approximate thickness of 2.5 cm (1 in) and place it underneath your head. Adjust the thickness as needed. Alternatively—for example, if you have a deep cervical spine curve—roll up a blanket or beach towel and place it behind your neck. Adjust the thickness of the roll so that your neck feels gently supported, but without putting pressure on your cervical spine. You may want to try different thicknesses, starting with a smaller roll to find your ideal configuration.

- If available, place an eye pillow, sleep mask or folded-up hand towel over your eyes.

- Place a block, folded-up blanket or towel or a bolster (the latter length or widthwise) on your belly to support a sense of groundedness.

SUGGESTIONS FOR PROPS

- Yoga or gymnastic mat (alternatively, you can practice this one on carpet as well).

- Yoga bolster, cushion or rolled-up beach towel to be placed under your knees.

- One or two blankets or beach towels (one to be folded up and be placed under the torso; one to be rolled up slightly to be used as neck support).

- Blanket, light cushion or bolster to be placed on the belly as additional, grounding weight.

- Eye pillow, sleep mask or folded-up hand towel to cover the eyes.

SUPPORTED CHILD'S POSE

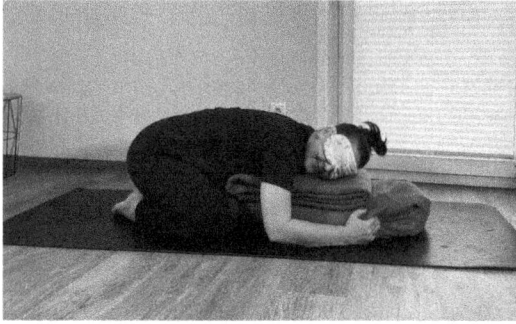

BACKGROUND AND RESEARCH FINDINGS

In this pose, the head and heart are placed on the same level, optimizing cardiovascular strain (Joshi, Raveendran and Arumugam, 2024). While you can practice child's pose without any props, adding blankets, bolsters and a sleep mask can support relaxation. It may take some time to settle into this pose and find the ideal configuration. Taking time to do so is encouraged for a maximum sense of relaxation and restoration.

DO THE PRACTICE

- Place a bolster lengthwise in the center of your mat.
- Kneel just behind the bolster, so you are facing it. Take your knees a bit wider than hip's width apart while keeping the feet/big toes together and sit back toward your heels.
- Lie down on the bolster, with your forearms resting comfortably on the mat (elbows approximately under the shoulders).
- Turn your head to whatever side feels more comfortable. You can change sides whenever you feel like it.
- Duration: you can remain as long as you like; five to ten minutes is recommended.

VARIATIONS

- Supporting/elevating your torso: place a folded-up blanket or beach towel on the bolster before lying down (size of the fold to be approximately the same as the bolster, so your head and torso can be equally supported).
- Supporting your knees: placing a folded-up blanket or towel in the hollows of your knees can help support discomfort from intense flexion in the knees. Make sure the blanket or towel is folded up in a soft enough fashion, so that the pressure on the knees and calves does not create discomfort.
- Supporting your ankles: roll up a blanket or towel (approximately 2.5–5 cm or 1–2 in, depending on your individual anatomy) and place it on the floor, underneath the front side of your ankles. This may help to keep your feet from falling asleep or reduce discomfort if your ankle range of motion does not agree with this position).
- If available, place a sleep mask over your eyes. An eye pillow or folded-up hand towel may work as well; however, they may slip around and in turn create an unsettling situation instead of supporting relaxation.

SUGGESTIONS FOR PROPS

- Yoga or gymnastic mat (alternatively, you could practice this one on carpet as well).
- Yoga bolster.
- One to three blankets or beach towels.
- Sleep mask to cover the eyes.

LEGS UP THE WALL POSE

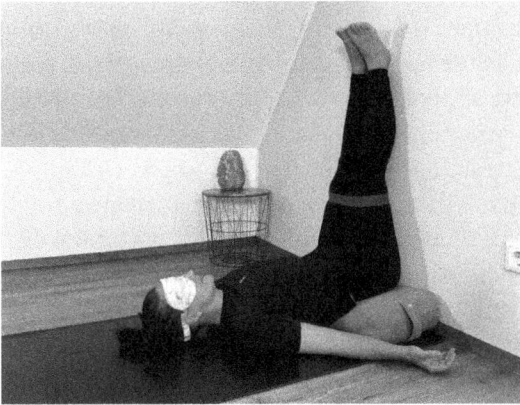

BACKGROUND AND RESEARCH FINDINGS

This pose can gently support lymphatic flow and venous return toward the heart (Joshi, Raveendran and Arumugam, 2024). It has to be noted that yoga inversions may be contraindicated—for example, they can increase intraocular pressure soon after starting and are therefore not recommended for individuals with glaucoma (Chetry *et al.*, 2023). Inverted yoga poses can furthermore result in increased blood pressure, which may be a consideration for some. However, supported legs up the wall pose is thought to put a relatively low risk of increased blood pressure compared to other inverted yoga poses, or may even decrease intraocular pressure (Joshi, Raveendran and Arumugam, 2024). It may take some time to settle into this pose and find the ideal configuration. Taking time to do so is encouraged for a maximum sense of relaxation and restoration.

DO THE PRACTICE

- Bring your mat to the wall, with the short edge touching the wall.
- Fold/stack one or two blankets to a size of about 50 cm long x 30 cm wide and 5–10 cm high (20 in x 12 in x 2–4 in) and place your stack next to you. You could also use a yoga bolster.
- Sit sideways with your hips close to the wall, knees bent.
- Swing your legs up the wall and work your buttocks toward the wall. If your range of motion in the back of the legs and low back does not allow for you to completely work your way toward the wall, bring your buttocks slightly away from the wall.
- Bend your knees and place the soles of your feet on the wall, lifting your buttocks a little to scoot your blanket/towel stack or bolster underneath your buttocks and hips.
- Lower your hips back down and re-straighten your legs as much as your individual range of motion allows. Find rest.
- Duration: you can remain as long as you like; five to ten minutes would be recommended.

VARIATIONS

- Placing a looped yoga belt around your thighs may allow you to relax more into the pose.
- If available, place an eye pillow, sleep mask or folded-up hand towel over your eyes.

SUGGESTIONS FOR PROPS

- Yoga or gymnastic mat (alternatively, you could practice this one on carpet as well).
- Wall space (alternatively, resting the legs on the back of a couch or armchair can work as well).
- One or two blankets or beach towels or a yoga bolster.
- One strap.
- Eye pillow, sleep mask or folded-up hand towel to cover the eyes.

SELF-MYOFASCIAL RELEASE (SMFR)

Self-myofascial release (sMFR) is a form of self-massage, applying self-induced mechanical stimulation of the tissue with devices such as foam rollers, myofascial release balls or yoga blocks (Russo *et al.*, 2023). Tennis balls can be a cost-effective alternative. Tools are available in different sizes, hardness and surface texture (Cheatham and Stull, 2018). Self-myofascial release is popularly applied with the intention of influencing the fascial system (Beardsley and Škarabot, 2015; Wilke *et al.*, 2020). sMFR is used by individuals in the leisure and health sector, in competitive and elite sports as part of short-term preparation for training or competition, as well as after sporting exertion to support regeneration (Wiewelhove *et al.*, 2019). Research particularly addresses the effectiveness of foam rolling in terms of mobility, athletic performance and pain perception (Skinner, Moss and Hammond, 2020; Grieve *et al.*, 2022; Martínez-Aranda *et al.*, 2024). Initial research furthermore suggests that sMFR may be helpful to alleviate stress and support individuals psychologically (see also text box "Rolling for relaxation?" in section 5.3): one study engaging 66 individuals with fibromyalgia reported lower levels of depression and anxiety as well as improved scores related to daily functioning and sleep quality after 40 sMFR sessions (Ceca *et al.*, 2020).

When using sMFR to positively target the nervous system, the focus is to create body awareness in a gentle manner. To achieve this, a before and after check can be applied (i.e. finding a specific posture or movement before and after rolling to compare bodily sensations). While research protocols often use a perceived intensity of around five to seven on a ten-step visual analogue scale (ten representing maximum discomfort) (Aboodarda, Spence and Button, 2015), working with lower intensities (e.g. three to five on a ten-scale) appears to be suitable when aiming to foster relaxation. Short durations of 30–90 seconds in one position or area are sufficient—there is no need to stay longer (Dębski, Białas and Gnat, 2019; Hughes and Ramer, 2019; Hendricks *et al.*, 2020). While there is no absolute "right" or "wrong" when it comes to positioning oneself on sMFR tools, pain sensations, tingling or numbness should be avoided (moving slightly on the tool may help; if that is not the case, stop the exercise). Whole-body tension or holding the breath can be further signs that the intensity is too high. Some body regions such as the front of the throat, inguinal area, the carpal tunnel area and direct work on bones (especially in people with osteopenia or osteoporosis) should be avoided. Furthermore, rolling cannot be recommended with open wounds, newly formed scars or fractures. Caution is indicated in individuals with myositis ossificans, osteomyelitis, local tissue inflammation, or a history of deep vein thrombosis (Bartsch *et al.*, 2021).

WORKING DOWN YOUR BACK

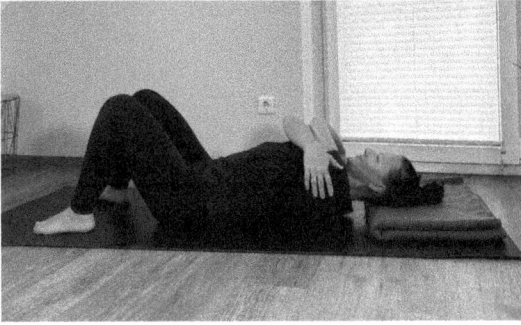

DO THE PRACTICE

- Ideas for check-in posture or movements: back thigh stretch in supine position (padangusthasana), child's pose (balasana), cat-cow movement.

- Take two myofascial release balls or tennis balls, ideally tied together in a small bag or tennis sock, so the spinous processes of the spine will not directly receive pressure from the balls.

- You can work your way down your back, from upper back (approximately at the top of the shoulder blades), mid back (approximately lower third of the shoulder blades), to the low back (where the lordotic curve is most prominent).

- Start in supine position, with the feet on the floor. Place the balls widthwise on your mat, and lie down on top of them (starting position in upper back as described above). Using a folded blanket or towel under the head to avoid hyperextension of the cervical spine is recommended.

- Take deep, relaxed breaths and let your weight sink into the balls.

- If you are comfortable and relaxed, you can initiate movement, possibly coordinating it with your breath. For example, bring your arms over head toward the floor as you inhale, and bring them back next to your pelvis as you exhale. Repeat for a few cycles, then remain resting on the balls, deepening the breath for a couple of rounds.

- Either roll up slightly on the balls or sit up briefly to move the balls further down toward the mid back position (described above). Proceed similarly as before; for incorporating movement, you may want to try alternating between arms opened wide to the side on your inhale, and crossing the arms in front of your chest (as if giving yourself a hug) on your exhale.

- Lastly, bring your balls to your low back. Make sure your low back is comfortable in this position. You may want to place the towel or blanket underneath your hips/sacrum to reduce lumbar curve and thereby decrease intensity. If this does not feel good in your low back, skip this last position. For movement, you may gently rock the knees side to side in this position.

- Pressing the feet into the mat and lifting the hips, take the balls out from underneath you. Lower your body back down and remain in a neutral supine resting position for a couple of resting breaths (or longer).

VARIATIONS

- Work standing against a wall, use softer balls, or add a blanket or towel on top of the balls to reduce intensity.

SUGGESTIONS FOR PROPS

- Yoga or gymnastic mat (alternatively, you could practice this one on carpet as well).
- Two myofascial release balls or tennis balls, ideally tied together in a small bag or tennis sock.
- Folded blanket or towel as head/low back support

FOREHEAD RELEASE

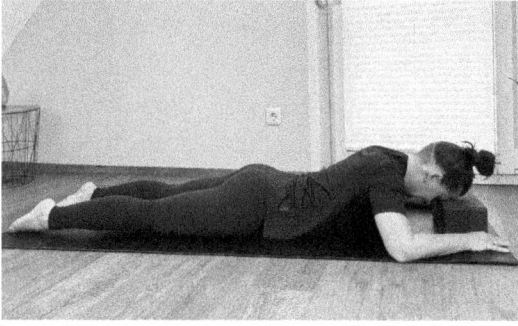

DO THE PRACTICE

- Place a yoga block on its lowest height on your mat.
- Lie prone on your mat, with the block under your forehead.
- Let your hands and forearm find a comfortable position, gently supporting your head and torso.
- Let your forehead rest into the block, making sure you find a comfortable position on the block. Take deep breaths and relax the face and neck.
- Start slowly rolling side to side, massaging the forehead and area between your eyebrows.

VARIATIONS

- Add a blanket or towel on top of the block to adjust (i.e. reduce) intensity.

SUGGESTIONS FOR PROPS

- Yoga or gymnastic mat (alternatively, you could practice this one on carpet as well).
- One yoga block, ideally a soft foam block. If working with a wooden block, add a blanket or towel on top of the block to decrease intensity.

Glossary

Aerobic performance	The ability to sustain prolonged exercise (e.g. endurance running) using oxygen-dependent energy systems. It relies on respiratory and cardiovascular efficiency.
Allopregnanolone	A neurosteroid derived from progesterone that influences brain function by modulating the activity of the neurotransmitter gamma-aminobutyric acid (GABA). It is thought to be involved in conditions like premenstrual dysphoric disorder (PMDD).
Amenorrhea	The absence of menstruation. Primary amenorrhea is present when a woman never begins menstruating; secondary amenorrhea describes the cessation of a previously regular menstrual cycle.
Anaerobic performance	The ability to perform short bursts of high-intensity exercise (e.g. sprinting, jumping) without relying on oxygen for energy production. Anaerobic performance primarily uses glycogen (carbohydrates) energy.
Androgens	A group of hormones, including testosterone, that are typically associated with male traits but also are important in female health. Androgens are involved in muscle growth, libido and fat distribution. Excess levels can be observed in conditions like polycystic ovary syndrome (PCOS).
Anovulation	The absence of ovulation during a menstrual cycle, where the ovary fails to release an egg. It can result in irregular or absent periods and is associated with hormonal imbalances, stress or excessive exercise.
Anterior cruciate ligament (ACL)	A ligament in the knee joint that stabilizes the knee during movement. Female athletes are at a higher risk of ACL injuries, partly due to biomechanical differences and hormonal fluctuations.
Anti-Müllerian hormone (AMH)	A hormone produced by ovarian follicles, reflective of a woman's ovarian follicle reserve. During reproductive years, AMH puts a brake on follicle stimulating hormone secretion, thereby limiting the number of maturing follicles each month.
Aromatase	An enzyme involved in a key step of estrogen production: the conversion of androgens into estrogens. Also known as estrogen synthase.
Bioidentical hormones	Hormones that are chemically identical to those produced by the human body.
Bone mineral density (BMD)	A measurement of the amount of minerals contained in bone. Estrogen helps maintain BMD, and its decline (e.g. related to menopause) can lead to an increased risk of osteoporosis and fractures.
Breathwork	An umbrella term for techniques employing deliberate control of the breath in order to promote mental, emotional and physical health. Breathwork techniques originate from different roots, ranging from Eastern traditions (e.g. pranayama, tai chi, qi gong), Eastern European practices (e.g. Buteyko method), medical communities (e.g. resonant frequency or coherent breathing), and communities looking for consciousness-expanding/psychedelic experiences (e.g. conscious connected breathing, holotropic breathing).

Cervix	The lower, narrow end of the uterus, connecting the uterus to the vagina.
Collagen	A structural protein that provides strength and elasticity to connective tissues.
Corpus albicans	Scar tissue within the ovary that is a remnant of ovulation. The corpus luteum degenerates into a scar if no fertilization takes place.
Corpus luteum	A temporary endocrine gland, which produces progesterone. It is created monthly by the remnants of the granulosa cells surrounding the dominant follicle after ovulation.
Cortisol	A steroid hormone produced by the adrenal glands. It plays an important role in regulating metabolism, immune function and recovery from exercise.
Decidua	A specialized layer of the uterine lining (endometrium), forming during pregnancy as the base of the placenta. It is expelled from the body after giving birth by bleeding and discharge, lasting approximately six weeks after childbirth (lochia).
Dysmenorrhea	Painful menstruation, often characterized by severe cramping in the lower abdomen.
Endogenous hormones	Hormones produced within the body.
Endometriosis	A chronic condition where tissue similar to the lining inside the uterus grows outside the uterus. Endometriosis can lead to hormonal imbalances, inflammation, menstrual irregularities, pain and infertility.
Endometrium	The inner lining or layer of the uterus.
ER knockout mice	Genetically engineered mice, which lack estrogen receptors (ER). These animal models are used in research to study the effects of estrogen deficiency.
Estradiol (oestradiol)	The most potent form of estrogen, which is predominant during a woman's reproductive years.
Estriol (oestriol)	A weaker form of estrogen (compared to estradiol) produced in significant amounts during pregnancy.
Estrogen	A female sex hormone responsible for the development and regulation of the female reproductive system. Estrogen levels fluctuate throughout the menstrual cycle as well as through a woman's lifespan. Different types of estrogen are estradiol, estriol and estrone.
Estrone (oestrone)	A type of estrogen, primarily produced in fat tissue after menopause. Estrone is a weaker form of estrogen compared to estradiol.
Ethinyl estrogen	An exogenous form of estrogen. The most widely used component of oral contraceptives.
Eumenorrhea	A normal, regular menstrual cycle, typically lasting 21–35 days. Eumenorrhea indicates balanced reproductive hormones, without significant irregularities or disruptions in the menstrual cycle.
Exercise	Physical activity with a specific external objective, such as performance or fitness goals.
Exogenous hormones	Hormones from an external source (i.e. not produced internally by the body). Oral contraceptives, menopausal hormone therapy and gender-affirming hormone treatment are examples.
Fallopian tube	Part of the female reproductive organs. Conduit between the ovaries and the uterus.
Fat oxidation	The process of breaking down fat stores for energy. Fat oxidization is influenced by estrogen, which enhances fat utilization.
Follicle	A small fluid-filled sac inside a woman's ovaries containing one immature egg (oocyte).
Follicle-stimulating hormone (FSH)	A hormone produced by the pituitary gland, promoting the growth and maturation of ovarian follicles in women. FSH levels rise during the follicular phase of the menstrual cycle, leading up to ovulation.

Follicular phase	The first phase of the menstrual cycle, beginning on the first day of menses. During this phase, follicle-stimulating hormone (FSH) promotes the development of ovarian follicles, and estrogen levels rise to prepare the body for ovulation.
Folliculogenesis	The maturation of ovarian follicles.
Fundus	The top (superior) part of the uterus. Its position (fundal height) is used to measure the progression of pregnancy.
Gamma-aminobutyric acid (GABA)	An inhibitory neurotransmitter.
Gender-affirming hormone treatment (GAHT)	The primary medical intervention for transgender people to facilitate secondary sex characteristics more aligned with an individual's gender identity. Feminizing GAHT is available for individuals identifying as female (transgender women), who were assigned male at birth; it typically comprises estradiol and anti-androgens. Masculinizing hormone treatment for transgender men, who were assigned female at birth, primarily involves testosterone.
Gonadotropin-releasing hormone (GnRH)	A hormone secreted by the hypothalamus that stimulates the pituitary gland to release luteinizing hormone (LH) and follicle-stimulating hormone (FSH).
Gonadotropins	Peptide hormones regulating ovarian and testicular function. Examples are luteinizing hormone and follicle stimulating hormone.
Human chorionic gonadotropin (hCG)	A hormone produced by the placenta during pregnancy. hCG levels are used to test for pregnancy.
Hyponatremia	A condition when the blood concentration of sodium is abnormally low.
Hypothalamic amenorrhea	A condition caused by the suppression of the hypothalamic-pituitary-ovarian (HPO) axis, which can be caused by stress, undernutrition or excessive exercise. Hypothalamic amenorrhea leads to the cessation of menses and can result in long-term reproductive and bone health issues.
Hypothalamic-pituitary-adrenal (HPA) axis	A hormonal axis and communication system between the hypothalamus, pituitary gland and adrenal glands, which regulates stress reaction, mood and immune function.
Hypothalamic-pituitary-ovarian (HPO) axis	A tightly regulated hormonal system involving the hypothalamus, pituitary gland and ovaries that controls the menstrual cycle and female reproductive function.
Insulin sensitivity	The body's ability to effectively use insulin to regulate blood glucose levels.
Lactation	The production and secretion of milk by the mammary glands.
Luteal phase	The second phase of the menstrual cycle, beginning after ovulation and lasting until onset of menstruation. The luteal phase is marked by a rise in progesterone, preparing the uterus for potential implantation of a fertilized egg.
Luteinizing hormone (LH)	A hormone produced by the pituitary gland that triggers ovulation.
Menarche	The first occurrence of menstruation.
Menopause	The permanent cessation of menstruation, marking the end of a woman's reproductive years. Menopause can only be determined retrospectively, after 12 consecutive months without a menstrual period. Hormonal changes related to menopause—primarily a decrease in estrogen and progesterone—can affect metabolism, bone density and cardiovascular health.
Menorrhagia	Excessively heavy or prolonged menstrual bleeding.

Meta-analysis	A statistical technique used to synthesize quantitative data from multiple independent studies on a given topic. By pooling data, it allows researchers to increase the sample size and improve the precision of estimates. Meta-analyses are used to shape treatment guidelines and health-related policies.
Mini pill	A type of progestin-only oral contraceptive. It is often prescribed for women for whom estrogen is contraindicated or who are breastfeeding/pumping.
Monophasic oral contraceptives (OCs)	A type of oral contraceptive that delivers the same fixed dose of estrogen and progestin throughout the entire active pill phase (typically 21 days), followed by a seven-day withdrawal phase. Monophasic oral contraceptives are the most used form of birth control.
Multiphasic oral contraceptives (OCs)	A type of oral contraceptive that delivers varying levels of hormones (estrogen and/or progestin) throughout the active pill cycle. Multiphasic OCs are designed to more closely mimic the natural fluctuations of the menstrual cycle compared to monophasic OCs.
Myometrium	The muscular tissue layer of the uterus.
Network meta-analysis	A statistical method comparing multiple treatments simultaneously by using a common comparator (e.g. if studies compare intervention A to intervention B, and intervention B to intervention C, a network meta-analysis can indirectly compare intervention A to intervention C, using a shared comparator (intervention B)).
Oocyte	An immature female egg cell.
Oral contraception	A form of birth control that involves taking pills containing synthetic hormones (estrogen and/or progestin). Oral contraceptives prevent pregnancy by suppressing ovulation, altering the uterine lining, and thickening cervical mucus.
Oral contraceptive (OC) consumption phase	The phase during the oral contraceptive (OC) cycle when active hormone pills (containing synthetic estrogen and/or progestin) are taken.
Oral contraceptive (OC) withdrawal phase	The phase of the oral contraceptive cycle when inactive pills are taken, leading to a withdrawal bleed. Also termed OC placebo phase.
Ovarian cycle	The development (i.e. growth and maturation) of an oocyte, including folliculogenesis, ovulation and formation of the corpus luteum and corpus albicans.
Ovariectomized rats	Female rats that have had their ovaries surgically removed, leading to a significant reduction in estrogen production. These animal models are used in research to mimic the effects of estrogen deficiency, similar to menopause in humans.
Ovulation	The release of a mature follicle from the ovary, triggered by a surge in luteinizing hormone (LH).
Perimenopause	The transition period from the time of onset of cycle irregularities to menopause.
Physical activity	Any bodily movement resulting in substantial increase in energy expenditure.
Phytoestrogens	Estrogen-like compounds derived from plants.
Polycystic ovary syndrome (PCOS)	A common condition in women of reproductive age, characterized by multiple small cysts on the ovaries, irregular menstrual cycles, and excess androgen levels.
Postpartum	The period following childbirth, during which the mother's body gradually returns to its pre-pregnancy state. Some consider the period from childbirth until six weeks postpartum; more recent views extend this period to 12 months after birth (Bø et al., 2016a).
Premenstrual dysphoric disorder (PMDD)	A severe form of premenstrual disorder, characterized by affective symptoms and functional impairment in the late luteal phase.

Premenstrual syndrome (PMS)	A group of physical and psychological symptoms that occur in the late luteal phase of the menstrual cycle. Common symptoms include mood swings, headaches and fatigue.
Primary follicle	A more developed stage of folliculogenesis. Also known as dominant follicle.
Primordial follicle	A structure enveloping an oocyte. The basic functional unit of female reproduction and starting point of folliculogenesis.
Progesterone	A hormone produced in the ovaries, particularly during the luteal phase of the menstrual cycle and pregnancy. Progesterone prepares the uterus for a fertilized egg and helps maintain early pregnancy.
Progestin	A synthetic form of progesterone used in hormonal contraception and hormone replacement therapy.
Randomized controlled trial (RCT)	A form of scientific experiment, that randomly assigns participants into an experimental or intervention group or a control group, thereby ensuring that the results of the trial are not biased by the way participants were selected for each group.
Relative Energy Deficiency in Sport (RED-S)	A syndrome affecting athletes who do not meet their energy needs relative to their energy expenditure, leading to a variety of health and performance issues. Previously known as the Female Athlete Triad.
Relaxin	A hormone that increases during pregnancy, promoting relaxation of ligaments and the softening of the cervix.
Restorative yoga	A practice combining passive yoga postures, relaxation and possibly meditation. It focuses on restoration and inner stillness, thereby aiming to positively target the stress response.
Satellite cells	Adult muscle stem cells playing a critical role in muscle repair and regeneration following exercise or injury.
Self-myofascial release (sMFR)	A form of self-massage, applying self-induced mechanical stimulation of the tissue with devices such as foam rollers, myofascial release balls, tennis balls or yoga blocks.
Serotonin	A neurotransmitter that helps regulate mood, emotions, sleep and appetite.
Substrate metabolism	The process by which the body uses different energy sources (substrates), such as carbohydrates, proteins and fats.
Systematic review	A structured and comprehensive synthesis of all relevant studies on a clearly defined topic. It follows a predefined protocol, aiming to minimize bias and provide a reliable overview of the available research.
Testosterone	A sex hormone more abundant in males, but also present in smaller amounts in females. It supports muscle growth, fat metabolism and bone density.
Thermoregulation	The body's process of maintaining physiologic core body temperature. Female athletes may experience fluctuations in thermoregulation due to hormonal changes, especially during the menstrual cycle and menopause.
$VO_{2\,max}$	The maximum amount of oxygen an individual can use during intense exercise. Used as a key marker of aerobic endurance and cardiovascular fitness.
Xenoestrogens	Compounds mimicking estrogen, that are not produced by the body.

References

Aboodarda, S.J., Spence, A.J. and Button, D.C. (2015) Pain pressure threshold of a muscle tender spot increases following local and non-local rolling massage. *BMC Musculoskeletal Disorders*, 16, p. 265. Available at: https://doi.org/10.1186/s12891-015-0729-5.

Ackerman, K.E. *et al.* (2011) Bone microarchitecture is impaired in adolescent amenorrheic athletes compared with eumenorrheic athletes and nonathletic controls. *Journal of Clinical Endocrinology Metabolism*, 96(10), pp. 3123-3133. Available at: https://doi.org/10.1210/jc.2011-1614.

Ackerman, K.E. *et al.* (2019) Low energy availability surrogates correlate with health and performance consequences of relative energy deficiency in sport. *British Journal of Sports Medicine*, 53(10), pp. 628-633. Available at: https://doi.org/10.1136/bjsports-2017-098958.

ACOG Committee Opinion No. 760: Dysmenorrhea and Endometriosis in the Adolescent (2018) *Obstetrics and Gynecology*, 132(6), pp. E249-E258. Available at: https://doi.org/10.1097/AOG.0000000000002978.

Adstrum, S. *et al.* (2017) Defining the fascial system. *Journal of Bodywork and Movement Therapies*, 21(1), pp. 173-177. Available at: https://doi.org/10.1016/j.jbmt.2016.11.003.

Agyapong, B. *et al.* (2023) Interventions to reduce stress and burnout among teachers: A scoping review. *International Journal of Environmental Research and Public Health*, 20(9), p. 5625. Available at: https://doi.org/10.3390/IJERPH20095625.

Ahmed, A. *et al.* (2018) Impact of intermittent fasting on human health: An extended review of metabolic cascades. *International Journal of Food Properties*, 21(1), pp. 2700-2713. Available at: https://doi.org/10.1080/10942912.2018.1560312.

Aksel, S. *et al.* (1976) Vasomotor symptoms, serum estrogens, and gonadotropin levels in surgical menopause. *American Journal of Obstetrics and Gynecology*, 126(2), pp. 165-169. Available at: https://doi.org/10.1016/0002-9378(76)90270-2.

Aksungar, F.B. *et al.* (2005) Effects of intermittent fasting on serum lipid levels, coagulation status and plasma homocysteine levels. *Annals of Nutrition & Metabolism*, 49(2), pp. 77-82. Available at: https://doi.org/10.1159/000084739.

Alberton, C.L. *et al.* (2019) Water-based exercises in pregnancy: Apparent weight in immersion and ground reaction force at third trimester. *Clinical Biomechanics*, 67, pp. 148-152. Available at: https://doi.org/10.1016/j.clinbiomech.2019.05.021.

Allen, A.M. *et al.* (2016) Determining menstrual phase in human biobehavioral research: A review with recommendations. *Experimental and Clinical Psychopharmacology*, 24(1), pp. 1-11. Available at: https://doi.org/10.1037/pha0000057.

Allshouse, A., Pavlovic, J. and Santoro, N. (2018) Menstrual cycle hormone changes associated with reproductive aging and how they may relate to symptoms. *Obstetrics and Gynecology Clinics of North America*, 45(4), p. 613. Available at: https://doi.org/10.1016/J.OGC.2018.07.004.

Alzueta, E. *et al.* (2022) Tracking sleep, temperature, heart rate, and daily symptoms across the menstrual cycle with the oura ring in healthy women. *International Journal of Women's Health*, 14, pp. 491-503. Available at: https://doi.org/10.2147/IJWH.S341917.

American Psychiatric Association (2013) *Diagnostic and Statistical Manual of Mental Disorders*. Fifth edition. Washington (DC).

Anagnostis, P. *et al.* (2015) Effects of menopause, gender and age on lipids and high-density lipoprotein cholesterol subfractions. *Maturitas*, 81(1), pp. 62-68. Available at: https://doi.org/10.1016/J.MATURITAS.2015.02.262.

Anderson, D.J. *et al.* (2020) Obesity, smoking, and risk of vasomotor menopausal symptoms: A pooled analysis of eight cohort studies. *American Journal of Obstetrics and Gynecology*, 222(5), pp. 478.e1-478.e17. Available at: https://doi.org/10.1016/J.AJOG.2019.10.103.

Andreano, J.M. and Cahill, L. (2010) Menstrual cycle modulation of medial temporal activity evoked by negative emotion. *NeuroImage*, 53(4), pp. 1286–1293. Available at: https://doi.org/10.1016/J.NEUROIMAGE.2010.07.011.

Andréen, L. *et al.* (2009) Sex steroid induced negative mood may be explained by the paradoxical effect mediated by GABAA modulators. *Psychoneuroendocrinology*, 34(8), pp. 1121–1132. Available at: https://doi.org/10.1016/J.PSYNEUEN.2009.02.003.

Ansari, M.S. and Almalki, M.H. (2016) Primary hypothyroidism with markedly high prolactin. *Frontiers in Endocrinology*, 7(APR), p. 166938. Available at: https://doi.org/10.3389/FENDO.2016.00035/BIBTEX.

Ansdell, P. *et al.* (2019) Menstrual cycle-associated modulations in neuromuscular function and fatigability of the knee extensors in eumenorrheic women. *Journal of Applied Physiology (Bethesda, Md.: 1985)*, 126(6), pp. 1701–1712. Available at: https://doi.org/10.1152/JAPPLPHYSIOL.01041.2018.

Arbour, M.W. *et al.* (2021) Clinical implications for women of a low-carbohydrate or ketogenic diet with intermittent fasting. *Nursing for Women's Health*, 25(2), pp. 139–151. Available at: https://doi.org/10.1016/J.NWH.2021.01.009.

Ardern, C.L. *et al.* (2016) Consensus statement on return to sport from the First World Congress in Sports Physical Therapy, Bern. *British Journal of Sports Medicine*, 50(14), pp. 853–864. doi: 10.1136/bjsports-2016-096278. Epub 2016 May 25. PMID: 27226389.

Armanini, D. *et al.* (2022) Controversies in the pathogenesis, diagnosis and treatment of PCOS: Focus on insulin resistance, inflammation, and hyperandrogenism. *International Journal of Molecular Sciences*, 23(8). Available at: https://doi.org/10.3390/IJMS23084110.

Armour, M. *et al.* (2019) Exercise for dysmenorrhoea. *The Cochrane Database of Systematic Reviews*, 9(9). Available at: https://doi.org/10.1002/14651858.CD004142.PUB4.

Armour, M. *et al.* (2020) Australian female athlete perceptions of the challenges associated with training and competing when menstrual symptoms are present. *International Journal of Sports Science and Coaching*, 15(3), pp. 316–323. Available at: https://doi.org/10.1177/1747954120916073.

Atema, V. *et al.* (2019) Efficacy of internet-based cognitive behavioral therapy for treatment-induced menopausal symptoms in breast cancer survivors: Results of a randomized controlled trial. *Journal of Clinical Oncology: Official Journal of the American Society of Clinical Oncology*, 37(10), pp. 809–822. Available at: https://doi.org/10.1200/JCO.18.00655.

Audet, M. *et al.* (2017) Women, weight, poverty and menopause: Understanding health practices in a context of chronic disease prevention. *Sociology of Health & Illness*, 39(8), pp. 1412–1426. Available at: https://doi.org/10.1111/1467-9566.12593.

Avery, N.D. *et al.* (1999) Fetal responses to maternal strength conditioning exercises in late gestation. *Canadian Journal of Applied Physiology = Revue Canadienne de Physiologie Appliquee*, 24(4), pp. 362–376. Available at: https://doi.org/10.1139/H99-028.

Avis, N.E. *et al.* (2015) Duration of menopausal vasomotor symptoms over the menopause transition. *JAMA Internal Medicine*, 175(4), pp. 531–539. Available at: https://doi.org/10.1001/JAMAINTERNMED.2014.8063.

Awad, E. *et al.* (2017) Efficacy of exercise on pelvic pain and posture associated with endometriosis: Within subject design. *Journal of Physical Therapy Science*, 29(12), p. 2112. Available at: https://doi.org/10.1589/JPTS.29.2112.

Ayers, B. *et al.* (2012) Effectiveness of group and self-help cognitive behavior therapy in reducing problematic menopausal hot flushes and night sweats (MENOS 2): A randomized controlled trial. *Menopause (New York, N.Y.)*, 19(7), pp. 749–759. Available at: https://doi.org/10.1097/GME.0B013E31823FE835.

Ayrim, A., Aktepe Keskin, E. and Özol, D. (2014) Pittsburgh Sleep Quality Index scores and their relationship with body measurements in late menopause patients. *Turkish Journal of Medical Sciences*, 44(5), pp. 799–803. Available at: https://doi.org/10.3906/SAG-1304-6.

Azizi, M. *et al.* (2022) The efficacy and safety of selective serotonin reuptake inhibitors and serotonin-norepinephrine reuptake inhibitors in the treatment of menopausal hot flashes: A systematic review of clinical trials. *Iranian Journal of Medical Sciences*, 47(3), pp. 173–193. Available at: https://doi.org/10.30476/IJMS.2020.87687.1817.

Azziz, R. *et al.* (2009) The Androgen Excess and PCOS Society criteria for the polycystic ovary syndrome: The complete task force report. *Fertility and Sterility*, 91(2), pp. 456–488. Available at: https://doi.org/10.1016/J.FERTNSTERT.2008.06.035.

Babbar, S. *et al.* (2016) Acute feTal behavioral Response to prenatal Yoga: A single, blinded, randomized controlled trial (TRY yoga). *American Journal of Obstetrics and Gynecology*, 214(3), pp. 399.e1–399.e8. Available at: https://doi.org/10.1016/J.AJOG.2015.12.032.

Bäckström, T. *et al.* (2011) Paradoxical effects of GABA-A modulators may explain sex steroid induced negative mood symptoms in some persons. *Neuroscience*, 191, pp. 46–54. Available at: https://doi.org/10.1016/J.NEUROSCIENCE.2011.03.061.

Badawy, Y. *et al.* (2024) The risk of depression in the menopausal stages: A systematic review and meta-analysis. *Journal of Affective Disorders*, 357, pp. 126–133. Available at: https://doi.org/10.1016/J.JAD.2024.04.041.

Bahar, A. *et al.* (2011) Hyperprolactinemia in association with subclinical hypothyroidism. *Caspian Journal of Internal Medicine*, 2(2), p. 229. Available at: https://pmc.ncbi.nlm.nih.gov/articles/PMC3766941.

Bahr, M.A. and Bahr, R. (2014) Jump frequency may contribute to risk of jumper's knee: A study of inter-individual and sex differences in a total of 11,943 jumps video recorded during training and matches in young elite volleyball players. *British Journal of Sports Medicine*, 48(17), pp. 1322–1326. Available at: https://doi.org/10.1136/BJSPORTS-2014-093593.

Baird, S. *et al.* (2022) Improving menstrual health literacy through life-skills programming in rural Ethiopia. *Frontiers in Global Women's Health*, 3, p. 838961. Available at: https://doi.org/10.3389/fgwh.2022.838961.

Baker, F.C., Lampio, L. *et al.* (2018) Sleep and sleep disorders in the menopausal transition. *Sleep Medicine Clinics*, 13(3), pp. 443–456. Available at: https://doi.org/10.1016/J.JSMC.2018.04.011.

Baker, F.C., De Zambotti, M. *et al.* (2018) Sleep problems during the menopausal transition: Prevalence, impact, and management challenges. *Nature and Science of Sleep*, 10, pp. 73–95. Available at: https://doi.org/10.2147/NSS.S125807.

Baker, F.C. *et al.* (2021) Effects of forehead cooling and supportive care on menopause-related sleep difficulties, hot flashes and menopausal symptoms: A pilot study. *Behavioral Sleep Medicine*, 19(5), pp. 615–628. Available at: https://doi.org/10.1080/15402002.2020.1826484.

Balachandar, V., Marciniak, J.L., Wall, O. and Balachandar, C. (2017) Effects of the menstrual cycle on lower-limb biomechanics, neuromuscular control, and anterior cruciate ligament injury risk: A systematic review. *Muscles, Ligaments and Tendons Journal*, 7(1), pp. 136–146. doi: 10.11138/mltj/2017.7.1.136.

Balban, M.Y. *et al.* (2023) Brief structured respiration practices enhance mood and reduce physiological arousal. *Cell Reports. Medicine*, 4(1). Available at: https://doi.org/10.1016/J.XCRM.2022.100895.

Bangasser, D.A. and Valentino, R.J. (2014) Sex differences in stress-related psychiatric disorders: Neurobiological perspectives. *Frontiers in Neuroendocrinology*, 35(3), pp. 303–319. Available at: https://doi.org/10.1016/j.yfrne.2014.03.008.

Barakat, R. *et al.* (2016) Exercise during pregnancy protects against hypertension and macrosomia: Randomized clinical trial. *American Journal of Obstetric Gynecology*, 214(5), pp. 649.e1–649.e8. Available at: https://doi.org/10.1016/j.ajog.2015.11.039.

Barnard, L. *et al.* (2007) Quality of life and psychological well being in polycystic ovary syndrome. *Human Reproduction*, 22(8), pp. 2279–2286. Available at: https://doi.org/10.1093/HUMREP/DEM108.

Bartkowiak-Wieczorek, J. *et al.* (2024) The dual faces of oestrogen: The impact of exogenous oestrogen on the physiological and pathophysiological functions of tissues and organs. *International Journal of Molecular Sciences*, 25(15). Available at: https://doi.org/10.3390/IJMS25158167.

Bartsch, K.M. *et al.* (2021) Expert consensus on the contraindications and cautions of foam rolling: An international Delphi study. *Journal of Clinical Medicine*, 10(22). Available at: https://doi.org/10.3390/JCM10225360.

Bayliss, D.A. and Millhorn, D.E. (1992) Central neural mechanisms of progesterone action: Application to the respiratory system. *Journal of Applied Physiology (Bethesda, Md.: 1985)*, 73(2), pp. 393–404. Available at: https://doi.org/10.1152/JAPPL.1992.73.2.393.

BC Collins, R.A.A.L.C.B.N.X.C.C. (2019) Estrogen regulates the satellite cell compartment in females. *Cell Reports*, 28, pp. 368–381.e6.

Beardsley, C. and Škarabot, J. (2015) Effects of self-myofascial release: A systematic review. *Journal of Bodywork and Movement Therapies*, 19(4), pp. 747–758. Available at: https://doi.org/10.1016/j.jbmt.2015.08.007.

Bedenk, J., Vrtačnik-Bokal, E. and Virant-Klun, I. (2020) The role of anti-Müllerian hormone (AMH) in ovarian disease and infertility. *Journal of Assisted Reproduction and Genetics*, 37(1), p. 89. Available at: https://doi.org/10.1007/S10815-019-01622-7.

Beezhold, B. *et al.* (2018) Vegans report less bothersome vasomotor and physical menopausal symptoms than omnivores. *Maturitas*, 112, pp. 12–17. Available at: https://doi.org/10.1016/J.MATURITAS.2018.03.009.

Beilock, S.L., Feltz, D.L. and Pivarnik, J.M. (2001) Training patterns of athletes during pregnancy and postpartum. *Research Quarterly for Exercise and Sport*, 72(1), pp. 39–46. Available at: https://doi.org/10.1080/02701367.2001.10608930.

Belenkaia, L.V. *et al.* (2019) Criteria, phenotypes and prevalence of polycystic ovary syndrome. *Minerva Ginecologica*, 71, pp. 211–223.

Bellemare, F., Jeanneret, A. and Couture, J. (2003) Sex differences in thoracic dimensions and configuration. *American Journal of Respiratory and Critical Care Medicine*, 168(3), pp. 305–312. Available at: https://doi.org/10.1164/RCCM.200208-876OC.

Bellofiore, N. *et al.* (2018) A missing piece: The spiny mouse and the puzzle of menstruating species. *Journal of Molecular Endocrinology*, 61(1), pp. R25–R41. Available at: https://doi.org/10.1530/JME-17-0278.

Beníčková, M., Gimunová, M. and Paludo, A.C. (2024) Effect of circadian rhythm and menstrual cycle on physical performance in women: A systematic review. *Frontiers in Physiology*, 15. Available at: https://doi.org/10.3389/FPHYS.2024.1347036.

Bennie, J.A. *et al.* (2019) The epidemiology of aerobic physical activity and muscle-strengthening activity guideline adherence among 383,928 U.S. adults. *International Journal of Behavioral Nutrition and Physical Activity*, 16(1). Available at: https://doi.org/10.1186/S12966-019-0797-2.

Bentley, T.G.K. *et al.* (2023) Breathing practices for stress and anxiety reduction: Conceptual framework of implementation guidelines based on a systematic review of the published literature. *Brain Sciences*, 13(12). Available at: https://doi.org/10.3390/BRAINSCI13121612/S1.

Beral, V. *et al.* (2015) Menopausal hormone use and ovarian cancer risk: Individual participant meta-analysis of 52 epidemiological studies. *Lancet (London, England)*, 385(9980), pp. 1835–1842. Available at: https://doi.org/10.1016/S0140-6736(14)61687-1.

Berbic, M. *et al.* (2009) Macrophage expression in endometrium of women with and without endometriosis. *Human Reproduction (Oxford, England)*, 24(2), pp. 325–332. Available at: https://doi.org/10.1093/HUMREP/DEN393.

Bernardi, L. *et al.* (2001) Breathing patterns and cardiovascular autonomic modulation during hypoxia induced by simulated altitude. *Journal of Hypertension*, 19(5), pp. 947–958. Available at: https://doi.org/10.1097/00004872-200105000-00016.

Beville, J.M. *et al.* (2014) Gender differences in college leisure time physical activity: Application of the theory of planned behavior and integrated behavioral model. *Journal of American College Health*, 62(3), pp. 173–184. Available at: https://doi.org/10.1080/07448481.2013.872648.

Bey, M.E., Marzilger, R., Hinkson, L., Arampatzis, A. and Legerlotz, K. (2019) Patellar tendon stiffness is not reduced during pregnancy. *Frontiers in Physiology*, 10, p. 334. doi: 10.3389/fphys.2019.00334.

Bhattacharya, S.M. and Jha, A. (2010) Prevalence and risk of depressive disorders in women with polycystic ovary syndrome (PCOS). *Fertility and Sterility*, 94(1), pp. 357–359. Available at: https://doi.org/10.1016/J.FERTNSTERT.2009.09.025.

Biggs, W. and Demuth, R. (2011) Premenstrual syndrome and premenstrual dysphoric disorder. *American Family Physician*, 84(8), pp. 918–924. Available at: www.aafp.org/pubs/afp/issues/2011/1015/p918.html (Accessed: 24 August 2024).

Bixo, M. *et al.* (1997) Progesterone, 5 α-pregnane-3,20-dione and 3 α-hydroxy-5 α-pregnane-20-one in specific regions of the human female brain in different endocrine states. *Brain Research*, 764(1–2), pp. 173–178. Available at: https://doi.org/10.1016/S0006-8993(97)00455-1.

Blagrove, R.C., Bruinvels, G. and Pedlar, C.R. (2020) Variations in strength-related measures during the menstrual cycle in eumenorrheic women: A systematic review and meta-analysis. *Journal of Science and Medicine in Sport*, 23(12), pp. 1220–1227. Available at: https://doi.org/10.1016/J.JSAMS.2020.04.022.

Bloom, M.S. *et al.* (2020) Adiposity is associated with anovulation independent of serum free testosterone: A prospective cohort study. *Paediatric and Perinatal Epidemiology* [Preprint].

Bluth, K., Roberson, P.N.E. and Girdler, S.S. (2017) Adolescent sex differences in response to a mindfulness intervention: A call for research. *Journal of Child and Family Studies*, 26(7), p. 1900. Available at: https://doi.org/10.1007/S10826-017-0696-6.

Bø, K. *et al.* (2016a) Exercise and pregnancy in recreational and elite athletes: 2016 evidence summary from the IOC expert group meeting, Lausanne. Part 1—exercise in women planning pregnancy and those who are pregnant. *British Journal of Sports Medicine*, 50(10), pp. 571–589. Available at: https://doi.org/10.1136/bjsports-2016-096218.

Bø, K. *et al.* (2016b) Exercise and pregnancy in recreational and elite athletes: 2016 evidence summary from the IOC expert group meeting, Lausanne. Part 2—the effect of exercise on the fetus, labour and birth. *British Journal of Sports Medicine*, 50(21), pp. 1297–1305. Available at: https://doi.org/10.1136/BJSPORTS-2016-096810.

Bø, K. *et al.* (2017) Exercise and pregnancy in recreational and elite athletes: 2016/17 evidence summary from the IOC Expert Group Meeting, Lausanne. Part 3—exercise in the postpartum period. *British Journal of Sports Medicine*, 51(21), pp. 1516–1525. Available at: https://doi.org/10.1136/BJSPORTS-2017-097964.

Bø, K. *et al.* (2018) Exercise and pregnancy in recreational and elite athletes: 2016/2017 evidence summary from the IOC expert group meeting, Lausanne. Part 5—recommendations for health professionals and active women. *British Journal of Sports Medicine*, 52(17), pp. 1080–1085. Available at: https://doi.org/10.1136/bjsports-2018-099351.

Bø, K. and Backe-Hansen, K.L. (2007) Do elite athletes experience low back, pelvic girdle and pelvic floor complaints during and after pregnancy? *Scandinavian Journal of Medicine & Science in Sports*, 17(5), pp. 480–487. Available at: https://doi.org/10.1111/j.1600-0838.2006.00599.x.

Boden, G. (1996) Fuel metabolism in pregnancy and in gestational diabetes mellitus. *Obstetrics and Gynecology Clinics of North America*, 23(1), pp. 1–10. Available at: https://doi.org/10.1016/S0889-8545(05)70241-2.

Boisseau, N. and Isacco, L. (2022) Substrate metabolism during exercise: Sexual dimorphism and women's specificities. *European Journal of Sport Science*, 22(5), pp. 672–683. Available at: https://doi.org/10.1080/17461391.2021.1943713.

Bondarev, D. et al. (2021) Physical performance during the menopausal transition and the role of physical activity. The Journals of Gerontology Series A: Biological Sciences and Medical Sciences, 76(9), p. 1587. Available at: https://doi.org/10.1093/GERONA/GLAA292.

Booyens, R.M. et al. (2022) To clot, or not to clot: The dilemma of hormone treatment options for menopause. Thrombosis Research, 218, pp. 99–111. Available at: https://doi.org/10.1016/J.THROMRES.2022.08.016.

Borenstein, J.E. et al. (2007) Differences in symptom scores and health outcomes in premenstrual syndrome. Journal of Women's Health (2002), 16(8), pp. 1139–1144. Available at: https://doi.org/10.1089/JWH.2006.0230.

Bosch de Basea, L. et al. (2024) Sex-dependent metabolic effects in diet-induced obese rats following intermittent fasting compared with continuous food restriction. Nutrients, 16(7). Available at: https://doi.org/10.3390/NU16071009.

Bouchard, S. et al. (2012) Using biofeedback while immersed in a stressful videogame increases the effectiveness of stress management skills in soldiers. PLOS One, 7(4). Available at: https://doi.org/10.1371/JOURNAL.PONE.0036169.

Boulant, J.A. (2000) Role of the preoptic-anterior hypothalamus in thermoregulation and fever. Clinical Infectious Diseases: An Official Publication of the Infectious Diseases Society of America, 31 Suppl. 5(SUPPL. 5). Available at: https://doi.org/10.1086/317521.

Boyd, A. et al. (2015) Gender differences in mental disorders and suicidality in Europe: Results from a large cross-sectional population-based study. Journal of Affective Disorders, 173, pp. 245–254. Available at: https://doi.org/10.1016/J.JAD.2014.11.002.

Boyle, R. et al. (2012) Pelvic floor muscle training for prevention and treatment of urinary and faecal incontinence in antenatal and postnatal women. Cochrane Database of Systematic Reviews (Online), 10, pp. CD007471–CD007471. Available at: https://doi.org/10.1002/14651858.CD007471.pub2.

Bozzini, B.N. et al. (2021) Evaluating the effects of oral contraceptive use on biomarkers and body composition during a competitive season in collegiate female soccer players. Journal of Applied Physiology (Bethesda, Md.: 1985), 130(6), pp. 1971–1982. Available at: https://doi.org/10.1152/JAPPLPHYSIOL.00818.2020.

Bridgeman, J.T. et al. (2010) Estrogen receptor expression in posterior tibial tendon dysfunction: A pilot study. Foot & Ankle International, 31(12), pp. 1081–1084. Available at: https://doi.org/10.3113/FAI.2010.1081.

Broderick, P.C. (2005) Mindfulness and coping with dysphoric mood: Contrasts with rumination and distraction. Cognitive Therapy and Research, 29(5), pp. 501–510. Available at: https://doi.org/10.1007/S10608-005-3888-0.

Brown, L. et al. (2024) Promoting good mental health over the menopause transition. The Lancet, 403(10430), pp. 969–983. Available at: https://pubmed.ncbi.nlm.nih.gov/38458216.

Brown, L.M. and Clegg, D.J. (2010) Central effects of estradiol in the regulation of food intake, body weight, and adiposity. The Journal of Steroid Biochemistry and Molecular Biology, 122(1–3), pp. 65–73. Available at: https://doi.org/10.1016/J.JSBMB.2009.12.005.

Brown, N., Knight, C.J. and Forrest, L.J. (2021) Elite female athletes' experiences and perceptions of the menstrual cycle on training and sport performance. Scandinavian Journal of Medicine & Science in Sports, 31(1), pp. 52–69. Available at: https://doi.org/10.1111/SMS.13818.

Brown, W.J., Heesch, K.C. and Miller, Y.D. (2009) Life events and changing physical activity patterns in women at different life stages. Annals of Behavioral Medicine: A Publication of the Society of Behavioral Medicine, 37(3), pp. 294–305. Available at: https://doi.org/10.1007/S12160-009-9099-2.

Brown, Z.A. et al. (2011) The phenotype of polycystic ovary syndrome ameliorates with aging. Fertility and Sterility, 96(5), pp. 1259–1265. Available at: https://doi.org/10.1016/J.FERTNSTERT.2011.09.002.

Bruinvels, G. et al. (2016) The prevalence and impact of heavy menstrual bleeding (menorrhagia) in elite and non-elite athletes. PLOS One, 11(2). Available at: https://doi.org/10.1371/JOURNAL.PONE.0149881.

Bruinvels, G. et al. (2017) Sport, exercise and the menstrual cycle: Where is the research? British Journal of Sports Medicine, 51(6), pp. 487–488. Available at: https://doi.org/10.1136/BJSPORTS-2016-096279.

Bruinvels, G., Hackney, A.C. and Pedlar, C.R. (2022) Menstrual cycle: The importance of both the phases and the transitions between phases on training and performance. Sports Medicine (Auckland, N.Z.), 52(7), pp. 1457–1460. Available at: https://doi.org/10.1007/S40279-022-01691-2.

Bruning, J.C. et al. (2000) Role of brain insulin receptor in control of body weight and reproduction. Science (New York, N.Y.), 289(5487), pp. 2122–2125. Available at: https://doi.org/10.1126/SCIENCE.289.5487.2122.

Buchanan, T.A. et al. (1990) Insulin sensitivity and B-cell responsiveness to glucose during late pregnancy in lean and moderately obese women with normal glucose tolerance or mild gestational diabetes. American Journal of Obstetrics and Gynecology, 162(4), pp. 1008–1014. Available at: https://doi.org/10.1016/0002-9378(90)91306-W.

Buckinx, F. and Aubertin-Leheudre, M. (2019) Menopause and high-intensity interval training: Effects on body composition and physical performance. *Menopause (New York, N.Y.)*, 26(11), pp. 1232–1233. Available at: https://doi.org/10.1097/GME.0000000000001433.

Bühlmayer, L. *et al.* (2017) Effects of mindfulness practice on performance-relevant parameters and performance outcomes in sports: A meta-analytical review. *Sports Medicine (Auckland, N.Z.)*, 47(11), pp. 2309–2321. Available at: https://doi.org/10.1007/S40279-017-0752-9.

Bühren, C., Gschwend, M. and Krumer, A. (2024) Expectations, gender, and choking under pressure: Evidence from alpine skiing. *Journal of Economic Psychology*, 100, p. 102692. Available at: https://doi.org/10.1016/J.JOEP.2023.102692.

Bulun, S.E. *et al.* (2019) Endometriosis. *Endocrine Reviews*, 40(4), p. 1048. Available at: https://doi.org/10.1210/ER.2018-00242.

Burger, H.G. *et al.* (2002) Hormonal changes in the menopause transition. *Recent Progress in Hormone Research*, 57, pp. 257–275. Available at: https://doi.org/10.1210/RP.57.1.257.

Burke, L.M. *et al.* (2018) Pitfalls of conducting and interpreting estimates of energy availability in free-living athletes. *International Journal of Sport Nutrition and Exercise Metabolism*, 28(4), pp. 350–363. Available at: https://doi.org/10.1123/IJSNEM.2018-0142.

Burney, R.O. and Giudice, L.C. (2012) Pathogenesis and pathophysiology of endometriosis. *Fertility and Sterility*, 98(3), pp. 511–519. Available at: https://doi.org/10.1016/J.FERTNSTERT.2012.06.029.

Burrows, M. and Bird, S.R. (2005) Velocity at VO2max and peak treadmill velocity are not influenced within or across the phases of the menstrual cycle. *European Journal of Applied Physiology*, 93(5–6), pp. 575–580. Available at: https://doi.org/10.1007/S00421-004-1272-5.

Burrows, M. and Peters, C.E. (2007) The influence of oral contraceptives on athletic performance in female athletes. *Sports Medicine (Auckland, N.Z.)*, 37(7), pp. 557–574. Available at: https://doi.org/10.2165/00007256-200737070-00001.

Byeon, K. *et al.* (2012) The response of the vena cava to abdominal breathing. *Journal of Alternative and Complementary Medicine (New York, N.Y.)*, 18(2), pp. 153–157. Available at: https://doi.org/10.1089/ACM.2010.0656.

Cabre, H.E. *et al.* (2024) Effects of the menstrual cycle and hormonal contraceptive use on metabolic outcomes, strength performance, and recovery: A narrative review. *Metabolites*, 14(7), p. 347. Available at: https://doi.org/10.3390/METABO14070347.

Cain, U. *et al.* (2021) Musculoskeletal injuries in pregnancy. *Seminars in Roentgenology*, 56(1), pp. 79–89. Available at: https://doi.org/10.1053/J.RO.2020.09.002.

Cakmak, B., Ribeiro, A.P. and Inanir, A. (2016) Postural balance and the risk of falling during pregnancy. *The Journal of Maternal-Fetal & Neonatal Medicine: The Official Journal of the European Association of Perinatal Medicine, the Federation of Asia and Oceania Perinatal Societies, the International Society of Perinatal Obstetricians*, 29(10), pp. 1623–1625. Available at: https://doi.org/10.3109/14767058.2015.1057490.

Capeless, E.L. and Clapp, J.F. (1991) When do cardiovascular parameters return to their preconception values? *American Journal of Obstetrics and Gynecology*, 165(4 Pt 1), pp. 883–886. Available at: https://doi.org/10.1016/0002-9378(91)90432-q.

Carmichael, M.A. *et al.* (2021) The impact of menstrual cycle phase on athletes' performance: A narrative review. *International Journal of Environmental Research and Public Health*, 18(4), pp. 1–24. Available at: https://doi.org/10.3390/IJERPH18041667.

Carmody, J.F. *et al.* (2011) Mindfulness training for coping with hot flashes: Results of a randomized trial. *Menopause (New York, N.Y.)*, 18(6), pp. 611–620. Available at: https://doi.org/10.1097/GME.0B013E318204A05C.

Carneiro, M.A.S. *et al.* (2022) Effects of resistance training at different loads on inflammatory biomarkers, muscle mass, muscular strength, and physical performance in postmenopausal women. *Journal of Strength and Conditioning Research*, 36(6), pp. 1582–1590. Available at: https://doi.org/10.1519/JSC.0000000000003768.

Cary, E. and Simpson, P. (2024) Premenstrual disorders and PMDD: A review. *Best Practice & Research Clinical Endocrinology & Metabolism*, 38(1), p. 101858. Available at: https://doi.org/10.1016/J.BEEM.2023.101858.

Casagrande, D. *et al.* (2015) Low back pain and pelvic girdle pain in pregnancy. *The Journal of the American Academy of Orthopaedic Surgeons*, 23(9), pp. 539–549. Available at: https://doi.org/10.5435/JAAOS-D-14-00248.

Casazza, G.A. *et al.* (2002) Effects of oral contraceptives on peak exercise capacity. *Journal of Applied Physiology (Bethesda, Md.: 1985)*, 93(5), pp. 1698–1702. Available at: https://doi.org/10.1152/JAPPLPHYSIOL.00622.2002.

Catalano, P.M. *et al.* (1991) Longitudinal changes in insulin release and insulin resistance in nonobese pregnant women. *American Journal of Obstetrics and Gynecology*, 165(6 Pt 1), pp. 1667–1672. Available at: https://doi.org/10.1016/0002-9378(91)90012-G.

Catalini, L. and Fedder, J. (2020) Characteristics of the endometrium in menstruating species: Lessons learned from the animal kingdom. *Biology of Reproduction*, 102(6), pp. 1160–1169. Available at: https://doi.org/10.1093/biolre/ioaa029.

Cauci, S., Francescato, M.P. and Curcio, F. (2017) Combined oral contraceptives increase high-sensitivity c-reactive protein but not haptoglobin in female athletes. *Sports Medicine (Auckland, N.Z.)*, 47(1), pp. 175–185. Available at: https://doi.org/10.1007/S40279-016-0534-9.

Ceca, D. *et al.* (2020) Effectiveness of a self-myofascial conditioning programme on pain, depression, anxiety and sleep quality in people with Fibromyalgia. *Cuadernos de Psicología del Deporte*, 20(1), pp. 147–465.

Chang, K.V. *et al.* (2017) Is sarcopenia associated with depression? A systematic review and meta-analysis of observational studies. *Age and Ageing*, 46(5), pp. 738–746. Available at: https://doi.org/10.1093/AGEING/AFX094.

Charlton, W.P.H., Coslett-Charlton, L.M. and Ciccotti, M.G. (2001) Correlation of estradiol in pregnancy and anterior cruciate ligament laxity. *Clinical Orthopaedics and Related Research*, 387(387), pp. 165–170. Available at: https://doi.org/10.1097/00003086-200106000-00022.

Cheatham, S.W. and Stull, K.R. (2018) Comparison of three different density type foam rollers on knee range of motion and pressure pain threshold: A randomized controlled trial. *International Journal of Sports Physical Therapy*, 13(3), pp. 474–482.

Chen, C.X. *et al.* (2018) Reasons women do not seek health care for dysmenorrhea. *Journal of Clinical Nursing*, 27(1–2), p. e301. Available at: https://doi.org/10.1111/JOCN.13946.

Chen, T.L. *et al.* (2021) Effectiveness of mindfulness-based interventions on quality of life and menopausal symptoms in menopausal women: A meta-analysis. *Journal of Psychosomatic Research*, 147. Available at: https://doi.org/10.1016/J.JPSYCHORES.2021.110515.

Chetry, D. *et al.* (2023) Effect of yoga on intra-ocular pressure in patients with glaucoma: A systematic review and meta-analysis. *Indian Journal of Ophthalmology*, 71(5), p. 1757. Available at: https://doi.org/10.4103/IJO.IJO_2054_22.

Cheung, A.S., Nolan, B.J. and Zwickl, S. (2023) Transgender health and the impact of aging and menopause. *Climacteric*, 26(3), pp. 256–262. Available at: https://doi.org/10.1080/13697137.2023.2176217.

Chidi-Ogbolu, N. and Baar, K. (2018) Effect of estrogen on musculoskeletal performance and injury risk. *Frontiers in Physiology*, 9, p. 1834. Available at: https://doi.org/10.3389/fphys.2018.01834.

Choudhry, D.N. *et al.* (2024) The effect of resistance training in reducing hot flushes in post-menopausal women: A meta-analysis. *Journal of Bodywork and Movement Therapies*, 39, pp. 335–342. Available at: https://doi.org/10.1016/J.JBMT.2024.03.018.

Christ, J.P. and Cedars, M.I. (2023) Current guidelines for diagnosing PCOS. *Diagnostics*, 13(6). Available at: https://doi.org/10.3390/DIAGNOSTICS13061113.

Christakis, M.K. *et al.* (2020) The effect of menopause on metabolic syndrome: Cross-sectional results from the Canadian Longitudinal Study on Aging. *Menopause (New York, N.Y.)*, 27(9), pp. 999–1009. Available at: https://doi.org/10.1097/GME.0000000000001575.

Chugh, M. *et al.* (2013) Women weigh in: Obese African American and White women's perspectives on physicians' roles in weight management. *Journal of the American Board of Family Medicine*, 26(4), pp. 421–428. Available at: https://doi.org/10.3122/JABFM.2013.04.120350.

Cienfuegos, S. *et al.* (2021) Changes in body weight and metabolic risk during time restricted feeding in premenopausal versus postmenopausal women. *Experimental Gerontology*, 154. Available at: https://doi.org/10.1016/J.EXGER.2021.111545.

Clapp, J.F. (1991) The changing thermal response to endurance exercise during pregnancy. *American Journal of Obstetrics and Gynecology*, 165(6 Pt 1), pp. 1684–1689. Available at: https://doi.org/10.1016/0002-9378(91)90015-J.

Clapp, J.F. (2000) Exercise during pregnancy: A clinical update. *Clinics in Sports Medicine*, 19(2), pp. 273–286. Available at: https://doi.org/10.1016/S0278-5919(05)70203-9.

Clapp, J.F. and Capeless, E. (1997) Cardiovascular function before, during, and after the first and subsequent pregnancies. *The American Journal of Cardiology*, 80(11), pp. 1469–1473. Available at: https://doi.org/10.1016/s0002-9149(97)00738-8.

Clarke, A.C. *et al.* (2021) Hormonal contraceptive use in football codes in Australia. *Frontiers in Sports and Active Living*, 3, p. 634866. Available at: https://doi.org/10.3389/FSPOR.2021.634866/BIBTEX.

Cohen, L.S. *et al.* (2002) Prevalence and predictors of premenstrual dysphoric disorder (PMDD) in older premenopausal women: The Harvard study of moods and cycles. *Journal of Affective Disorders*, 70(2), pp. 125–132. Available at: https://doi.org/10.1016/S0165-0327(01)00458-X.

Cole, A. (2015) *What Happens When You Get Your Period in Space?* Available at: www.npr.org/sections/health-shots/2015/09/17/441160250/what-happens-when-you-get-your-period-in-space?t=1661864580065.

Coleman, E. *et al.* (2022) Standards of Care for the Health of Transgender and Gender Diverse People, Version 8. *International Journal of Transgender Health*, 23(Suppl 1), pp. S1–S259. Available at: https://doi.org/10.1080/26895269.2022.2100644.

Colenso-Semple, L.M. *et al.* (2023) Current evidence shows no influence of women's menstrual cycle phase on acute strength performance or adaptations to resistance exercise training. *Frontiers in Sports and*

Active Living, 5. Available at: https://doi.org/10.3389/FSPOR.2023.1054542.

Composto, J. *et al.* (2021) Thermal comfort intervention for hot-flash related insomnia symptoms in perimenopausal and postmenopausal-aged women: An exploratory study. *Behavioral Sleep Medicine*, 19(1), pp. 38–47. Available at: https://doi.org/10.1080/15402002.2019.1699100.

Conder, R., Zamani, R. and Akrami, M. (2019) The biomechanics of pregnancy: A systematic review. *Journal of Functional Morphology and Kinesiology*, 4(4). Available at: https://doi.org/10.3390/JFMK4040072.

Cong, J. *et al.* (2015) Structural and functional changes in maternal left ventricle during pregnancy: A three-dimensional speckle-tracking echocardiography study. *Cardiovascular Ultrasound*, 13(1). Available at: https://doi.org/10.1186/1476-7120-13-6.

Cook, C.J., Kilduff, L.P. and Crewther, B.T. (2018) Basal and stress-induced salivary testosterone variation across the menstrual cycle and linkage to motivation and muscle power. *Scandinavian Journal of Medicine and Science in Sports*, 28(4), pp. 1345–1353. Available at: https://doi.org/10.1111/SMS.13041.

Corrigan, L. *et al.* (2022) The characteristics and effectiveness of pregnancy yoga interventions: A systematic review and meta-analysis. *BMC Pregnancy and Childbirth*, 22(1). Available at: https://doi.org/10.1186/S12884-022-04474-9.

Cortés-Montaña, D. *et al.* (2023) Impact of pre-storage melatonin application on the standard, sensory, and bioactive quality of early sweet cherry. *Foods (Basel, Switzerland)*, 12(8). Available at: https://doi.org/10.3390/FOODS12081723.

Costello, J.T., Bieuzen, F. and Bleakley, C.M. (2014) Where are all the female participants in Sports and Exercise Medicine research? *European Journal of Sport Science*, 14(8), pp. 847–851. Available at: https://doi.org/10.1080/17461391.2014.911354.

Cotto, J.H. *et al.* (2010) Gender effects on drug use, abuse, and dependence: A special analysis of results from the National Survey on Drug Use and Health. *Gender Medicine*, 7(5), pp. 402–413. Available at: https://doi.org/10.1016/J.GENM.2010.09.004.

Crain, D.A. *et al.* (2008) Female reproductive disorders: The roles of endocrine-disrupting compounds and developmental timing. *Fertility and Sterility*, 90(4), pp. 911–940. Available at: https://doi.org/10.1016/J.FERTNSTERT.2008.08.067.

Crewther, B.T. *et al.* (2011) Two emerging concepts for elite athletes: The short-term effects of testosterone and cortisol on the neuromuscular system and the dose-response training role of these endogenous hormones. *Sports Medicine*, 41(2), pp. 103–123. Available at: https://doi.org/10.2165/11539170-000000000-00000.

Csapo, A.I., Pulkkinen, M.O. and Wiest, W.G. (1973) Effects of luteectomy and progesterone replacement therapy in early pregnant patients. *American Journal of Obstetrics and Gynecology*, 115(6), pp. 759–765. Available at: https://doi.org/10.1016/0002-9378(73)90517-6.

Cui, J., Shen, Y. and Li, R. (2013) Estrogen synthesis and signaling pathways during aging: From periphery to brain. *Trends in Molecular Medicine*, 19(3), pp. 197–209. Available at: https://doi.org/10.1016/j.molmed.2012.12.007.

Curtis, K., Weinrib, A. and Katz, J. (2012) Systematic review of yoga for pregnant women: Current status and future directions. *Evidence-Based Complementary and Alternative Medicine: eCAM*, 2012. Available at: https://doi.org/10.1155/2012/715942.

Dalgaard, L.B. *et al.* (2019) Influence of oral contraceptive use on adaptations to resistance training. *Frontiers in Physiology*, 10. Available at: https://doi.org/10.3389/FPHYS.2019.00824.

Dam, T.V. *et al.* (2022) Muscle performance during the menstrual cycle correlates with psychological well-being, but not fluctuations in sex hormones. *Medicine and Science in Sports and Exercise*, 54(10), pp. 1678–1689. Available at: https://doi.org/10.1249/MSS.0000000000002961.

Danhauer, S.C. *et al.* (2009) Restorative yoga for women with breast cancer: Findings from a randomized pilot study. *Psycho-oncology*, 18(4), pp. 360–368. Available at: https://doi.org/10.1002/PON.1503.

Davies, J. and Kadir, R.A. (2017) Heavy menstrual bleeding: An update on management. *Thrombosis Research*, 151 Suppl 1, pp. S70–S77. Available at: https://doi.org/10.1016/S0049-3848(17)30072-5.

Davis, S.R. *et al.* (2023) The 2023 Practitioner's Toolkit for Managing Menopause. *Climacteric*, 26(6), pp. 517–536. Available at: https://doi.org/10.1080/13697137.2023.2258783.

Déa, C.A. *et al.* (2024) Sexual function, quality of life, anxiety, and depression in women of reproductive age using hormonal, nonhormonal, and no contraceptive methods. *The Journal of Sexual Medicine*, 21(8), pp. 683–690. Available at: https://doi.org/10.1093/JSXMED/QDAE060.

Dębski, P., Białas, E. and Gnat, R. (2019) The parameters of foam rolling, self-myofascial release treatment: A review of the literature. *Biomedical Human Kinetics*, 11(1), pp. 36–46. Available at: https://doi.org/10.2478/BHK-2019-0005.

Deeks, A.A., Gibson-Helm, M.E. and Teede, H.J. (2010) Anxiety and depression in polycystic ovary syndrome: A comprehensive investigation. *Fertility and Sterility*, 93(7), pp. 2421–2423. Available at: https://doi.org/10.1016/J.FERTNSTERT.2009.09.018.

Defreyne, J., Van de Bruaene, L.D.L., Rietzschel, E., Van Schuylenbergh, J. and T'Sjoen, G.G.R. (2019) Effects of gender-affirming hormones on lipid, metabolic, and cardiac surrogate blood markers in transgender persons. *Clinical Chemistry*, 65(1), pp. 119–134. doi: 10.1373/clinchem.2018.288241. PMID: 30602477.

Delamater, L. and Santoro, N. (2018) Management of the perimenopause. *Clinical Obstetrics and Gynecology*, 61(3), pp. 419–432. Available at: https://doi.org/10.1097/GRF.0000000000000389.

Dewey, K.G. (no date) Effects of maternal caloric restriction and exercise during lactation. *Journal of Nutrition*, 128(2 Suppl), pp. 386s–9.

Dewey, K.G. *et al.* (1994) A randomized study of the effects of aerobic exercise by lactating women on breast-milk volume and composition. *New England Journal of Medicine*, 330(7), pp. 449–453. Available at: https://doi.org/10.1056/nejm199402173300701.

D'Hooghe, T.M. and Debrock, S. (2002) Endometriosis, retrograde menstruation and peritoneal inflammation in women and in baboons. *Human Reproduction Update*, 8(1), pp. 84–88. Available at: https://doi.org/10.1093/HUMUPD/8.1.84.

Diamanti-Kandarakis, E. and Dunaif, A. (2012) Insulin resistance and the polycystic ovary syndrome revisited: An update on mechanisms and implications. *Endocrine Reviews*, 33(6), pp. 981–1030. Available at: https://doi.org/10.1210/ER.2011-1034.

Diaz, A., Laufer, M.R. and Breech, L.L. (2006) Menstruation in girls and adolescents: Using the menstrual cycle as a vital sign. *Pediatrics*, 118(5), pp. 2245–2250. Available at: https://doi.org/10.1542/peds.2006-2481.

Dick, T.E. *et al.* (2014) Increased cardio-respiratory coupling evoked by slow deep breathing can persist in normal humans. *Respiratory Physiology & Neurobiology*, 0, p. 99. Available at: https://doi.org/10.1016/J.RESP.2014.09.013.

Dieli-Conwright, C. *et al.* (2009a) Hormone therapy attenuates exercise-induced skeletal muscle damage in postmenopausal women. *Journal of Applied Physiology*, 107, pp. 853–858.

Dieli-Conwright, C.M. *et al.* (2009b) Influence of hormone replacement therapy on eccentric exercise induced myogenic gene expression in postmenopausal women. *Journal of Applied Physiology*, 107(5), pp. 1381–1388. Available at: https://doi.org/10.1152/JAPPLPHYSIOL.00590.2009.

Diffey, B. *et al.* (1997) The effect of oral contraceptive agents on the basal metabolic rate of young women. *British Journal of Nutrition*, 77(6), pp. 853–862. Available at: https://doi.org/10.1079/BJN19970084.

Diwadkar, V.A., Murphy, E.R. and Freedman, R.R. (2014) Temporal sequencing of brain activations during naturally occurring thermoregulatory events. *Cerebral Cortex (New York, N.Y.: 1991)*, 24(11), pp. 3006–3013. Available at: https://doi.org/10.1093/CERCOR/BHT155.

Dong, J. and Rees, D.A. (2023) Polycystic ovary syndrome: Pathophysiology and therapeutic opportunities. *BMJ Medicine*, 2(1), p. e000548. Available at: https://doi.org/10.1136/BMJMED-2023-000548.

Donnell-Fink, L.A. *et al.* (2015) Effectiveness of knee injury and anterior cruciate ligament tear prevention programs: A meta-analysis. *PLOS One*, 10(12). Available at: https://doi.org/10.1371/JOURNAL.PONE.0144063.

Dougherty, D.M. *et al.* (1997) The influence of menstrual-cycle phase on the relationship between testosterone and aggression. *Physiology and Behavior*, 62(2), pp. 431–435. Available at: https://doi.org/10.1016/S0031-9384(97)88991-3.

Dozières-Puyravel, B. *et al.* (2018) Ketogenic diet therapies in France: State of the use in 2018. *Epilepsy and Behavior*, 86, pp. 204–206. Available at: https://doi.org/10.1016/j.yebeh.2018.05.031.

Dragoman, M.V. (2014) The combined oral contraceptive pill: Recent developments, risks and benefits. *Best Practice & Research. Clinical Obstetrics & Gynaecology*, 28(6), pp. 825–834. Available at: https://doi.org/10.1016/J.BPOBGYN.2014.06.003.

Dreon, D.M., Slavin, J.L. and Phinney, S.D. (2003) Oral contraceptive use and increased plasma concentration of C-reactive protein. *Life Sciences*, 73(10), pp. 1245–1252. Available at: https://doi.org/10.1016/S0024-3205(03)00425-9.

DuBois, L.Z. *et al.* (2024) Gender minority stress and diurnal cortisol profiles among transgender and gender diverse people in the United States. *Hormones and Behavior*, 159, p. 105473. Available at: https://doi.org/10.1016/J.YHBEH.2023.105473.

Duckitt, K. (2010) Managing perimenopausal menorrhagia. *Maturitas*, 66(3), pp. 251–256. Available at: https://doi.org/10.1016/J.MATURITAS.2010.03.013.

Dumas, G.A. and Reid, J.G. (1997) Laxity of knee cruciate ligaments during pregnancy. *The Journal of Orthopaedic and Sports Physical Therapy*, 26(1), pp. 2–6. Available at: https://doi.org/10.2519/JOSPT.1997.26.1.2.

Dupuit, M., Maillard, F. *et al.* (2020) Effect of high intensity interval training on body composition in women before and after menopause: A meta-analysis. *Experimental Physiology*, 105(9), pp. 1470–1490. Available at: https://doi.org/10.1113/EP088654.

Dupuit, M., Rance, M. *et al.* (2020) Moderate-intensity continuous training or high-intensity interval training with or without resistance training for altering body composition in postmenopausal women. *Medicine and Science in Sports and Exercise*, 52(3), pp. 736–745. Available at: https://doi.org/10.1249/MSS.0000000000002162.

Durlinger, A.L.L. *et al.* (2002) Anti-Müllerian hormone inhibits initiation of primordial follicle growth in the mouse ovary. *Endocrinology*, 143(3), pp.

1076–1084. Available at: https://doi.org/10.1210/ENDO.143.3.8691.

Eck, L.H. *et al.* (1997) Differences in macronutrient selections in users and nonusers of an oral contraceptive. *American Journal of Clinical Nutrition*, 65(2), pp. 419–424. Available at: https://doi.org/10.1093/AJCN/65.2.419.

Edwards, A.C. *et al.* (2022) Oral contraceptive use and risk of suicidal behavior among young women. *Psychological Medicine*, 52(9), pp. 1710–1717. Available at: https://doi.org/10.1017/S0033291720003475.

Egli, T. *et al.* (2011) Influence of age, sex, and race on college students' exercise motivation of physical activity. *Journal of American College Health*, 59(5), pp. 399–406. Available at: https://doi.org/10.1080/07448481.2010.513074.

Ekenros, L. *et al.* (2013) Oral contraceptives do not affect muscle strength and hop performance in active women. *Clinical Journal of Sport Medicine: Official Journal of the Canadian Academy of Sport Medicine*, 23(3), pp. 202–207. Available at: https://doi.org/10.1097/JSM.0B013E3182625A51.

Ekkekakis, P., Hall, E.E. and Petruzzello, S.J. (2008) The relationship between exercise intensity and affective responses demystified: To crack the 40-year-old nut, replace the 40-year-old nutcracker! *Annals of Behavioral Medicine*, 35(2), pp. 136–149. Available at: https://doi.org/10.1007/S12160-008-9025-Z.

El-Hemaidi, I., Gharaibeh, A. and Shehata, H. (2007) Menorrhagia and bleeding disorders. *Current Opinion in Obstetrics & Gynecology*, 19(6), pp. 513–520. Available at: https://doi.org/10.1097/GCO.0B013E3282F1DDBE.

Elkins, G. *et al.* (2008) Randomized trial of a hypnosis intervention for treatment of hot flashes among breast cancer survivors. *Journal of Clinical Oncology: Official Journal of the American Society of Clinical Oncology*, 26(31), pp. 5022–5026. Available at: https://doi.org/10.1200/JCO.2008.16.6389.

Elkins, G.R. *et al.* (2013) Clinical hypnosis in the treatment of postmenopausal hot flashes: A randomized controlled trial. *Menopause (New York, N.Y.)*, 20(3), pp. 291–298. Available at: https://doi.org/10.1097/GME.0B013E31826CE3ED.

Elliott, K.J., Cable, N.T. and Reilly, T. (2005) Does oral contraceptive use affect maximum force production in women? *British Journal of Sports Medicine*, 39(1), pp. 15–19. Available at: https://doi.org/10.1136/BJSM.2003.009886.

Elliott-Sale, K. and Hicks, K. (2018) Hormonal-Based Contraception and the Exercising Female. In J. Forsyth and C.M. Roberts (eds), *The Exercising Female*. Taylor & Francis. Available at: https://researchportal.northumbria.ac.uk/en/publications/hormonal-based-contraception-and-the-exercising-female (Accessed: 5 August 2024).

Elliott-Sale, K.J. *et al.* (2020) The effects of oral contraceptives on exercise performance in women: A systematic review and meta-analysis. *Sports Medicine (Auckland, N.Z.)*, 50(10), pp. 1785–1812. Available at: https://doi.org/10.1007/S40279-020-01317-5.

Elliott-Sale, K.J. *et al.* (2021) Methodological considerations for studies in sport and exercise science with women as participants: A working guide for standards of practice for research on women. *Sports Medicine (Auckland, N.Z.)*, 51(5), p. 843. Available at: https://doi.org/10.1007/S40279-021-01435-8.

Emiliano, A.B. *et al.* (2022) Sex-specific differences in metabolic outcomes after sleeve gastrectomy and intermittent fasting in obese middle-aged mice. *American Journal of Physiology: Endocrinology and Metabolism*, 323(1), pp. E107–E121. Available at: https://pubmed.ncbi.nlm.nih.gov/35658544.

Ensari, I. *et al.* (2022) Associations between physical exercise patterns and pain symptoms in individuals with endometriosis: A cross-sectional mHealth-based investigation. *BMJ Open*, 12(7). Available at: https://doi.org/10.1136/BMJOPEN-2021-059280.

Entin, P.L. and Coffin, L. (2004) Physiological basis for recommendations regarding exercise during pregnancy at high altitude. *High Altitude Medicine & Biology*, 5(3), pp. 321–334. Available at: https://doi.org/10.1089/HAM.2004.5.321.

Erdélyi, A. *et al.* (2023) The importance of nutrition in menopause and perimenopause: A review. *Nutrients*, 16(1). Available at: https://doi.org/10.3390/NU16010027.

Eriksson, E. (2014) SSRIs probably counteract premenstrual syndrome by inhibiting the serotonin transporter. *Journal of Psychopharmacology (Oxford, England)*, 28(2), pp. 173–174. Available at: https://doi.org/10.1177/0269881113512910.

Eston, R.G. and Burke, E.J. (1984) Effects of the menstrual cycle on selected responses to short constant-load exercise. *Journal of Strategic Marketing*, 2(2), pp. 145–153. Available at: https://doi.org/10.1080/02640418408729710.

Evans, S. *et al.* (2019) Psychological and mind-body interventions for endometriosis: A systematic review. *Journal of Psychosomatic Research*, 124. Available at: https://doi.org/10.1016/J.JPSYCHORES.2019.109756.

Fahs, D. *et al.* (2023) Polycystic ovary syndrome: Pathophysiology and controversies in diagnosis. *Diagnostics*, 13(9), p. 1559. Available at: https://doi.org/10.3390/DIAGNOSTICS13091559.

Falcone, T. and Flyckt-Rebecca, R. (2018) Clinical management of endometriosis. *Obstetrics and Gynecology*, 131(3), pp. 557–571. Available at: https://doi.org/10.1097/AOG.0000000000002469.

Falcone, T. and Lebovic, D.I. (2011) Clinical management of endometriosis. *Obstetrics and Gynecology*, 118(3), pp. 691–705. Available at: https://doi.org/10.1097/AOG.0B013E31822ADFD1.

Fatouros, I.G. and Jamurtas, A.Z. (2016) Insights into the molecular etiology of exercise-induced inflammation: Opportunities for optimizing performance. *Journal of Inflammation Research*, 9, pp. 175–186. Available at: https://doi.org/10.2147/JIR.S114635.

Fede, C. *et al.* (2016) Hormone receptor expression in human fascial tissue. *European Journal of Histochemistry*, 60(4), p. 2710. Available at: https://doi.org/10.4081/ejh.2016.2710.

Fede, C. *et al.* (2019) Sensitivity of the fasciae to sex hormone levels: Modulation of collagen-I, collagen-III and fibrillin production. *PLOS One*, 14(9), p. e0223195. Available at: https://doi.org/10.1371/journal.pone.0223195.

Fede, C. *et al.* (2022) The effects of aging on the intramuscular connective tissue. *International Journal of Molecular Sciences*, 23(19), p. 11061. Available at: https://doi.org/10.3390/IJMS231911061.

Feldt-Rasmussen, U. and Mathiesen, E.R. (2011) Endocrine disorders in pregnancy: Physiological and hormonal aspects of pregnancy. *Best Practice & Research Clinical Endocrinology & Metabolism*, 25(6), pp. 875–884. Available at: https://doi.org/10.1016/J.BEEM.2011.07.004.

Fenlon, D. *et al.* (2020) Effectiveness of nurse-led group CBT for hot flushes and night sweats in women with breast cancer: Results of the MENOS4 randomised controlled trial. *Psycho-oncology*, 29(10), p. 1514. Available at: https://doi.org/10.1002/PON.5432.

Ferreira, L. *et al.* (2024) Effects of exercise programs on cardiorespiratory fitness and arterial stiffness on postmenopausal women: A systematic review study. *Maturitas*, 181. Available at: https://doi.org/10.1016/J.MATURITAS.2024.107917.

Fieril, K.P. *et al.* (2014) Experiences of exercise during pregnancy among women who perform regular resistance training: A qualitative study. *Physical Therapy*, 94(8), pp. 1135–1143. Available at: https://doi.org/10.2522/PTJ.20120432.

Figueiredo, B.G.D. de *et al.* (2021) Mapping changes in women's visual functions during the menstrual cycle: Narrative review. *Sao Paulo Medical Journal (Revista Paulista de Medicina)*, 139(6), pp. 662–674. Available at: https://doi.org/10.1590/1516-3180.2020.0474.R2.03052021.

Filicori, M., Butler, J.P. and Crowley, W.F.J. (1984) Neuroendocrine regulation of the corpus luteum in the human: Evidence for pulsatile progesterone secretion. *The Journal of Clinical Investigation*, 73(6), pp. 1638–1647. Available at: https://doi.org/10.1172/JCI111370.

Findlay, R.J. *et al.* (2020) How the menstrual cycle and menstruation affect sporting performance: Experiences and perceptions of elite female rugby players. *British Journal of Sports Medicine*, 54(18), pp. 1108–1113. Available at: https://doi.org/10.1136/BJSPORTS-2019-101486.

Fisher, J.P. *et al.* (2017) A minimal dose approach to resistance training for the older adult; the prophylactic for aging. *Experimental Gerontology*, 99, pp. 80–86. Available at: https://doi.org/10.1016/J.EXGER.2017.09.012.

Fiurašková, K. *et al.* (2022) Oral contraceptive use during relationship formation and current relationship satisfaction: Testing the congruency hypothesis in couples attending pregnancy and fertility clinics. *Psychoneuroendocrinology*, 135. Available at: https://doi.org/10.1016/J.PSYNEUEN.2021.105451.

Forsyth, J.J. and Reilly, T. (2008) The effect of menstrual cycle on 2000-m rowing ergometry performance. *European Journal of Sport Science*, 8, pp. 351–357.

Foy, M.R. *et al.* (1999) 17β-estradiol enhances NMDA receptor-mediated EPSPs and long-term potentiation. *Journal of Neurophysiology*, 81(2), pp. 925–929. Available at: https://doi.org/10.1152/JN.1999.81.2.925.

Franklin, R.M., Ploutz-Snyder, L. and Kanaley, J.A. (2009) Longitudinal changes in abdominal fat distribution with menopause. *Metabolism: Clinical and Experimental*, 58(3), pp. 311–315. Available at: https://doi.org/10.1016/J.METABOL.2008.09.030.

Fréchou, M. *et al.* (2020) Dose-dependent and long-term cerebroprotective effects of intranasal delivery of progesterone after ischemic stroke in male mice. *Neuropharmacology*, 170, p. 108038. Available at: https://doi.org/10.1016/j.neuropharm.2020.108038.

Fréchou, M. *et al.* (2021) Sex differences in the cerebroprotection by Nestorone intranasal delivery following stroke in mice. *Neuropharmacology*, 198, p. 108760. Available at: https://doi.org/10.1016/j.neuropharm.2021.108760.

Freedman, R.R. (2014) Menopausal hot flashes: Mechanisms, endocrinology, treatment. *The Journal of Steroid Biochemistry and Molecular Biology*, 142, pp. 115–120. Available at: https://doi.org/10.1016/J.JSBMB.2013.08.010.

Freedman, R.R. *et al.* (2006) Cortical activation during menopausal hot flashes. *Fertility and Sterility*, 85(3), pp. 674–678. Available at: https://doi.org/10.1016/J.FERTNSTERT.2005.08.026.

Freeman, E.W. (2015) Depression in the menopause transition: Risks in the changing hormone milieu as observed in the general population. *Women's Midlife Health*, 1(1). Available at: https://doi.org/10.1186/S40695-015-0002-Y.

Freeman, M.E. *et al.* (2000) Prolactin: Structure, function, and regulation of secretion. *Physiological*

Reviews, 80(4), pp. 1523–1631. Available at: https://doi.org/10.1152/physrev.2000.80.4.1523.

Fuss, J. *et al.* (2019) Does sex hormone treatment reverse the sex-dependent stress regulation? A longitudinal study on hypothalamus-pituitary-adrenal (HPA) axis activity in transgender individuals. *Psychoneuroendocrinology*, 104, pp. 228–237. Available at: https://doi.org/10.1016/J.PSYNEUEN.2019.02.023.

Gallicchio, L. *et al.* (2005) Body mass, estrogen levels, and hot flashes in midlife women. *American Journal of Obstetrics and Gynecology*, 193(4), pp. 1353–1360. Available at: https://doi.org/10.1016/J.AJOG.2005.04.001.

Gallicchio, L. *et al.* (2006) Cigarette smoking, estrogen levels, and hot flashes in midlife women. *Maturitas*, 53(2), pp. 133–143. Available at: https://doi.org/10.1016/J.MATURITAS.2005.03.007.

Gangestad, S.W., Caldwell Hooper, A.E. and Eaton, M.A. (2012) On the function of placental corticotropin-releasing hormone: A role in maternal-fetal conflicts over blood glucose concentrations. *Biological Reviews of the Cambridge Philosophical Society*, 87(4), pp. 856–873. Available at: https://doi.org/10.1111/J.1469-185X.2012.00226.X.

Gangestad, S.W. and Dinh, T. (2022) Women's estrus and extended sexuality: Reflections on empirical patterns and fundamental theoretical issues. *Frontiers in Psychology*, 13, p. 900737. Available at: https://doi.org/10.3389/fpsyg.2022.900737.

Gangestad, S.W. and Thornhill, R. (2008) Human oestrus. *Proceedings. Biological Sciences*, 275(1638), pp. 991–1000. Available at: https://doi.org/10.1098/rspb.2007.1425.

Gariépy, G., Honkaniemi, H. and Quesnel-Vallée, A. (2016) Social support and protection from depression: Systematic review of current findings in Western countries. *The British Journal of Psychiatry: The Journal of Mental Science*, 209(4), pp. 284–293. Available at: https://doi.org/10.1192/BJP.BP.115.169094.

Gavin, N.I. *et al.* (2005) Perinatal depression: A systematic review of prevalence and incidence. *Obstetrics & Gynecology*, 106(5 Pt 1), pp. 1071–1083. Available at: https://doi.org/10.1097/01.aog.0000183597.31630.db.

Gavrilov, S.G. (2017) Vulvar varicosities: Diagnosis, treatment, and prevention. *International Journal of Women's Health*, 9, pp. 463–475. Available at: https://doi.org/10.2147/IJWH.S126165.

Gehlert, S. *et al.* (2009) The prevalence of premenstrual dysphoric disorder in a randomly selected group of urban and rural women. *Psychological Medicine*, 39(1), pp. 129–136. Available at: https://doi.org/10.1017/S003329170800322X.

Georgakis, M.K. *et al.* (2016) Association of age at menopause and duration of reproductive period with depression after menopause: A systematic review and meta-analysis. *JAMA Psychiatry*, 73(2), pp. 139–149. Available at: https://doi.org/10.1001/JAMAPSYCHIATRY.2015.2653.

Geraci, A. *et al.* (2021) Sarcopenia and menopause: The role of estradiol. *Frontiers in Endocrinology*, 12. Available at: https://doi.org/10.3389/FENDO.2021.682012.

Getahun, D. *et al.* (2018) Cross-sex hormones and acute cardiovascular events in transgender persons: A cohort study. *Annals of Internal Medicine*, 169(4), pp. 205–213. Available at: https://doi.org/10.7326/M17-2785.

Gharahdaghi, N. *et al.* (2020) Links between testosterone, oestrogen, and the growth hormone/insulin-like growth factor axis and resistance exercise muscle adaptations. *Frontiers in Physiology*, 11, p. 621226. Available at: https://doi.org/10.3389/fphys.2020.621226.

Ghoumari, A.M. *et al.* (2020) Roles of progesterone, testosterone and their nuclear receptors in central nervous system myelination and remyelination. *International Journal of Molecular Sciences*, 21(9). Available at: https://doi.org/10.3390/ijms21093163.

Gibbs, J.C. *et al.* (2014) Low bone density risk is higher in exercising women with multiple triad risk factors. *Medicine & Science in Sports & Exercise*, 46(1), pp. 167–176. Available at: https://doi.org/10.1249/mss.0b013e3182a03b8b.

Giersch, G.E.W. *et al.* (2020) Fluid balance and hydration considerations for women: Review and future directions. *Sports Medicine*, 50(2), pp. 253–261. Available at: https://doi.org/10.1007/S40279-019-01206-6.

Gilson, G.J. *et al.* (1997) Changes in hemodynamics, ventricular remodeling, and ventricular contractility during normal pregnancy: A longitudinal study. *Obstetrics and Gynecology*, 89(6), pp. 957–962. Available at: https://doi.org/10.1016/S0029-7844(97)85765-1.

Gimunová, M. *et al.* (2022) The prevalence of menstrual cycle disorders in female athletes from different sports disciplines: A rapid review. *International Journal of Environmental Research and Public Health*, 19(21). Available at: https://doi.org/10.3390/IJERPH192114243.

Girard, O., Brocherie, F. and Bishop, D.J. (2015) Sprint performance under heat stress: A review. *Scandinavian Journal of Medicine and Science in Sports*, 25(S1), pp. 79–89. Available at: https://doi.org/10.1111/SMS.12437.

Gluppe, S., Engh, M.E. and Bø, K. (2021) What is the evidence for abdominal and pelvic floor muscle training to treat diastasis recti abdominis postpartum? A systematic review with meta-analysis. *Brazilian Journal of Physical Therapy*, 25(6), pp. 664–675. Available at: https://doi.org/10.1016/j.bjpt.2021.06.006.

Golden, N.H. and Carlson, J.L. (2008) The pathophysiology of amenorrhea in the adolescent. *Annals of* the New York Academy of Sciences, 1135, pp. 163–178. Available at: https://doi.org/10.1196/annals.1429.014.

Goldsmith, L.T. and Weiss, G. (2009) Relaxin in human pregnancy. Annals of the New York Academy of Sciences, 1160, pp. 130–135. Available at: https://doi.org/10.1111/J.1749-6632.2008.03800.X.

Goldštajn, M.Š. et al. (2023) Effects of transdermal versus oral hormone replacement therapy in postmenopause: A systematic review. Archives of Gynecology and Obstetrics, 307(6), pp. 1727–1745. Available at: https://doi.org/10.1007/S00404-022-06647-5.

Gordon, D. et al. (2013) The effects of menstrual cycle phase on the development of peak torque under isokinetic conditions. Isokinetics and Exercise Science, 21(4), pp. 285–291. Available at: https://doi.org/10.3233/IES-130499.

Gordon, J.L. et al. (2019) Estradiol fluctuation, sensitivity to stress, and depressive symptoms in the menopause transition: A pilot study. Frontiers in Psychology, 10(JUN). Available at: https://doi.org/10.3389/FPSYG.2019.01319.

Gooren, L.J., Giltay, E.J. and Bunck, M.C. (2008) Long-term treatment of transsexuals with cross-sex hormones: Extensive personal experience. Journal of Clinical Endocrinology & Metabolism, 93(1), pp. 19–25. doi: 10.1210/jc.2007-1809.

Gracia, C.R. et al. (2009) Allopregnanolone levels before and after selective serotonin reuptake inhibitor treatment of premenstrual symptoms. Journal of Clinical Psychopharmacology, 29(4), pp. 403–405. Available at: https://doi.org/10.1097/JCP.0B013E3181AD8825.

Grandner, M.A. et al. (2015) Insomnia symptoms predict physical and mental impairments among postmenopausal women. Sleep Medicine, 16(3), pp. 317–318. Available at: https://doi.org/10.1016/J.SLEEP.2015.01.002.

Gray, A.M., Gugala, Z. and Baillargeon, J.G. (2016) Effects of oral contraceptive use on anterior cruciate ligament injury epidemiology. Medicine & Science in Sports & Exercise, 48(4), pp. 648–654. Available at: https://doi.org/10.1249/MSS.0000000000000806.

Green, S.M. et al. (2019) Cognitive behavior therapy for menopausal symptoms (CBT-Meno): A randomized controlled trial. Menopause (New York, N.Y.), 26(9), pp. 972–980. Available at: https://doi.org/10.1097/GME.0000000000001363.

Greenhall, M. et al. (2021) Influence of the menstrual cycle phase on marathon performance in recreational runners. International Journal of Sports Physiology and Performance, 16(4), pp. 601–604. Available at: https://doi.org/10.1123/IJSPP.2020-0238.

Grieve, R. et al. (2022) The effects of foam rolling on ankle dorsiflexion range of motion in healthy adults: A systematic literature review. Journal of Bodywork and Movement Therapies, 30, pp. 53–59. Available at: https://doi.org/10.1016/J.JBMT.2022.01.006.

Grimes, C. et al. (2023) Postreproductive female killer whales reduce socially inflicted injuries in their male offspring. Current Biology, 33(15), pp. 3250–3256.e4. Available at: https://doi.org/10.1016/J.CUB.2023.06.039.

Gröpel, P. and Mesagno, C. (2019) Choking interventions in sports: A systematic review. International Review of Sport and Exercise Psychology, 12(1), pp. 176–201. Available at: https://doi.org/10.1080/1750984X.2017.1408134.

Gu, Y. et al. (2022) Life modifications and PCOS: Old story but new tales. Frontiers in Endocrinology, 13. Available at: https://doi.org/10.3389/FENDO.2022.808898.

Ha, B. et al. (2023) Effects of nonpharmacological interventions on sleep quality and insomnia in perimenopausal and postmenopausal women: A meta-analysis. Healthcare, 11(3). Available at: https://doi.org/10.3390/HEALTHCARE11030327.

Haakstad, L.A.H. and Bø, K. (2011) Effect of regular exercise on prevention of excessive weight gain in pregnancy: A randomised controlled trial. European Journal of Contraception and Reproductive Health Care, 16(2), pp. 116–125. Available at: https://doi.org/10.3109/13625187.2011.560307.

Haisenleder, D.J. et al. (1991) A pulsatile gonadotropin-releasing hormone stimulus is required to increase transcription of the gonadotropin subunit genes: Evidence for differential regulation of transcription by pulse frequency in vivo. Endocrinology, 128(1), pp. 509–517. Available at: https://doi.org/10.1210/ENDO-128-1-509.

Hale, G.E. et al. (2007) Endocrine features of menstrual cycles in middle and late reproductive age and the menopausal transition classified according to the Staging of Reproductive Aging Workshop (STRAW) staging system. Journal of Clinical Endocrinology and Metabolism, 92(8), pp. 3060–3067. Available at: https://doi.org/10.1210/JC.2007-0066.

Hale, G.E. et al. (2009) Atypical estradiol secretion and ovulation patterns caused by luteal out-of-phase (LOOP) events underlying irregular ovulatory menstrual cycles in the menopausal transition. Menopause (New York, N.Y.), 16(1), pp. 50–59. Available at: https://doi.org/10.1097/GME.0B013E31817EE0C2.

Hale, G.E. and Burger, H.G. (2009) Hormonal changes and biomarkers in late reproductive age, menopausal transition and menopause. Best Practice and Research: Clinical Obstetrics and Gynaecology, 23(1), pp. 7–23. Available at: https://doi.org/10.1016/J.BPOBGYN.2008.10.001.

Hale, G.E., Robertson, D.M. and Burger, H.G. (2014) The perimenopausal woman: Endocrinology and management. Journal of Steroid Biochemistry and

Molecular Biology, 142, pp. 121-131. Available at: https://doi.org/10.1016/J.JSBMB.2013.08.015.

Hall, H.R. and Jolly, K. (2014) Women's use of complementary and alternative medicines during pregnancy: A cross-sectional study. *Midwifery*, 30(5), pp. 499-505. Available at: https://doi.org/10.1016/J.MIDW.2013.06.001.

Hall, K.D. (2017) A review of the carbohydrate–insulin model of obesity. *European Journal of Clinical Nutrition*, 71(3), pp. 323-326. Available at: https://doi.org/10.1038/ejcn.2016.260.

Hamidovic, A. *et al.* (2020) Higher circulating cortisol in the follicular vs. luteal phase of the menstrual cycle: A meta-analysis. *Frontiers in Endocrinology*, 11, pp. 1-12. Available at: https://doi.org/10.3389/FENDO.2020.00311.

Handy, A.B. *et al.* (2023) Reduction in genital sexual arousal varies by type of oral contraceptive pill. *The Journal of Sexual Medicine*, 20(8), pp. 1094-1102. Available at: https://doi.org/10.1093/JSXMED/QDAD072.

Hansen, K.R. *et al.* (2008) A new model of reproductive aging: The decline in ovarian non-growing follicle number from birth to menopause. *Human Reproduction (Oxford, England)*, 23(3), pp. 699-708. Available at: https://doi.org/10.1093/HUMREP/DEM408.

Hansen, M. *et al.* (2008) Ethinyl oestradiol administration in women suppresses synthesis of collagen in tendon in response to exercise. *The Journal of Physiology*, 586(12), pp. 3005-3016. Available at: https://doi.org/10.1113/JPHYSIOL.2007.147348.

Hansen, M. *et al.* (2011) Effect of administration of oral contraceptives on the synthesis and breakdown of myofibrillar proteins in young women. *Scandinavian Journal of Medicine and Science in Sports*, 21(1), pp. 62-72. Available at: https://doi.org/10.1111/J.1600-0838.2009.01002.X.

Hansen, M. and Kjaer, M. (2014) Influence of sex and estrogen on musculotendinous protein turnover at rest and after exercise. *Exercise and Sport Sciences Reviews*, 42(4), pp. 183-192. Available at: https://doi.org/10.1249/JES.0000000000000026.

Hantsoo, L. and Epperson, C.N. (2020) Allopregnanolone in premenstrual dysphoric disorder (PMDD): Evidence for dysregulated sensitivity to GABA-A receptor modulating neuroactive steroids across the menstrual cycle. *Neurobiology of Stress*, 12. Available at: https://doi.org/10.1016/J.YNSTR.2020.100213.

Hardy, C. *et al.* (2018) Self-help cognitive behavior therapy for working women with problematic hot flushes and night sweats (MENOS@Work): A multicenter randomized controlled trial. *Menopause (New York, N.Y.)*, 25(5), pp. 508-519. Available at: https://doi.org/10.1097/GME.0000000000001048.

Harlow, S.D. (2000) Menstruation and Menstrual Disorders: The Epidemiology of Menstruation and Menstrual Dysfunction. In M. Goldman and M. Hatch (eds), *Women and Health*. San Diego, CA: Academic Press, pp. 99-113.

Harlow, S.D. *et al.* (2012) Executive summary of the Stages of Reproductive Aging Workshop + 10: Addressing the unfinished agenda of staging reproductive aging. *Menopause (New York, N.Y.)*, 19(4), pp. 387-395. Available at: https://doi.org/10.1097/GME.0B013E31824D8F40.

Harlow, S.D. and Ephross, S.A. (1995) Epidemiology of menstruation and its relevance to women's health. *Epidemiologic Reviews*, 17(2), pp. 265-286. Available at: https://doi.org/10.1093/oxfordjournals.epirev.a036193.

Hawkins, S.M. and Matzuk, M.M. (2008) The menstrual cycle: Basic biology. *Annals of the New York Academy of Sciences*, 1135, pp. 10-18. Available at: https://doi.org/10.1196/annals.1429.018.

Heck, A.L. and Handa, R.J. (2019) Sex differences in the hypothalamic–pituitary–adrenal axis' response to stress: An important role for gonadal hormones. *Neuropsychopharmacology*, 44(1), pp. 45-58. Available at: https://doi.org/10.1038/S41386-018-0167-9.

Heenan, A.P. and Wolfe, L.A. (2000) Plasma acid-base regulation above and below ventilatory threshold in late gestation. *Journal of Applied Physiology (Bethesda, Md.: 1985)*, 88(1), pp. 149-157. Available at: https://doi.org/10.1152/JAPPL.2000.88.1.149.

Heeren, A. and Philippot, P. (2011) Changes in ruminative thinking mediate the clinical benefits of mindfulness: Preliminary findings. *Mindfulness*, 2(1), pp. 8-13. Available at: https://doi.org/10.1007/S12671-010-0037-Y.

Heim, C. and Binder, E.B. (2012) Current research trends in early life stress and depression: Review of human studies on sensitive periods, gene-environment interactions, and epigenetics. *Experimental Neurology*, 233(1), pp. 102-111. Available at: https://doi.org/10.1016/J.EXPNEUROL.2011.10.032.

Heldring, N. *et al.* (2007) Estrogen receptors: How do they signal and what are their targets. *Physiological Reviews*, 87(3), pp. 905-931. Available at: https://doi.org/10.1152/physrev.00026.2006.

Hendrick, V., Altshuler, L.L. and Suri, R. (1998) Hormonal changes in the postpartum and implications for postpartum depression. *Psychosomatics*, 39(2), pp. 93-101. Available at: https://doi.org/10.1016/S0033-3182(98)71355-6.

Hendricks, S. *et al.* (2020) Effects of foam rolling on performance and recovery: A systematic review of the literature to guide practitioners on the use of foam rolling. *Journal of Bodywork and Movement*

Therapies, 24(2), pp. 151–174. Available at: https://doi.org/10.1016/j.jbmt.2019.10.019.

Herber-Gast, G.C.M. and Mishra, G.D. (2013) Fruit, Mediterranean-style, and high-fat and -sugar diets are associated with the risk of night sweats and hot flushes in midlife: Results from a prospective cohort study. *The American Journal of Clinical Nutrition*, 97(5), pp. 1092–1099. Available at: https://doi.org/10.3945/AJCN.112.049965.

Herman, J.P. *et al.* (2003) Central mechanisms of stress integration: Hierarchical circuitry controlling hypothalamo-pituitary-adrenocortical responsiveness. *Frontiers in Neuroendocrinology*, 24(3), pp. 151–180. Available at: https://doi.org/10.1016/J.YFRNE.2003.07.001.

Hermesch, A.C. *et al.* (2024) Oxytocin: Physiology, pharmacology, and clinical application for labor management. *American Journal of Obstetrics and Gynecology*, 230(3S), pp. S729–S739. Available at: https://doi.org/10.1016/J.AJOG.2023.06.041.

Herzberg, S.D. *et al.* (2017) The effect of menstrual cycle and contraceptives on ACL injuries and laxity: A systematic review and meta-analysis. *Orthopaedic Journal of Sports Medicine*, 5(7). Available at: https://doi.org/10.1177/2325967117718781.

Hickey, M. *et al.* (2024) An empowerment model for managing menopause. *Lancet (London, England)*, 403(10430), pp. 947–957. Available at: https://doi.org/10.1016/S0140-6736(23)02799-X.

Himelein, M.J. and Thatcher, S.S. (2006) Depression and body image among women with polycystic ovary syndrome. *Journal of Health Psychology*, 11(4), pp. 613–625. Available at: https://doi.org/10.1177/1359105306065021.

Hirshfield, A.N. (1997) Overview of ovarian follicular development: Considerations for the toxicologist. *Environmental and Molecular Mutagenesis*, 29(1), pp. 10–15.

Hoffkling, A., Obedin-Maliver, J. and Sevelius, J. (2017) From erasure to opportunity: A qualitative study of the experiences of transgender men around pregnancy and recommendations for providers. *BMC Pregnancy and Childbirth*, 17(Suppl 2). Available at: https://doi.org/10.1186/S12884-017-1491-5.

Hoffman, J.R. *et al.* (2009) Position stand on androgen and human growth hormone use. *Journal of Strength and Conditioning Research*, 23(5 Suppl), pp. S1–S59. Available at: https://doi.org/10.1519/JSC.0b013e31819df2e6.

Holmes, G.B. and Lin, J. (2006) Etiologic factors associated with symptomatic Achilles tendinopathy. *Foot & Ankle International*, 27(11), pp. 952–959. Available at: https://doi.org/10.1177/107110070602701115.

Holmes, K. *et al.* (2021) Adolescent menstrual health literacy in low, middle and high-income countries: A narrative review. *International Journal of Environmental Research and Public Health*, 18(5). Available at: https://doi.org/10.3390/ijerph18052260.

Hopper, S.I. *et al.* (2019) Effectiveness of diaphragmatic breathing for reducing physiological and psychological stress in adults: A quantitative systematic review. *JBI Database of Systematic Reviews and Implementation Reports*, 17(9), pp. 1855–1876. Available at: https://doi.org/10.11124/JBISRIR-2017-003848.

Hoyenga, K.B. and Hoyenga, K.T. (1982) Gender and energy balance: Sex differences in adaptations for feast and famine. *Physiology & Behavior*, 28(3), pp. 545–563. Available at: https://doi.org/10.1016/0031-9384(82)90153-6.

Huang, A.J. *et al.* (2010) An intensive behavioral weight loss intervention and hot flushes in women. *Archives of Internal Medicine*, 170(13), pp. 1161–1167. Available at: https://doi.org/10.1001/ARCHINTERNMED.2010.162.

Hughes, G.A. and Ramer, L.M. (2019) Duration of myofascial rolling for optimal recovery, range of motion, and performance: A systematic review of the literature. *International Journal of Sports Physical Therapy*, 14(6), pp. 845–859.

Hughesdon, P.E. (1982) Morphology and morphogenesis of the Stein-Leventhal ovary and of so-called "hyperthecosis." *Obstetrical & Gynecological Survey*, 37(2), pp. 59–77. Available at: https://doi.org/10.1097/00006254-198202000-00001.

Hunter, M. and Rendall, M. (2007) Bio-psycho-socio-cultural perspectives on menopause. *Best Practice & Research Clinical Obstetrics & Gynaecology*, 21(2), pp. 261–274. Available at: https://doi.org/10.1016/J.BPOBGYN.2006.11.001.

Hunter, M.S. *et al.* (2002) A randomized comparison of psychological (cognitive behavior therapy), medical (fluoxetine) and combined treatment for women with premenstrual dysphoric disorder. *Journal of Psychosomatic Obstetrics and Gynaecology*, 23(3), pp. 193–199. Available at: https://doi.org/10.3109/01674820209074672.

Hutchins, K.P. *et al.* (2021) Female (under) representation in exercise thermoregulation research. *Sports Medicine—Open*, 7(1). Available at: https://doi.org/10.1186/S40798-021-00334-6.

Hylan, T.R., Sundell, K. and Judge, R. (1999) The impact of premenstrual symptomatology on functioning and treatment-seeking behavior: Experience from the United States, United Kingdom, and France. *Journal of Women's Health and Gender-Based Medicine*, 8(8), pp. 1043–1052. Available at: https://doi.org/10.1089/JWH.1.1999.8.1043.

Ibrahim, S., Jarefors, E., Nel, D.G., Vollmer, L., Groenewald, C.A. and Odendaal, H.J. (2015) Effect of maternal position and uterine activity on periodic maternal heart rate changes before elective cesarean section at term. *Acta Obstetrica et Gynecologica Scandinavica*, 94(12), pp. 1359–1366. doi: 10.1111/aogs.12763.

Inge, P. *et al.* (2022) Exercise after pregnancy. *Australian Journal of General Practice*, 51(3), pp. 117–121. Available at: https://doi.org/10.31128/AJGP-09-21-6181.

Islam, H. *et al.* (2022) An update on polycystic ovary syndrome: A review of the current state of knowledge in diagnosis, genetic etiology, and emerging treatment options. *Women's Health*, 18. Available at: https://pubmed.ncbi.nlm.nih.gov/35972046.

Itriyeva, K. (2022) The normal menstrual cycle. *Current Problems in Pediatric and Adolescent Health Care*, 52(5), p. 101183. Available at: https://doi.org/10.1016/j.cppeds.2022.101183.

Jacobson, B.H. and Lentz, W. (1998) Perception of physical variables during four phases of the menstrual cycle. *Perceptual and Motor Skills*, 87(2), pp. 565–566. doi: 10.2466/pms.1998.87.2.565.

Jagadeesh, N. *et al.* (2021) Risk factors of ACL injury. *Arthroscopy* [Preprint]. Available at: https://doi.org/10.5772/INTECHOPEN.99952.

Jain, S. *et al.* (2007) A randomized controlled trial of mindfulness meditation versus relaxation training: Effects on distress, positive states of mind, rumination, and distraction. *Annals of Behavioral Medicine*, 33(1), pp. 11–21. doi: 10.1207/s15324796abm3301_2.

James, A.H. *et al.* (2009) Von Willebrand disease and other bleeding disorders in women: Consensus on diagnosis and management from an international expert panel. *American Journal of Obstetrics and Gynecology*, 201(1), pp. 12.e1–12.e8. Available at: https://doi.org/10.1016/J.AJOG.2009.04.024.

James, A.H. *et al.* (2011) Evaluation and management of acute menorrhagia in women with and without underlying bleeding disorders: Consensus from an international expert panel. *European Journal of Obstetrics & Gynecology and Reproductive Biology*, 158(2), pp. 124–134. Available at: https://doi.org/10.1016/J.EJOGRB.2011.04.025.

Janse De Jonge, X., Thompson, B. and Han, A. (2019) Methodological recommendations for menstrual cycle research in sports and exercise. *Medicine & Science in Sports & Exercise*, 51(12), pp. 2610–2617. Available at: https://doi.org/10.1249/MSS.0000000000002073.

Janse De Jonge, X.A.K. (2003) Effects of the menstrual cycle on exercise performance. *Sports Medicine*, 33(11), pp. 833–851. Available at: https://doi.org/10.2165/00007256-200333110-00004.

Janse De Jonge, X.A.K. *et al.* (2012) Exercise performance over the menstrual cycle in temperate and hot, humid conditions. *Medicine & Science in Sports &*

Exercise, 44(11), pp. 2190–2198. Available at: https://doi.org/10.1249/MSS.0B013E3182656F13.

Janssen, I. *et al.* (2015) Variations in jump height explain the between-sex difference in patellar tendon loading during landing. *Scandinavian Journal of Medicine & Science in Sports*, 25(2), pp. 265–272. Available at: https://doi.org/10.1111/SMS.12172.

Jarrell, J. (2018) The significance and evolution of menstruation. *Best Practice & Research. Clinical Obstetrics & Gynaecology*, 50, pp. 18–26. Available at: https://doi.org/10.1016/J.BPOBGYN.2018.01.007.

Javert, C.T. (1952) The spread of benign and malignant endometrium in the lymphatic system with a note on coexisting vascular involvement. *American Journal of Obstetrics and Gynecology*, 64(4), pp. 780–806. Available at: https://doi.org/10.1016/S0002-9378(16)38796-8.

Jeffreys, R.M., Stepanchak, W., Lopez, B., Hardis, J. and Clapp, J.F. 3rd. (2006) Uterine blood flow during supine rest and exercise after 28 weeks of gestation. *BJOG*, 113(11), pp. 1239–1247. doi: 10.1111/j.1471-0528.2006.01056.x.

Jensen, M.D. and Levine, J. (1998) Effects of oral contraceptives on free fatty acid metabolism in women. *Metabolism: Clinical and Experimental*, 47(3), pp. 280–284. Available at: https://doi.org/10.1016/S0026-0495(98)90257-8.

Jerman, L.F. and Hey-Cunningham, A.J. (2015) The role of the lymphatic system in endometriosis: A comprehensive review of the literature. *Biology of Reproduction*, 92(3). Available at: https://doi.org/10.1095/BIOLREPROD.114.124313.

JF, C. (2009) Is exercise during pregnancy related to preterm birth? *Clinical Journal of Sport Medicine: Official Journal of the Canadian Academy of Sport Medicine*, 19(3), p. 241. Available at: https://doi.org/10.1097/JSM.0B013E3181A5FBFA.

Ji, M.-X. and Yu, Q. (2015) Primary osteoporosis in postmenopausal women. *Chronic Diseases and Translational Medicine*, 1(1), p. 9. Available at: https://doi.org/10.1016/J.CDTM.2015.02.006.

Jones, E.E. (1995) Androgenic effects of oral contraceptives: Implications for patient compliance. *The American Journal of Medicine*, 98(1A). Available at: https://doi.org/10.1016/S0002-9343(99)80069-2.

Jose, A. *et al.* (2022) Impact of relaxation therapy on premenstrual symptoms: A systematic review. *Journal of Education and Health Promotion*, 11(1). Available at: https://doi.org/10.4103/JEHP.JEHP_586_22.

Joshi, A.M., Raveendran, A.V. and Arumugam, M. (2024) Therapeutic role of yoga in hypertension. *World Journal of Methodology*, 14(1). Available at: https://doi.org/10.5662/WJM.V14.I1.90127.

Joswig, M. *et al.* (1999) Postmenopausal hormone replacement therapy and the vascular wall: Mechanisms of

17 beta-estradiol's effects on vascular biology. *Experimental and Clinical Endocrinology & Diabetes: Official Journal, German Society of Endocrinology [and] German Diabetes Association*, 107(8), pp. 477–487. Available at: https://doi.org/10.1055/S-0029-1232556.

Jubanyik, K.J. and Comite, F. (1997) Extrapelvic endometriosis. *Obstetrics and Gynecology Clinics of North America*, 24(2), pp. 411–440. Available at: https://doi.org/10.1016/S0889-8545(05)70311-9.

Julian, R. *et al.* (2017) The effects of menstrual cycle phase on physical performance in female soccer players. *PLOS One*, 12(3). Available at: https://doi.org/10.1371/JOURNAL.PONE.0173951.

Kadian, S. and O'Brien, S. (2012) Classification of premenstrual disorders as proposed by the International Society for Premenstrual Disorders. *Menopause International*, 18(2), pp. 43–47. Available at: https://doi.org/10.1258/Ml.2012.012017.

Kalra, S. *et al.* (2022) Impact of physical activity on physical and mental health of postmenopausal women: A systematic review. *Journal of Clinical and Diagnostic Research* [Preprint]. Available at: https://doi.org/10.7860/JCDR/2022/52302.15974.

Kanbour, S.A. and Dobs, A.S. (2022) Hyperandrogenism in women with polycystic ovarian syndrome: Pathophysiology and controversies. *Androgens*, 3(1), pp. 22–30. Available at: https://doi.org/10.1089/andro.2021.0020.

Karvonen-Gutierrez, C. and Kim, C. (2016) Association of mid-life changes in body size, body composition and obesity status with the menopausal transition. *Healthcare (Basel, Switzerland)*, 4(3). Available at: https://doi.org/10.3390/HEALTHCARE4030042.

Kelsey, T.W. *et al.* (2011) A validated model of serum anti-Müllerian hormone from conception to menopause. *PLOS One*, 6(7). Available at: https://doi.org/10.1371/JOURNAL.PONE.0022024.

Kerin, J. (1982) Ovulation detection in the human. *Clinical Reproduction and Fertility*, pp. 27–54.

Kerksick, C.M. and Leutholtz, B. (2005) Nutrient administration and resistance training. *Journal of the International Society of Sports Nutrition*, 2(1). Available at: https://doi.org/10.1186/1550-2783-2-1-50.

Khadilkar, S.S. (2019) Musculoskeletal disorders and menopause. *Journal of Obstetrics and Gynecology of India*, 69(2), pp. 99–103. Available at: https://doi.org/10.1007/S13224-019-01213-7.

Khalafi, M. *et al.* (2023) Influence of exercise type and duration on cardiorespiratory fitness and muscular strength in post-menopausal women: A systematic review and meta-analysis. *Frontiers in Cardiovascular Medicine*, 10. Available at: https://doi.org/10.3389/FCVM.2023.1190187.

Khan-Dawood, F.S. *et al.* (1989) Human corpus luteum secretion of relaxin, oxytocin, and progesterone. *The Journal of Clinical Endocrinology and Metabolism*, 68(3), pp. 627–631. Available at: https://doi.org/10.1210/jcem-68-3-627.

Kim, J.J. *et al.* (2019) Prevalence of insulin resistance in Korean women with polycystic ovary syndrome according to various homeostasis model assessment for insulin resistance cutoff values. *Fertility and Sterility*, 112(5), pp. 959–966.e1. Available at: https://doi.org/10.1016/J.FERTNSTERT.2019.06.035.

Kimm, S.Y.S. *et al.* (2001) Effects of race, cigarette smoking, and use of contraceptive medications on resting energy expenditure in young women. *American Journal of Epidemiology*, 154(8), pp. 718–724. Available at: https://doi.org/10.1093/AJE/154.8.718.

Kingsberg, S.A. *et al.* (2023) Global view of vasomotor symptoms and sleep disturbance in menopause: A systematic review. *Climacteric: Journal of the International Menopause Society*, 26(6), pp. 537–549. Available at: https://doi.org/10.1080/13697137.2023.2256658.

Kingston, T. *et al.* (2007) Mindfulness-based cognitive therapy for residual depressive symptoms. *Psychology and Psychotherapy: Theory, Research and Practice*, 80(2), pp. 193–203. Available at: https://doi.org/10.1348/147608306X116016.

Kishali, N.F., Kiyici, F., Burmaoglu, G., Tas, M., Paktas, Y. and Ertan, F. (2010) Some performance parameter changes during menstrual cycle periods of athletes and non-athletes. *Ovidius University Annals, Series Physical Education and Sport/Science, Movement and Health*, 10(1), pp. 46+. https://link.gale.com/apps/doc/A234570222/AONE?u=anon~202b4674&sid=googleScholar&xid=86513dfd.

Kissow, J. *et al.* (2022) Effects of follicular and luteal phase-based menstrual cycle resistance training on muscle strength and mass. *Sports Medicine*, 52(12), pp. 2813–2819. Available at: https://doi.org/10.1007/S40279-022-01679-Y/FIGURES/3.

Kitajima, Y. and Ono, Y. (2016) Estrogens maintain skeletal muscle and satellite cell functions. *Journal of Endocrinology*, 229(3), pp. 267–275. Available at: https://doi.org/10.1530/JOE-15-0476.

Klein, D.A., Paradise, S.L. and Reeder, R.M. (2019) Amenorrhea: A systematic approach to diagnosis and management. *American Family Physician*, 100(1), pp. 39–48. Available at: www.aafp.org/pubs/afp/issues/2019/0701/p39.html (Accessed: 23 August 2024).

Klein, N.A. *et al.* (2002) Is the short follicular phase in older women secondary to advanced or accelerated dominant follicle development? *The Journal of Clinical Endocrinology and Metabolism*, 87(12), pp. 5746–5750. Available at: https://doi.org/10.1210/JC.2002-020622.

Kloss, J.D., Tweedy, K. and Gilrain, K. (2004) Psychological factors associated with sleep disturbance among perimenopausal women. *Behavioral Sleep Medicine*, 2(4), pp. 177–190. Available at: https://doi.org/10.1207/S15402010BSM0204_1.

Klusmann, H. et al. (2022) HPA axis activity across the menstrual cycle: A systematic review and meta-analysis of longitudinal studies. *Frontiers in Neuroendocrinology*, 66. Available at: https://doi.org/10.1016/J.YFRNE.2022.100998.

Klusmann, H. et al. (2023) Menstrual cycle-related changes in HPA axis reactivity to acute psychosocial and physiological stressors: A systematic review and meta-analysis of longitudinal studies. *Neuroscience & Biobehavioral Reviews*, 150, p. 105212. Available at: https://doi.org/10.1016/J.NEUBIOREV.2023.105212.

Knight, M.G. et al. (2021) Weight regulation in menopause. *Menopause (New York, N.Y.)*, 28(8), pp. 960–965. Available at: https://doi.org/10.1097/GME.0000000000001792.

Ko, S.H. and Jung, Y. (2021) Energy metabolism changes and dysregulated lipid metabolism in postmenopausal women. *Nutrients*, 13(12). Available at: https://doi.org/10.3390/NU13124556.

Kodoth, V., Scaccia, S. and Aggarwal, B. (2022) Adverse changes in body composition during the menopausal transition and relation to cardiovascular risk: A contemporary review. *Women's Health Reports*, 3(1), p. 573. Available at: https://doi.org/10.1089/WHR.2021.0119.

Kolář, P. et al. (2009) Analysis of diaphragm movement during tidal breathing and during its activation while breath holding using MRI synchronized with spirometry. *Physiological Research*, 58(3), pp. 383–392. Available at: https://doi.org/10.33549/PHYSIOLRES.931376.

Kolte, A.M. et al. (2015) Depression and emotional stress is highly prevalent among women with recurrent pregnancy loss. *Human Reproduction (Oxford, England)*, 30(4), pp. 777–782. Available at: https://doi.org/10.1093/HUMREP/DEV014.

Konopka, J.A., Hsue, L.J. and Dragoo, J.L. (2019) Effect of oral contraceptives on soft tissue injury risk, soft tissue laxity, and muscle strength: A systematic review of the literature. *Orthopaedic Journal of Sports Medicine*, 7(3). Available at: https://doi.org/10.1177/2325967119831061.

Kovacs, C.S. and Ralston, S.H. (2015) Presentation and management of osteoporosis presenting in association with pregnancy or lactation. *Osteoporosis International*, 26(9), pp. 2223–2241. Available at: https://doi.org/10.1007/s00198-015-3149-3.

Kraemer, W.J. and Ratamess, N.A. (2005) Hormonal responses and adaptations to resistance exercise and training. *Sports Medicine (Auckland, N.Z.)*, 35(4), pp. 339–361. Available at: https://doi.org/10.2165/00007256-200535040-00004.

Kraemer, W.J., Ratamess, N.A. and Nindl, B.C. (2017) Recovery responses of testosterone, growth hormone, and IGF-1 after resistance exercise. *Journal of Applied Physiology (Bethesda, Md.: 1985)*, 122(3), pp. 549–558. Available at: https://doi.org/10.1152/japplphysiol.00599.2016.

Kraft, M.Z. et al. (2024) Symptoms of mental disorders and oral contraception use: A systematic review and meta-analysis. *Frontiers in Neuroendocrinology*, 72. Available at: https://doi.org/10.1016/J.YFRNE.2023.101111.

Kravitz, H.M. et al. (2008) Sleep disturbance during the menopausal transition in a multi-ethnic community sample of women. *Sleep*, 31(7), p. 979. Available at: https://doi.org/10.5665/sleep/31.7.979.

Kriengsinyos, W. et al. (2004) Phase of menstrual cycle affects lysine requirement in healthy women. *American Journal of Physiology: Endocrinology and Metabolism*, 287(3), 50–53. Available at: https://doi.org/10.1152/AJPENDO.00262.2003.

Kuhl, H. (2005) Breast cancer risk in the WHI study: The problem of obesity. *Maturitas*, 51(1), pp. 83–97. Available at: https://doi.org/10.1016/J.MATURITAS.2005.02.018.

Kwa, M. et al. (2016) The intestinal microbiome and estrogen receptor-positive female breast cancer. *Journal of the National Cancer Institute*, 108(8). Available at: https://doi.org/10.1093/JNCI/DJW029.

Kwon, R. et al. (2020) A systematic review: The effects of yoga on pregnancy. *European Journal of Obstetrics, Gynecology, and Reproductive Biology*, 250, pp. 171–177. Available at: https://doi.org/10.1016/J.EJOGRB.2020.03.044.

Lahey, B.B. et al. (1999) Developmental epidemiology of the disruptive behavior disorders. *Handbook of Disruptive Behavior Disorders*, pp. 23–48. Available at: https://doi.org/10.1007/978-1-4615-4881-2_2.

Lalioti, A. et al. (2024) Common misconceptions about diet and breast cancer: An unclear issue to dispel. *Cancers*, 16(2). Available at: https://doi.org/10.3390/CANCERS16020306.

Lamceva, J., Uljanovs, R. and Strumfa, I. (2023) The main theories on the pathogenesis of endometriosis. *International Journal of Molecular Sciences*, 24(5), p. 4254. Available at: https://doi.org/10.3390/IJMS24054254.

Lamont, L.S., Lemon, P.W.R. and Bruot, B.C. (1987) Menstrual cycle and exercise effects on protein catabolism. *Medicine & Science in Sports & Exercise*, 19(2), pp. 106–110. Available at: https://doi.org/10.1249/00005768-198704000-00007.

Langer, R.D. et al. (2021) Hormone replacement therapy—where are we now? *Climacteric*, 24(1), pp. 3–10.

Available at: https://doi.org/10.1080/13697137.2020.1851183.

Lankila, H. et al. (2024) Associations of menopausal status and eating behaviour with subjective measures of sleep. Journal of Sleep Research [Preprint]. Available at: https://doi.org/10.1111/JSR.14155.

Lantto, I. et al. (2015) Epidemiology of Achilles tendon ruptures: Increasing incidence over a 33-year period. Scandinavian Journal of Medicine & Science in Sports, 25(1), pp. e133–e138. Available at: https://doi.org/10.1111/SMS.12253.

Larson, A. et al. (2020) Oestradiol affects skeletal muscle mass, strength and satellite cells following repeated injuries. Experimental Physiology, 105, pp. 1700–1707.

Leaf, A. et al. (2024) International society of sports nutrition position stand: Ketogenic diets. Journal of the International Society of Sports Nutrition, 21(1). Available at: https://doi.org/10.1080/15502783.2024.2368167.

Lebrun, C.M. et al. (1995) Effects of menstrual cycle phase on athletic performance. Medicine and Science in Sports and Exercise, 27(3), pp. 437–444. Available at: https://doi.org/10.1249/00005768-199503000-00022.

Lebrun, C.M. et al. (2003) Decreased maximal aerobic capacity with use of a triphasic oral contraceptive in highly active women: A randomised controlled trial. British Journal of Sports Medicine, 37(4), pp. 315–320. Available at: https://doi.org/10.1136/BJSM.37.4.315.

Lefevre, N. et al. (2013) Anterior cruciate ligament tear during the menstrual cycle in female recreational skiers. Orthopaedics & Traumatology, Surgery & Research, 99(5), pp. 571–575. Available at: https://doi.org/10.1016/J.OTSR.2013.02.005.

Legerlotz, K. and Hansen, M. (2020) Editorial: Female Hormones: Effect on Musculoskeletal Adaptation and Injury Risk. Frontiers in Physiology, 11, p. 628. Available at: https://doi.org/10.3389/FPHYS.2020.00628.

Lewiecki, E.M. et al. (2016) Best practices for dual-energy x-ray absorptiometry measurement and reporting: International Society for Clinical Densitometry Guidance. Journal of Clinical Densitometry, 19(2), pp. 127–140. Available at: https://doi.org/10.1016/J.JOCD.2016.03.003.

Li, J. et al. (2024) Prevalence and associated factors of depression in postmenopausal women: A systematic review and meta-analysis. BMC Psychiatry, 24(1). Available at: https://doi.org/10.1186/S12888-024-05875-0.

Li, X. et al. (2023) Effect of pregnancy on female gait characteristics: A pilot study based on portable gait analyzer and induced acceleration analysis. Frontiers in Physiology, 14. Available at: https://doi.org/10.3389/FPHYS.2023.1034132.

Lian, Ø.B., Engebretsen, L. and Bahr, R. (2005) Prevalence of jumper's knee among elite athletes from different sports: A cross-sectional study. The American Journal of Sports Medicine, 33(4), pp. 561–567. Available at: https://doi.org/10.1177/0363546504270454.

Liang, G. et al. (2024) Menopause-associated depression: Impact of oxidative stress and neuroinflammation on the central nervous system: A review. Biomedicines, 12(1). Available at: https://doi.org/10.3390/BIOMEDICINES12010184.

Light, A.D. et al. (2014) Transgender men who experienced pregnancy after female-to-male gender transitioning. Obstetric Gynecology, 124(6), pp. 1120–1127. Available at: https://doi.org/10.1097/aog.0000000000000540.

Liguori, F., Saraiello, E. and Calella, P. (2023) Premenstrual syndrome and premenstrual dysphoric disorder's impact on quality of life, and the role of physical activity. Medicina (Kaunas, Lithuania), 59(11). Available at: https://doi.org/10.3390/MEDICINA59112044.

Lim, C.E.D. et al. (2019) Acupuncture for polycystic ovarian syndrome. The Cochrane Database of Systematic Reviews, 7(7). Available at: https://doi.org/10.1002/14651858.CD007689.PUB4.

Lin, S. et al. (2021) Does the weight loss efficacy of alternate day fasting differ according to sex and menopausal status? Nutrition, Metabolism, and Cardiovascular Diseases: NMCD, 31(2), pp. 641–649. Available at: https://doi.org/10.1016/J.NUMECD.2020.10.018.

Lindqvist, P.G. et al. (2003) Thermal response to submaximal exercise before, during and after pregnancy: A longitudinal study. The Journal of Maternal-Fetal & Neonatal Medicine: The Official Journal of the European Association of Perinatal Medicine, the Federation of Asia and Oceania Perinatal Societies, the International Society of Perinatal Obstetricians, 13(3), pp. 152–156. Available at: https://doi.org/10.1080/jmf.13.3.152.156.

Liu, Yang et al. (2019) Menopausal hormone replacement therapy and the risk of ovarian cancer: A meta-analysis. Frontiers in Endocrinology, 10, p. 801. Available at: https://doi.org/10.3389/FENDO.2019.00801/FULL.

Liu, Yanghui et al. (2019) Associations of Resistance Exercise with Cardiovascular Disease Morbidity and Mortality. Medicine & Science in Sports & Exercise, 51(3), pp. 499–508. Available at: https://doi.org/10.1249/MSS.0000000000001822.

Lizneva, D. et al. (2016) Criteria, prevalence, and phenotypes of polycystic ovary syndrome. Fertility and Sterility, 106, pp. 6–15.

Logue, C.M. and Moos, R.H. (1988) Positive perimenstrual changes: Toward a new perspective on the menstrual cycle. Journal of Psychosomatic

Research, 32(1), pp. 31–40. Available at: https://doi.org/10.1016/0022-3999(88)90086-4.

Long, J.L. *et al.* (2022) The more you know, the less you stress: Menstrual health literacy in schools reduces menstruation-related stress and increases self-efficacy for very young adolescent girls in Mexico. *Frontiers in Global Women's Health*, 3, p. 859797. Available at: https://doi.org/10.3389/fgwh.2022.859797.

Lontay, B. *et al.* (2015) Pregnancy and smoothelin-like protein 1 (SMTNL1) deletion promote the switching of skeletal muscle to a glycolytic phenotype in human and mice. *The Journal of Biological Chemistry*, 290(29), pp. 17985–17998. Available at: https://doi.org/10.1074/JBC.M115.658120.

Loucks, A.B. (2004) Energy balance and body composition in sports and exercise. *Journal of Sports Sciences*, 22(1), pp. 1–14. Available at: https://doi.org/10.1080/0264041031000140518.

Lovejoy, J.C. *et al.* (2008) Increased visceral fat and decreased energy expenditure during the menopausal transition. *International Journal of Obesity (2005)*, 32(6), pp. 949–958. Available at: https://doi.org/10.1038/IJO.2008.25.

Lovelady, C.A., Lonnerdal, B. and Dewey, K.G. (1990) Lactation performance of exercising women. *American Journal of Clinical Nutrition*, 52(1), pp. 103–109. Available at: https://doi.org/10.1093/ajcn/52.1.103.

Lowe, D.A., Baltgalvis, K.A. and Greising, S.M. (2010) Mechanisms behind estrogen's beneficial effect on muscle strength in females. *Exercise and Sport Sciences Reviews*, 38(2), pp. 61–67. Available at: https://doi.org/10.1097/JES.0B013E3181D496BC.

Lu, C.B. *et al.* (2020) Musculoskeletal pain during the menopausal transition: A systematic review and meta-analysis. *Neural Plasticity*, 2020. Available at: https://doi.org/10.1155/2020/8842110.

Ludwig, B., Roy, B. and Dwivedi, Y. (2019) Role of HPA and the HPG axis interaction in testosterone-mediated learned helpless behavior. *Molecular Neurobiology*, 56(1), pp. 394–405. Available at: https://doi.org/10.1007/S12035-018-1085-X.

Maccagnano, C. *et al.* (2013) Ureteral endometriosis: Proposal for a diagnostic and therapeutic algorithm with a review of the literature. *Urologia Internationalis*, 91(1), pp. 1–9. Available at: https://doi.org/10.1159/000345140.

MacDonald, T. *et al.* (2016) Transmasculine individuals' experiences with lactation, chestfeeding, and gender identity: A qualitative study. *BMC Pregnancy Childbirth*, 16(1), p. 106. Available at: https://doi.org/10.1186/s12884-016-0907-y.

Macklon, N.S. and Fauser, B.C. (2001a) Follicle-stimulating hormone and advanced follicle development in the human. *Archives of Medical Research*, 32(6), pp. 595–600. Available at: https://doi.org/10.1016/s0188-4409(01)00327-7.

Macklon, N.S. and Fauser, B.C. (2001b) Follicle-stimulating hormone and advanced follicle development in the human. *Archives of Medical Research*, 32(6), pp. 595–600. Available at: https://doi.org/10.1016/s0188-4409(01)00327-7.

MacLeod, S. *et al.* (2018) Practical non-pharmacological intervention approaches for sleep problems among older adults. *Geriatric Nursing (New York, N.Y.)*, 39(5), pp. 506–512. Available at: https://doi.org/10.1016/J.GERINURSE.2018.02.002.

Madanmohan *et al.* (2002) Modulation of cold pressor-induced stress by shavasan in normal adult volunteers. *Indian Journal of Physiology and Pharmacology*, 46(3), pp. 307–312.

Madhra, M. *et al.* (2014) Abnormal uterine bleeding: Advantages of formal classification to patients, clinicians and researchers. *Acta Obstetricia et Gynecologica Scandinavica*, 93(7), pp. 619–625. Available at: https://doi.org/10.1111/AOGS.12390.

Maffiuletti, N.A. *et al.* (2016) Rate of force development: Physiological and methodological considerations. *European Journal of Applied Physiology*, 116(6), pp. 1091–1116. Available at: https://doi.org/10.1007/S00421-016-3346-6.

Maged, A.M. *et al.* (2018) Effect of swimming exercise on premenstrual syndrome. *Archives of Gynecology and Obstetrics*, 297(4), pp. 951–959. Available at: https://doi.org/10.1007/S00404-018-4664-1.

Magon, N. and Kalra, S. (2011) The orgasmic history of oxytocin: Love, lust, and labor. *Indian Journal of Endocrinology and Metabolism*, 15(Suppl 3), pp. S156–161. Available at: https://doi.org/10.4103/2230-8210.84851.

Maijala, A. *et al.* (2019) Nocturnal finger skin temperature in menstrual cycle tracking: Ambulatory pilot study using a wearable Oura ring. *BMC Women's Health*, 19(1), p. 150. Available at: https://doi.org/10.1186/s12905-019-0844-9.

Maity, S. *et al.* (2022) Academic and social impact of menstrual disturbances in female medical students: A systematic review and meta-analysis. *Frontiers in Medicine*, p. 821908. Available at: https://doi.org/10.3389/fmed.2022.821908.

Majewski, M., Susanne, H. and Klaus, S. (2006) Epidemiology of athletic knee injuries: A 10-year study. *The Knee*, 13(3), pp. 184–188. Available at: https://doi.org/10.1016/J.KNEE.2006.01.005.

Makadon, H. *et al.* (2015) *Fenway Guide to Lesbian, Gay, Bisexual, and Transgender Health*. Sheridan Books.

Makarem, N. *et al.* (2019) Association of sleep characteristics with cardiovascular health among women and differences by race/ethnicity and menopausal status: Findings from the American Heart Association

Go Red for Women Strategically Focused Research Network. *Sleep Health*, 5(5), pp. 501–508. Available at: https://doi.org/10.1016/J.SLEH.2019.05.005.

Mallhi, T.H. *et al.* (2018) Managing hot flushes in menopausal women: A review. *Journal of the College of Physicians and Surgeons Pakistan*, 28(6), pp. 460–465. Available at: https://doi.org/10.29271/JCPSP.2018.06.460.

Mallinson, R.J. and De Souza, M.J. (2014) Current perspectives on the etiology and manifestation of the "silent" component of the Female Athlete Triad. *International Journal of Women's Health*, 6(1), pp. 451–467. Available at: https://doi.org/10.2147/IJWH.S38603.

Management of osteoporosis in postmenopausal women: The 2021 position statement of The North American Menopause Society (2021) *Menopause (New York, N.Y.)*, 28(9), pp. 973–997. Available at: https://doi.org/10.1097/GME.0000000000001831.

Mann, E. *et al.* (2011) A randomised controlled trial of a cognitive behavioural intervention for women who have menopausal symptoms following breast cancer treatment (MENOS 1): Trial protocol. *BMC Cancer*, 11. Available at: https://doi.org/10.1186/1471-2407-11-44.

Manore, M.M. (2002) Dietary recommendations and athletic menstrual dysfunction. *Sports Medicine (Auckland, N.Z.)*, 32(14), pp. 887–901. Available at: https://doi.org/10.2165/00007256-200232140-00002.

Manson, J.E. and Kaunitz, A.M. (2016) Menopause management: Getting clinical care back on track. *New England Journal of Medicine*, 374(9), pp. 803–806. Available at: https://doi.org/10.1056/NEJMP1514242/SUPPL_FILE/NEJMP1514242_DISCLOSURES.PDF.

Marnach, M.L. *et al.* (2003) Characterization of the relationship between joint laxity and maternal hormones in pregnancy. *Obstetrics & Gynecology*, 101(2), pp. 331–335. Available at: https://doi.org/10.1016/S0029-7844(02)02447-X.

Marquardt, R.M. *et al.* (2019) Progesterone and estrogen signaling in the endometrium: What goes wrong in endometriosis? *International Journal of Molecular Sciences*, 20(15). Available at: https://doi.org/10.3390/IJMS20153822.

Marsh, W.K. *et al.* (2017) Lifelong estradiol exposure and risk of depressive symptoms during the transition to menopause and postmenopause. *Menopause (New York, N.Y.)*, 24(12), p. 1351. Available at: https://doi.org/10.1097/GME.0000000000000929.

Marshall, J. (1963) Thermal changes in the normal menstrual cycle. *British Medical Journal*, 1(5323), pp. 102–104. Available at: https://doi.org/10.1136/BMJ.1.5323.102.

Martin, D. *et al.* (2018) Period prevalence and perceived side effects of hormonal contraceptive use and the menstrual cycle in elite athletes. *International*

Journal of Sports Physiology and Performance, 13(7), pp. 926–932. Available at: https://doi.org/10.1123/IJSPP.2017-0330.

Martínez-Aranda, L.M. *et al.* (2024) Effects of self-myofascial release on athletes' physical performance: A systematic review. *Journal of Functional Morphology and Kinesiology*, 9(1), p. 20. Available at: https://doi.org/10.3390/JFMK9010020.

Masters, A. *et al.* (2014) Melatonin, the hormone of darkness: From sleep promotion to Ebola treatment. *Brain Disorders & Therapy*, 4(1). Available at: https://doi.org/10.4172/2168-975X.1000151.

Mathy, A. *et al.* (2024) The oral contraceptive cycle and its influences on maximal and submaximal endurance parameters in elite handball players. *Frontiers in Physiology*, 15. Available at: https://doi.org/10.3389/FPHYS.2024.1305895.

McClung, J.M., Davis, J.M., Wilson, M.A., Goldsmith, E.C. and Carson, J.A. (2006) Estrogen status and skeletal muscle recovery from disuse atrophy. *Journal of Applied Physiology*, 100, pp. 2012–2023. doi: 10.1152/japplphysiol.01583.2005.

McCurdy, A.P., Boulé, N.G. and Sivak, A. (no date) Effects of exercise on mild-to-moderate depressive symptoms in the postpartum period: A meta-analysis. *Obstetrics and Gynecology*, 129, pp. 1087–1097.

McEwen, B.S. (2001) Invited review: Estrogens effects on the brain: Multiple sites and molecular mechanisms. *Journal of Applied Physiology (Bethesda, Md.: 1985)*, 91(6), pp. 2785–2801. Available at: https://doi.org/10.1152/JAPPL.2001.91.6.2785.

McGhee, D.E. *et al.* (2013) Bra-breast forces generated in women with large breasts while standing and during treadmill running: Implications for sports bra design. *Applied Ergonomics*, 44(1), pp. 112–118. Available at: https://doi.org/10.1016/j.apergo.2012.05.006.

McKenna, K.A. and Fogleman, C.D. (2021) Dysmenorrhea. *American Family Physician*, 104(2), pp. 164–170. Available at: www.aafp.org/pubs/afp/issues/2021/0800/p164.html (Accessed: 23 August 2024).

McMahon, G. and Cook, J. (2024) Female tendons are from Venus and male tendons are from Mars, but does it matter for tendon health? *Sports Medicine (Auckland, N.Z.)* [Preprint]. Available at: https://doi.org/10.1007/S40279-024-02056-7.

McNamara, A., Harris, R. and Minahan, C. (2022) "That time of the month" …for the biggest event of your career! Perception of menstrual cycle on performance of Australian athletes training for the 2020 Olympic and Paralympic Games. *BMJ Open Sport & Exercise Medicine*, 8(2). Available at: https://doi.org/10.1136/BMJSEM-2021-001300.

McNulty, K.L. *et al.* (2020) The effects of menstrual cycle phase on exercise performance in eumenorrheic women: A systematic review and meta-analysis.

Sports Medicine, 50(10), pp. 1813–1827. Available at: https://doi.org/10.1007/S40279-020-01319-3.

Meier, R.K. (2018) Polycystic ovary syndrome. *Journal of Clinical Nursing*, 53, pp. 407–420.

Meignié, A. *et al.* (2021) The effects of menstrual cycle phase on elite athlete performance: A critical and systematic review. *Frontiers in Physiology*, 12. Available at: https://doi.org/10.3389/FPHYS.2021.654585.

Meng, X. *et al.* (2017) Dietary sources and bioactivities of melatonin. *Nutrients*, 9(4). Available at: https://doi.org/10.3390/NU9040367.

Mense, S. (2019) Innervation of the thoracolumbar fascia. *European Journal of Translational Myology*, 29(3), p. 8297. Available at: https://doi.org/10.4081/ejtm.2019.8297.

Mesen, T.B. and Young, S.L. (2015) Progesterone and the luteal phase: A requisite to reproduction. *Obstetrics and Gynecology Clinics of North America*, 42(1), pp. 135–151. Available at: https://doi.org/10.1016/j.ogc.2014.10.003.

Messinisi, I.E. (2006) Ovarian feedback, mechanism of action and possible clinical implications. *Human Reproduction Update*, 12(5), pp. 557–571. Available at: https://doi.org/10.1093/HUMUPD/DML020.

Meulenberg, P.M.M. *et al.* (1987) The effect of oral contraceptives on plasma-free and salivary cortisol and cortisone. *Clinica Chimica Acta; International Journal of Clinical Chemistry*, 165(2–3), pp. 379–385. Available at: https://doi.org/10.1016/0009-8981(87)90183-5.

Mihm, M., Gangooly, S. and Muttukrishna, S. (2011) The normal menstrual cycle in women. *Animal Reproduction Science*, 124(3–4), pp. 229–236. Available at: https://doi.org/10.1016/j.anireprosci.2010.08.030.

Milne, J.A., Howie, A.D. and Pack, A.I. (1978) Dyspnoea during normal pregnancy. *British Journal of Obstetrics and Gynaecology*, 85(4), pp. 260–263. Available at: https://doi.org/10.1111/J.1471-0528.1978.TB10497.X.

Minahan, C. *et al.* (2015) The influence of estradiol on muscle damage and leg strength after intense eccentric exercise. *European Journal of Applied Physiology*, 115(7), pp. 1493–1500. Available at: https://doi.org/10.1007/S00421-015-3133-9.

Mira, T.A.A. *et al.* (2018) Systematic review and meta-analysis of complementary treatments for women with symptomatic endometriosis. *International Journal of Gynaecology and Obstetrics: The Official Organ of the International Federation of Gynaecology and Obstetrics*, 143(1), pp. 2–9. Available at: https://doi.org/10.1002/IJGO.12576.

Mishra, G.D. *et al.* (2024) Optimising health after early menopause. *Lancet (London, England)*, 403(10430), pp. 958–968. Available at: https://doi.org/10.1016/S0140-6736(23)02800-3.

Mitchell, R.A. *et al.* (2018) Sex differences in respiratory muscle activation patterns during high-intensity exercise in healthy humans. *Respiratory Physiology & Neurobiology*, 247, pp. 57–60. Available at: https://doi.org/10.1016/J.RESP.2017.09.002.

Miyoshi, Y. (2019) Restorative yoga for occupational stress among Japanese female nurses working night shift: Randomized crossover trial. *Journal of Occupational Health*, 61(6), pp. 508–516. Available at: https://doi.org/10.1002/1348-9585.12080.

Mohamed, S. and Hunter, M.S. (2018) Transgender women's experiences and beliefs about hormone therapy through and beyond mid-age: An exploratory UK study. *The International Journal of Transgenderism*, 20(1), pp. 98–107. Available at: https://doi.org/10.1080/15532739.2018.1493626.

Mohebbi, R. *et al.* (2023) Exercise training and bone mineral density in postmenopausal women: An updated systematic review and meta-analysis of intervention studies with emphasis on potential moderators. *Osteoporosis International*, 34(7), pp. 1145–1178. Available at: https://doi.org/10.1007/S00198-023-06682-1.

Moholdt, T. *et al.* (2023) Randomised controlled trial of exercise training during lactation on breast milk composition in breastfeeding people with overweight/obesity: A study protocol for the MILKSHAKE trial. *BMJ Open Sport & Exercise Medicine*, 9(4). Available at: https://doi.org/10.1136/BMJSEM-2023-001751.

Money, A. *et al.* (2024) The impact of physical activity and exercise interventions on symptoms for women experiencing menopause: Overview of reviews. *BMC Women's Health*, 24(1), p. 399. Available at: https://doi.org/10.1186/S12905-024-03243-4.

Mooventhan, A. (2019) A comprehensive review on scientific evidence-based effects (including adverse effects) of yoga for normal and high-risk pregnancy-related health problems. *Journal of Bodywork and Movement Therapies*, 23(4), pp. 721–727. Available at: https://doi.org/10.1016/J.JBMT.2019.03.005.

Moran, A. *et al.* (2007) Estradiol replacement reverses ovariectomy-induced muscle contractile and myosin dysfunction in mature female mice. *Journal of Applied Physiology*, 102, pp. 1387–1393.

Mosconi, L. *et al.* (2024) In vivo brain estrogen receptor density by neuroendocrine aging and relationships with cognition and symptomatology. *Scientific Reports*, 14(1), pp. 1–15. Available at: https://doi.org/10.1038/s41598-024-62820-7.

Mottola, M.F. (2002) Exercise in the postpartum period: Practical applications. *Current Sports Medicine Reports*, 1(6), pp. 362–368. Available at: https://doi.org/10.1249/00149619-200212000-00010.

Mottola, M.F. *et al.* (2006) VO2peak prediction and exercise prescription for pregnant women. *Medicine & Science in Sports & Exercise*, 38(8), pp.

1389–1395. Available at: https://doi.org/10.1249/01.MSS.0000228940.09411.9C.

Mottola, M.F. and Christopher, P.D. (1991) Effects of maternal exercise on liver and skeletal muscle glycogen storage in pregnant rats. *Journal of Applied Physiology (Bethesda, Md.: 1985)*, 71(3), pp. 1015–1019. Available at: https://doi.org/10.1152/JAPPL.1991.71.3.1015.

Mountjoy, M. *et al.* (2018) IOC consensus statement on relative energy deficiency in sport (RED-S): 2018 update. *British Journal of Sports Medicine*, 52(11), pp. 687–697. Available at: https://doi.org/10.1136/BJSPORTS-2018-099193.

Mountjoy, M. *et al.* (2023) 2023 International Olympic Committee's (IOC) consensus statement on Relative Energy Deficiency in Sport (REDs). *British Journal of Sports Medicine*, 57(17), pp. 1073–1098. Available at: https://doi.org/10.1136/BJSPORTS-2023-106994.

Mukherjee, P., Mishra, S. and Ray, S. (2014) Menstrual characteristics of adolescent athletes: A study from West Bengal, India. *Collegium Antropologicum* [Preprint].

Mumford, S.L. and Kim, K. (2018) Subtle changes in menstrual cycle function: Pieces of the puzzle. *Paediatric and Perinatal Epidemiology*, 32(3), pp. 235–236. Available at: https://doi.org/10.1111/ppe.12470.

Munro, M.G. *et al.* (2018) The two FIGO systems for normal and abnormal uterine bleeding symptoms and classification of causes of abnormal uterine bleeding in the reproductive years: 2018 revisions. *International Journal of Gynaecology and Obstetrics: The Official Organ of the International Federation of Gynaecology and Obstetrics*, 143(3), pp. 393–408. Available at: https://doi.org/10.1002/IJGO.12666.

Munro, M.G. *et al.* (2022) The FIGO ovulatory disorders classification system. *International Journal of Gynaecology and Obstetrics: The Official Organ of the International Federation of Gynaecology and Obstetrics*, 159(1), pp. 1–20. Available at: https://doi.org/10.1002/IJGO.14331.

Myer, G.D. *et al.* (2008) The effects of generalized joint laxity on risk of anterior cruciate ligament injury in young female athletes. *The American Journal of Sports Medicine*, 36(6), pp. 1073–1080. Available at: https://doi.org/10.1177/0363546507313572.

Myllyaho, M.M. *et al.* (2021) Hormonal contraceptive use does not affect strength, endurance, or body composition adaptations to combined strength and endurance training in women. *Journal of Strength and Conditioning Research*, 35(2), pp. 449–457. Available at: https://doi.org/10.1519/JSC.0000000000002713.

Nagy, B. *et al.* (2021) Key to life: Physiological role and clinical implications of progesterone. *International Journal of Molecular Sciences*, 22(20). Available at: https://doi.org/10.3390/ijms222011039.

Najmabadi, S. *et al.* (2020) Menstrual bleeding, cycle length, and follicular and luteal phase lengths in women without known subfertility: A pooled analysis of three cohorts. *Paediatric and Perinatal Epidemiology*, 34(3), pp. 318–327. Available at: https://doi.org/10.1111/ppe.12644.

Nandi, A. *et al.* (2014) Polycystic ovary syndrome. *Endocrinology and Metabolism Clinics of North America*, 43, pp. 123–147.

Nattiv, A. *et al.* (2007) American College of Sports Medicine position stand: The female athlete triad. *Medicine and Science in Sports and Exercise*, 39(10), pp. 1867–1882. Available at: https://doi.org/10.1249/mss.0b013e318149f111.

Nayman, S. *et al.* (2023) Associations of premenstrual symptoms with daily rumination and perceived stress and the moderating effects of mindfulness facets on symptom cyclicity in premenstrual syndrome. *Archives of Women's Mental Health*, 26(2), pp. 167–176. Available at: https://doi.org/10.1007/S00737-023-01304-5.

Nelson, L.R. and Bulun, S.E. (2001) Estrogen production and action. *Journal of the American Academy of Dermatology*, 45(3 Suppl), pp. S116–124. Available at: https://doi.org/10.1067/mjd.2001.117432.

Nelson, S.M. *et al.* (2023) Anti-Müllerian hormone for the diagnosis and prediction of menopause: A systematic review. *Human Reproduction Update*, 29(3), pp. 327–346. Available at: https://doi.org/10.1093/HUMUPD/DMAC045.

Ní Chéileachair, F., McGuire, B.E. and Durand, H. (2022) Coping with dysmenorrhea: A qualitative analysis of period pain management among students who menstruate. *BMC Women's Health*, 22(1). Available at: https://doi.org/10.1186/S12905-022-01988-4.

Nichols, A.W. *et al.* (2008) Effects of combination oral contraceptives on strength development in women athletes. *Journal of Strength and Conditioning Research*, 22(5), pp. 1625–1632. Available at: https://doi.org/10.1519/JSC.0B013E31817AE1F3.

De Nicola, A.F. *et al.* (2022) Progesterone and allopregnanolone neuroprotective effects in the Wobbler Mouse Model of amyotrophic lateral sclerosis. *Cellular and Molecular Neurobiology*, 42(1), pp. 23–40. Available at: https://doi.org/10.1007/s10571-021-01118-y.

Niering, M. *et al.* (2024) The influence of menstrual cycle phases on maximal strength performance in healthy female adults: A systematic review with meta-analysis. *Sports (Basel, Switzerland)*, 12(1). Available at: https://doi.org/10.3390/SPORTS12010031.

Nillni, Y.I. *et al.* (2018) Treatment of depression, anxiety, and trauma-related disorders during the perinatal period: A systematic review. HHS Public Access. *Clinical Psychology Review*, 66, pp. 136–148. Available at: https://doi.org/10.1016/j.cpr.2018.06.004.

Nisolle, M. and Donnez, J. (1997) Peritoneal endometriosis, ovarian endometriosis, and adenomyotic nodules of the rectovaginal septum are three different entities. *Fertility and Sterility*, 68(4), pp. 585–596. Available at: https://doi.org/10.1016/S0015-0282(97)00191-X.

Nolan, D. *et al.* (2023) The effect of hormonal contraceptive use on skeletal muscle hypertrophy, power and strength adaptations to resistance exercise training: A systematic review and multilevel meta-analysis. *Sports Medicine*, 54(1), pp. 105–125. Available at: https://doi.org/10.1007/S40279-023-01911-3.

Nota, N.M. *et al.* (2019) Occurrence of acute cardiovascular events in transgender individuals receiving hormone therapy: Results from a large cohort study. *Circulation*, 139(11), pp. 1461–1462. Available at: https://doi.org/10.1161/CIRCULATIONAHA.118.038584.

Novella, S. *et al.* (2019) Mechanisms underlying the influence of oestrogen on cardiovascular physiology in women. *The Journal of Physiology*, 597(19), pp. 4873–4886. Available at: https://doi.org/10.1113/JP278063.

Obedin-Maliver, J. and Makadon, H.J. (2015) Transgender men and pregnancy. *Obstetric Medicine*, 9(1), pp. 4–8. Available at: https://doi.org/10.1177/1753495x15612658.

O'Brien, P.M.S. *et al.* (2011) Towards a consensus on diagnostic criteria, measurement and trial design of the premenstrual disorders: The ISPMD Montreal consensus. *Archives of Women's Mental Health*, 14(1), pp. 13–21. Available at: https://doi.org/10.1007/S00737-010-0201-3.

O'Connor, P.J. *et al.* (2011) Safety and efficacy of supervised strength training adopted in pregnancy. *Journal of Physical Activity & Health*, 8(3), pp. 309–320. Available at: https://doi.org/10.1123/JPAH.8.3.309.

Oladosu, F.A., Tu, F.F. and Hellman, K.M. (2018) Nonsteroidal anti-inflammatory drug resistance in dysmenorrhea: Epidemiology, causes, and treatment. *American Journal of Obstetrics and Gynecology*, 218(4), pp. 390–400. Available at: https://doi.org/10.1016/J.AJOG.2017.08.108.

O'Neill, M.E. *et al.* (1992) Accuracy of Borg's ratings of perceived exertion in the prediction of heart rates during pregnancy. *British Journal of Sports Medicine*, 26(2), pp. 121–124. Available at: https://doi.org/10.1136/BJSM.26.2.121.

Osborn, E. *et al.* (2021) Suicidality in women with Premenstrual Dysphoric Disorder: A systematic literature review. *Archives of Women's Mental Health*, 24(2), pp. 173–184. Available at: https://doi.org/10.1007/s00737-020-01054-8.

Ossewaarde, L. *et al.* (2010) Neural mechanisms underlying changes in stress-sensitivity across the menstrual cycle. *Psychoneuroendocrinology*, 35(1), pp. 47–55. Available at: https://doi.org/10.1016/J.PSYNEUEN.2009.08.011.

Ouzounian, J.G. and Elkayam, U. (2012) Physiologic changes during normal pregnancy and delivery. *Cardiology Clinics*, 30(3), pp. 317–329. Available at: https://doi.org/10.1016/J.CCL.2012.05.004.

Oxfeldt, M. *et al.* (2022) Sex hormones and satellite cell regulation in women. *Translational Sports Medicine*, 2022, pp. 1–12. Available at: https://doi.org/10.1155/2022/9065923.

Oxfeldt, M. *et al.* (2024) Influence of menstrual cycle phase and oral contraceptive phase on exercise performance in endurance-trained females. *The Journal of Sports Medicine and Physical Fitness*, 64(3), pp. 236–247. Available at: https://doi.org/10.23736/S0022-4707.23.15458-2.

Oyelowo, T. (2007) *Mosby's Guide to Women's Health*. St. Louis, Missouri: Mosby Elsevier.

Palagini, L. *et al.* (2019) The key role of insomnia and sleep loss in the dysregulation of multiple systems involved in mood disorders: A proposed model. *Journal of Sleep Research*, 28(6). Available at: https://doi.org/10.1111/JSR.12841.

Pallavi, L.C., Souza, U.J.D. and Shivaprakash, G. (2017) Assessment of musculoskeletal strength and levels of fatigue during different phases of menstrual cycle in young adults. *Journal of Clinical and Diagnostic Research*, 11(2), pp. CC11–CC13. Available at: https://doi.org/10.7860/JCDR/2017/24316.9408.

Pandey, A. and Huq, N. (2017) Acute and sub-acute hemodynamic effects of restorative yoga. *Journal of the American College of Cardiology*, 69(11), p. 1735. Available at: https://doi.org/10.1016/S0735-1097(17)35124-0.

De Paoli, M., Zakharia, A. and Werstuck, G.H. (2021) The role of estrogen in insulin resistance: A review of clinical and preclinical data. *American Journal of Pathology*, 191(9), pp. 1490–1498. Available at: https://doi.org/10.1016/j.ajpath.2021.05.011.

Paquin, D., Kato, D. and Kim, P. (2020) A mathematical model for the effects of grandmothering on human longevity. *Mathematical Biosciences and Engineering: MBE*, 17(4), pp. 3175–3189. Available at: https://doi.org/10.3934/MBE.2020180.

Park, H.S. and Lee, K.U. (2003) Postmenopausal women lose less visceral adipose tissue during a weight reduction program. *Menopause (New York, N.Y.)*, 10(3), pp. 222–227. Available at: https://doi.org/10.1097/00042192-200310030-00009.

Park, J.K. *et al.* (2013) Body fat distribution after menopause and cardiovascular disease risk factors: Korean National Health and Nutrition Examination Survey 2010. *Journal of Women's Health (2002)*, 22(7), pp. 587–594. Available at: https://doi.org/10.1089/JWH.2012.4035.

Parker, E.A. *et al.* (2022) Do relaxin levels impact hip injury incidence in women? A scoping review. *Frontiers in Endocrinology*, p. 827512. Available at: https://doi.org/10.3389/fendo.2022.827512.

Paschou, S.A. *et al.* (2019) Diabetes in menopause: Risks and management. *Current Vascular Pharmacology*, 17(6), pp. 556–563. Available at: https://doi.org/10.2174/1570161116666180625124405.

Patra, S. *et al.* (2023) A review on phytoestrogens: Current status and future direction. *Phytotherapy Research: PTR*, 37(7), pp. 3097–3120. Available at: https://doi.org/10.1002/PTR.7861.

Pavan, P.G. *et al.* (2014) Painful connections: Densification versus fibrosis of fascia. *Current Pain and Headache Reports*, 18(8). Available at: https://doi.org/10.1007/s11916-014-0441-4.

Pearce, E. *et al.* (2020) Exercise for premenstrual syndrome: A systematic review and meta-analysis of randomised controlled trials. *BJGP Open*, 4(3). Available at: https://doi.org/10.3399/BJGPOPEN20X101032.

Pellegrino, A., Tiidus, P.M. and Vandenboom, R. (2022) Mechanisms of estrogen influence on skeletal muscle: Mass, regeneration, and mitochondrial function. *Sports Medicine (Auckland, N.Z.)*, 52(12), pp. 2853–2869. Available at: https://doi.org/10.1007/S40279-022-01733-9.

Persons, P.A. *et al.* (2024) Weight gain during midlife: Does race/ethnicity influence risk? *Maturitas*, 185. Available at: https://doi.org/10.1016/J.MATURITAS.2024.108013.

Peters, B.A. *et al.* (2022) Spotlight on the gut microbiome in menopause: Current insights. *International Journal of Women's Health*, 14, pp. 1059–1072. Available at: https://doi.org/10.2147/IJWH.S340491.

Peters, C. and Burrows, M. (2006) Androgenicity of the progestin in oral contraceptives does not affect maximal leg strength. *Contraception*, 74(6), pp. 487–491. Available at: https://doi.org/10.1016/J.CONTRACEPTION.2006.08.005.

Petrofsky, J. and Lee, H. (2015) Greater reduction of balance as a result of increased plantar fascia elasticity at ovulation during the menstrual cycle. *The Tohoku Journal of Experimental Medicine*, 237(3), pp. 219–226. Available at: https://doi.org/10.1620/tjem.237.219.

Petrov Fieril, K., Glantz, A. and Fagevik Olsen, M. (2015) The efficacy of moderate-to-vigorous resistance exercise during pregnancy: A randomized controlled trial. *Acta Obstetricia et Gynecologica Scandinavica*, 94(1), pp. 35–42. Available at: https://doi.org/10.1111/AOGS.12525.

Petrovic, D. *et al.* (2016) Association between walking, dysphoric mood and anxiety in late pregnancy: A cross-sectional study. *Psychiatry Research*, 246, pp. 360–363. Available at: https://doi.org/10.1016/j.psychres.2016.10.009.

Phillips, S.K. *et al.* (1996) Changes in maximal voluntary force of human adductor pollicis muscle during the menstrual cycle. *Journal of Physiology*, 496(2), pp. 551–557. Available at: https://doi.org/10.1113/JPHYSIOL.1996.SP021706.

Pickar, J.H. and Baber, R.J. (2021) Managing the menopause: The question of evidence. *Climacteric*, 24(1), pp. 1–2. Available at: https://doi.org/10.1080/13697137.2020.1826127.

Pivarnik, J.M. (1996) Cardiovascular responses to aerobic exercise during pregnancy and postpartum. *Seminars in Perinatology*, 20(4), pp. 242–249. Available at: https://doi.org/10.1016/S0146-0005(96)80017-6.

Pivarnik, J.M. *et al.* (1992) Menstrual cycle phase affects temperature regulation during endurance exercise. *Journal of Applied Physiology*, 72(2), pp. 543–548. Available at: https://doi.org/10.1152/JAPPL.1992.72.2.543.

Pletzer, B. *et al.* (2019) The cycling brain: Menstrual cycle related fluctuations in hippocampal and fronto-striatal activation and connectivity during cognitive tasks. *Neuropsychopharmacology*, 44(11), pp. 1867–1875. Available at: https://doi.org/10.1038/S41386-019-0435-3.

Poitras, M. *et al.* (2024) Bloody stressed! A systematic review of the associations between adulthood psychological stress and menstrual cycle irregularity. *Neuroscience & Biobehavioral Reviews*, 163, p. 105784. Available at: https://doi.org/10.1016/J.NEUBIOREV.2024.105784.

Pöllänen, E. *et al.* (2010) Power training and postmenopausal hormone therapy affect transcriptional control of specific co-regulated gene clusters in skeletal muscle. *Age*, 32(3), pp. 347–363. Available at: https://doi.org/10.1007/S11357-010-9140-1.

Poromaa, I.S. and Gingnell, M. (2014) Menstrual cycle influence on cognitive function and emotion processing from a reproductive perspective. *Frontiers in Neuroscience*, 8(Nov). Available at: https://doi.org/10.3389/FNINS.2014.00380.

Potteiger, J., Welch, J. and Byrne, J. (1993) From parturition to marathon: A 16-wk study of an elite runner. *Medicine & Science in Sports & Exercise*, 25(6), pp. 673–677.

Poyatos-León, R., García-Hermoso, A. and Sanabria-Martínez, G. (no date) Effects of exercise-based interventions on postpartum depression: A meta-analysis of randomized controlled trials. *Birth*, 44, pp. 200–208.

Practice Bulletin No. 128 (2012) *Obstetrics & Gynecology*, 120(1), pp. 197–206. Available at: https://doi.org/10.1097/AOG.0B013E318262E320.

Prado, R.C.R. *et al.* (2021a) Menstrual cycle, psychological responses, and adherence to physical exercise: Viewpoint of a possible barrier. *Frontiers in*

Psychology, 12. Available at: https://doi.org/10.3389/FPSYG.2021.525943.

Prado, R.C.R. *et al.* (2021b) The effect of menstrual cycle and exercise intensity on psychological and physiological responses in healthy eumenorrheic women. *Physiology and Behavior*, 232. Available at: https://doi.org/10.1016/J.PHYSBEH.2020.113290.

Prasad, D. *et al.* (2021) Suicidal risk in women with premenstrual syndrome and premenstrual dysphoric disorder: A systematic review and meta-analysis. *Journal of Women's Health (2002)*, 30(12), pp. 1693–1707. Available at: https://doi.org/10.1089/jwh.2021.0185.

Prior, J.C. *et al.* (1987) Conditioning exercise decreases premenstrual symptoms: A prospective, controlled 6-month trial. *Fertility and Sterility*, 47(3), pp. 402–408. Available at: https://doi.org/10.1016/S0015-0282(16)59045-1.

Prior, J.C. *et al.* (2015) Ovulation prevalence in women with spontaneous normal-length menstrual cycles: A population-based cohort from HUNT3, Norway. *PLOS One*, 10(8), p. e0134473. Available at: https://doi.org/10.1371/journal.pone.0134473.

Prodromos, C.C. *et al.* (2007) A meta-analysis of the incidence of anterior cruciate ligament tears as a function of gender, sport, and a knee injury-reduction regimen. *Arthroscopy: The Journal of Arthroscopic & Related Surgery: Official Publication of the Arthroscopy Association of North America and the International Arthroscopy Association*, 23(12). Available at: https://doi.org/10.1016/J.ARTHRO.2007.07.003.

Pu, D. *et al.* (2017) Metabolic syndrome in menopause and associated factors: A meta-analysis. *Climacteric: The Journal of the International Menopause Society*, 20(6), pp. 583–591. Available at: https://doi.org/10.1080/13697137.2017.1386649.

Pugsley, Z. and Ballard, K. (2007) Management of endometriosis in general practice: The pathway to diagnosis. *The British Journal of General Practice*, 57(539), pp. 470–476.

Qiao, M. *et al.* (2012) Prevalence of premenstrual syndrome and premenstrual dysphoric disorder in a population-based sample in China. *European Journal of Obstetrics, Gynecology, and Reproductive Biology*, 162(1), pp. 83–86. Available at: https://doi.org/10.1016/J.EJOGRB.2012.01.017.

Quint, C. (2021) *Be Period Positive*. New York: Penguin Random House.

Rababa'h, A.M., Matani, B.R. and Yehya, A. (2022) An update of polycystic ovary syndrome: Causes and therapeutics options. *Heliyon*, 8(10). Available at: https://doi.org/10.1016/J.HELIYON.2022.E11010.

Rael, B. *et al.* (2021) Menstrual cycle phases influence on cardiorespiratory response to exercise in endurance-trained females. *International Journal of Environmental Research and Public Health*, 18(3), pp. 1–12. Available at: https://doi.org/10.3390/IJERPH18030860.

Rahmioglu, N. *et al.* (2023) The genetic basis of endometriosis and comorbidity with other pain and inflammatory conditions. *Nature Genetics*, 55(3), pp. 423–436. Available at: https://doi.org/10.1038/s41588-023-01323-z.

Rahr-Wagner, L. *et al.* (2014) Is the use of oral contraceptives associated with operatively treated anterior cruciate ligament injury? A case-control study from the Danish Knee Ligament Reconstruction Registry. *The American Journal of Sports Medicine*, 42(12), pp. 2897–2905. Available at: https://doi.org/10.1177/0363546514557240.

Ramin-Wright, A. *et al.* (2018) Fatigue: A symptom in endometriosis. *Human Reproduction (Oxford, England)*, 33(8), pp. 1459–1465. Available at: https://doi.org/10.1093/HUMREP/DEY115.

Ravichandran, H. and Janakiraman, B. (2022) Effect of aerobic exercises in improving premenstrual symptoms among healthy women: A systematic review of randomized controlled trials. *International Journal of Women's Health*, 14, pp. 1105–1114. Available at: https://doi.org/10.2147/IJWH.S371193.

Rechichi, C. and Dawson, B. (2009) Effect of oral contraceptive cycle phase on performance in team sport players. *Journal of Science and Medicine in Sport*, 12(1), pp. 190–195. Available at: https://doi.org/10.1016/J.JSAMS.2007.10.005.

Regehr, C., Glancy, D. and Pitts, A. (2013) Interventions to reduce stress in university students: A review and meta-analysis. *Journal of Affective Disorders*, 148(1), pp. 1–11. Available at: https://doi.org/10.1016/J.JAD.2012.11.026.

Rehbein, E. *et al.* (2021) Shaping of the female human brain by sex hormones: A review. *Neuroendocrinology*, 111(3), pp. 183–206. Available at: https://doi.org/10.1159/000507083.

Reif, A. *et al.* (2021) Strength performance across the oral contraceptive cycle of team sport athletes: A cross-sectional study. *Frontiers in Physiology*, 12. Available at: https://doi.org/10.3389/FPHYS.2021.658994.

Ren, B. and Zhu, Y. (2022) A new perspective on thyroid hormones: Crosstalk with reproductive hormones in females. *International Journal of Molecular Sciences*, 23(5), p. 2708. Available at: https://doi.org/10.3390/IJMS23052708.

Ribeiro, M.M., Andrade, A. and Nunes, I. (2021) Physical exercise in pregnancy: Benefits, risks and prescription. *Journal of Perinatal Medicine*, 50(1), pp. 4–17. Available at: https://doi.org/10.1515/JPM-2021-0315.

Richette, P., Corvol, M. and Bardin, T. (2003) Estrogens, cartilage, and osteoarthritis. *Joint Bone Spine*, 70(4), pp. 257–262. Available at: https://doi.org/10.1016/S1297-319X(03)00067-8.

Ritz, P. *et al.* (2008) Influence of gender and body composition on hydration and body water spaces. *Clinical Nutrition (Edinburgh, Scotland)*, 27(5), pp. 740–746. Available at: https://doi.org/10.1016/J.CLNU.2008.07.010.

Robakis, T. *et al.* (2019) Hormonal contraceptives and mood: Review of the literature and implications for future research. *Current Psychiatry Reports*, 21(7). Available at: https://doi.org/10.1007/S11920-019-1034-Z.

Roberts, S.C. *et al.* (2014) Partner choice, relationship satisfaction, and oral contraception: The congruency hypothesis. *Psychological Science*, 25(7), pp. 1497–1503. Available at: https://doi.org/10.1177/0956797614532295.

Robinson, D.P. and Klein, S.L. (2012) Pregnancy and pregnancy-associated hormones alter immune responses and disease pathogenesis. *Hormones and Behavior*, 62(3), p. 263. Available at: https://doi.org/10.1016/J.YHBEH.2012.02.023.

Rodrigues-Denize, N., Zolnikov, B.T.R. and Furio, F. (2024) A systematic review on the physical, mental, and occupational effects of exercise on pregnant women. *Dialogues in Health*, 4. Available at: https://doi.org/10.1016/J.DIALOG.2024.100181.

Rogers, A. *et al.* (2002) Circulating estradiol and osteoprotegerin as determinants of bone turnover and bone density in postmenopausal women. *The Journal of Clinical Endocrinology and Metabolism*, 87(10), pp. 4470–4475. Available at: https://doi.org/10.1210/JC.2002-020396.

Rojiani, R. *et al.* (2017) Women benefit more than men in response to college-based meditation training. *Frontiers in Psychology*, 8(APR), p. 254657. Available at: https://doi.org/10.3389/FPSYG.2017.00551/BIBTEX.

Romei, M. *et al.* (2010) Effects of gender and posture on thoraco-abdominal kinematics during quiet breathing in healthy adults. *Respiratory Physiology & Neurobiology*, 172(3), pp. 184–191. Available at: https://doi.org/10.1016/J.RESP.2010.05.018.

Romero-Parra, N. *et al.* (2021) Exercise-induced muscle damage during the menstrual cycle: A systematic review and meta-analysis. *Journal of Strength and Conditioning Research*, 35(2), pp. 549–561. Available at: https://doi.org/10.1519/JSC.0000000000003878.

Rosenfeld, C.S. (2017) Sex-dependent differences in voluntary physical activity. *Journal of Neuroscience Research*, 95(1–2), pp. 279–290. Available at: https://doi.org/10.1002/JNR.23896.

Rossmanith, W.G. and Ruebberdt, W. (2009) What causes hot flushes? The neuroendocrine origin of vasomotor symptoms in the menopause. *Gynecological Endocrinology*, 25(5), pp. 303–314. Available at: https://doi.org/10.1080/09513590802632514.

Röttger, S. *et al.* (2021) The effectiveness of combat tactical breathing as compared with prolonged exhalation. *Applied Psychophysiology and Biofeedback*, 46(1), pp. 19–28. Available at: https://doi.org/10.1007/S10484-020-09485-W.

Rubinow, D.R. and Roy Byrne, P. (1984) Premenstrual syndromes: Overview from a methodologic perspective. *The American Journal of Psychiatry*, 141(2), pp. 163–172. Available at: https://doi.org/10.1176/AJP.141.2.163.

Russo, L. *et al.* (2023) Self-myofascial release of the foot plantar surface: The effects of a single exercise session on the posterior muscular chain flexibility after one hour. *International Journal of Environmental Research and Public Health*, 20(2). Available at: https://doi.org/10.3390/IJERPH20020974.

Russo, M.A., Santarelli, D.M. and O'Rourke, D. (2017) The physiological effects of slow breathing in the healthy human. *Breathe (Sheffield, England)*, 13(4), pp. 298–309. Available at: https://doi.org/10.1183/20734735.009817.

Rzewuska, A.M. *et al.* (2023) Gonadotropin-releasing hormone antagonists—A new hope in endometriosis treatment? *Journal of Clinical Medicine*, 12(3), p. 1008. Available at: https://doi.org/10.3390/JCM12031008/S1.

Saadia, Z. (2020) Follicle stimulating hormone (LH: FSH) ratio in polycystic ovary syndrome (PCOS): Obese vs. non-obese women. *Medical Archives*, 74(4), p. 289. Available at: https://doi.org/10.5455/MEDARH.2020.74.289-293.

Sabin-Farrell, R. and Slade, P. (1999) Reconceptualizing pre-menstrual emotional symptoms as phasic differential responsiveness to stressors. *Journal of Reproductive and Infant Psychology*, 17(4), pp. 381–390. Available at: https://doi.org/10.1080/02646839908404603.

Sadeghi, M.R. (2022) Polycystic ovarian syndrome and endometriosis as two evil extremes of health continuum. *Journal of Reproduction & Infertility*, 23(1), p. 1. Available at: https://doi.org/10.18502/JRI.V23I1.8445.

Sady, M.A. *et al.* (1990) Cardiovascular response to maximal cycle exercise during pregnancy and at two and seven months post partum. *American Journal of Obstetrics and Gynecology*, 162(5), pp. 1181–1185. Available at: https://doi.org/10.1016/0002-9378(90)90012-v.

Saei Ghare Naz, M., Rostami Dovom, M. and Ramezani Tehrani, F. (2020) The menstrual disturbances in endocrine disorders: A narrative review. *International Journal of Endocrinology and Metabolism*, 18(4), p. e106694. Available at: https://doi.org/10.5812/ijem.106694.

Saha, R. *et al.* (2015) Heritability of endometriosis. *Fertility and Sterility*, 104(4), pp. 947–952. Available at: https://doi.org/10.1016/j.fertnstert.2015.06.035.

Salvesen, K.A., Hem, E. and Sundgot-Borgen, J. (2012) Fetal wellbeing may be compromised during strenuous exercise among pregnant elite athletes. *British Journal of Sports Medicine*, 46(4), pp. 279–283. Available at: https://doi.org/10.1136/BJSM.2010.080259.

Sampson, J.A. (1927) Metastatic or embolic endometriosis, due to the menstrual dissemination of endometrial tissue into the venous circulation. *The American Journal of Pathology*, 3(2), p. 93. Available at: www.ncbi.nlm.nih.gov/pmc/articles/PMC1931779 (Accessed: 26 August 2024).

Sampson, J.A. (1940) The development of the implantation theory for the origin of peritoneal endometriosis. *American Journal of Obstetrics and Gynecology*, 40(4), pp. 549–557. Available at: https://doi.org/10.1016/S0002-9378(40)91238-8.

Sanchez, B.N. *et al.* (2024) Sex differences in energy metabolism: A female-oriented discussion. *Sports Medicine (Auckland, N.Z.)* [Preprint]. Available at: https://doi.org/10.1007/S40279-024-02063-8.

Sandhu, S.K. and Hampson, G. (2011) The pathogenesis, diagnosis, investigation and management of osteoporosis. *Journal of Clinical Pathology*, 64(12), pp. 1042–1050. Available at: https://doi.org/10.1136/JCP.2010.077842.

Sanghavi, M. and Rutherford, J.D. (2014) Cardiovascular physiology of pregnancy. *Circulation*, 130(12), pp. 1003–1008. Available at: https://doi.org/10.1161/CIRCULATIONAHA.114.009029.

Santoro, N. *et al.* (1996) Characterization of reproductive hormonal dynamics in the perimenopause. *The Journal of Clinical Endocrinology and Metabolism*, 81(4), pp. 1495–1501. Available at: https://doi.org/10.1210/JCEM.81.4.8636357.

Santoro, N. *et al.* (2003) Impaired folliculogenesis and ovulation in older reproductive aged women. *The Journal of Clinical Endocrinology and Metabolism*, 88(11), pp. 5502–5509. Available at: https://doi.org/10.1210/JC.2002-021839.

Santoro, N. *et al.* (2008) Factors related to declining luteal function in women during the menopausal transition. *The Journal of Clinical Endocrinology and Metabolism*, 93(5), pp. 1711–1721. Available at: https://doi.org/10.1210/JC.2007-2165.

Santoro, N. and Randolph, J.F. (2011) Reproductive hormones and the menopause transition. *Obstetrics and Gynecology Clinics of North America*, 38(3), pp. 455–466. Available at: https://doi.org/10.1016/J.OGC.2011.05.004.

dos Santos Andrade, M. *et al.* (2012) Isokinetic hamstrings-to-quadriceps peak torque ratio: The influence of sport modality, gender, and angular velocity. *Journal of Sports Sciences*, 30(6), pp. 547–553. Available at: https://doi.org/10.1080/02640414.2011.644249.

Santos, R.M. and Santos, C.R. (2024) Gender differences in the determinants of choking under pressure: Evidence from penalty kicks in soccer. *Social Science Quarterly*, 105(4), pp. 1296–1307. Available at: https://doi.org/10.1111/SSQU.13415.

Sarwar, R., Niclos, B.B. and Rutherford, O.M. (1996) Changes in muscle strength, relaxation rate and fatiguability during the human menstrual cycle. *The Journal of Physiology*, 493(Pt 1), p. 267. Available at: https://doi.org/10.1113/JPHYSIOL.1996.SP021381.

Sassarini, D.J. (2016) Depression in midlife women. *Maturitas*, 94, pp. 149–154. Available at: https://doi.org/10.1016/J.MATURITAS.2016.09.004.

Sassarini, J. *et al.* (2011) Vascular function and cardiovascular risk factors in women with severe flushing. *Clinical Endocrinology*, 74(1), pp. 97–103. Available at: https://doi.org/10.1111/J.1365-2265.2010.03921.X.

Savage, K.J. and Clarkson, P.M. (2002) Oral contraceptive use and exercise-induced muscle damage and recovery. *Contraception*, 66(1), pp. 67–71. Available at: https://doi.org/10.1016/S0010-7824(02)00320-7.

Sayegh, R. *et al.* (1995) The effect of a carbohydrate-rich beverage on mood, appetite, and cognitive function in women with premenstrual syndrome. *Obstetrics and Gynecology*, 86(4 Pt 1), pp. 520–528. Available at: https://doi.org/10.1016/0029-7844(95)00246-N.

Schaffir, J., Worly, B.L. and Gur, T.L. (2016) Combined hormonal contraception and its effects on mood: A critical review. *The European Journal of Contraception & Reproductive Health Care: The Official Journal of the European Society of Contraception*, 21(5), pp. 347–355. Available at: https://doi.org/10.1080/13625187.2016.1217327.

Schantz, J.S., Fernandez, C.S.P. and Anne Marie, Z.J. (2021) Menstrual cycle tracking applications and the potential for epidemiological research: A comprehensive review of the literature. *Current Epidemiology Reports*, 8(1), pp. 9–19. Available at: https://doi.org/10.1007/s40471-020-00260-3.

Schaumberg, M.A. *et al.* (2018) Use of oral contraceptives to manipulate menstruation in young, physically active women. *International Journal of Sports Physiology and Performance*, 13(1), pp. 82–87. Available at: https://doi.org/10.1123/IJSPP.2016-0689.

Scherr, J. *et al.* (2013) Associations between Borg's rating of perceived exertion and physiological measures of exercise intensity. *European Journal of Applied Physiology*, 113(1), pp. 147–155. Available at: https://doi.org/10.1007/S00421-012-2421-X.

Schleip, R. (2003) Fascial plasticity: A new neurobiological explanation. Part 2. *Journal of Bodywork and Movement Therapies*, 7(2), pp. 104–116. Available at: https://doi.org/10.1016/S1360-8592(02)00076-1.

Schleip, R., Hedley, G. and Yucesoy, C.A. (2019) Fascial nomenclature: Update on related consensus process. *Clinical Anatomy (New York, N.Y.)*, 32(7), pp. 929–933. Available at: https://doi.org/10.1002/ca.23423.

Schmalenberger, K.M. *et al.* (2021) How to study the menstrual cycle: Practical tools and recommendations. *Psychoneuroendocrinology*, 123. Available at: https://doi.org/10.1016/J.PSYNEUEN.2020.104895.

Schmidt, P.J. and Rubinow, D.R. (1991) Menopause-related affective disorders: A justification for further study. *American Journal of Psychiatry*, 148(7), pp. 844–852. Available at: https://doi.org/10.1176/AJP.148.7.844.

Schneider, M.B. *et al.* (1999) Menstrual and premenstrual issues in female military cadets: A unique population with significant concerns. *Journal of Pediatric and Adolescent Gynecology*, 12(4), pp. 195–201. Available at: https://doi.org/10.1016/S1083-3188(99)00025-X.

Schöne, B. *et al.* (2018) Mindful breath awareness meditation facilitates efficiency gains in brain networks: A steady-state visually evoked potentials study. *Scientific Reports*, 8(1), pp. 1–10. Available at: https://doi.org/10.1038/s41598-018-32046-5.

Schumacher, S. *et al.* (2019) HPA axis regulation in post-traumatic stress disorder: A meta-analysis focusing on potential moderators. *Neuroscience and Biobehavioral Reviews*, 100, pp. 35–57. Available at: https://doi.org/10.1016/J.NEUBIOREV.2019.02.005.

Schwartz, B.I. *et al.* (2022) Experiences with menses in transgender and gender nonbinary adolescents. *Journal of Pediatric and Adolescent Gynecology*, 35(4), pp. 450–456. Available at: https://doi.org/10.1016/J.JPAG.2022.01.015.

Schwartz, B.I., Bear, B. and Kazak, A.E. (2023) Menstrual management choices in transgender and gender diverse adolescents. *Journal of Adolescent Health*, 72(2), pp. 207–213. Available at: https://doi.org/10.1016/J.JADOHEALTH.2022.09.023.

Seely, E.W. *et al.* (1999) Estradiol with or without progesterone and ambulatory blood pressure in postmenopausal women. *Hypertension (Dallas, Tex.: 1979)*, 33(5), pp. 1190–1194. Available at: https://doi.org/10.1161/01.HYP.33.5.1190.

Seyedahmadi, M. *et al.* (2022) What are gender differences in lower limb muscle activity during jump-landing tasks? A systematic review and meta-analysis. *BMC Sports Science, Medicine & Rehabilitation*, 14(1). Available at: https://doi.org/10.1186/S13102-022-00469-3.

Sharma, K. *et al.* (2022) A retrospective analysis of three focused attention meditation techniques: Mantra, breath, and external-point meditation. *Cureus*, 14(3). Available at: https://doi.org/10.7759/CUREUS.23589.

Shideler, S.E. *et al.* (1989) Ovarian-pituitary hormone interactions during the perimenopause. *Maturitas*, 11(4), pp. 331–339. Available at: https://doi.org/10.1016/0378-5122(89)90029-7.

Shim, J.Y., Laufer, M.R. and Grimstad, F.W. (2020) Dysmenorrhea and endometriosis in transgender adolescents. *Journal of Pediatric and Adolescent Gynecology*, 33(5), pp. 524–528. Available at: https://doi.org/10.1016/J.JPAG.2020.06.001.

Shu, X.O. *et al.* (2009) Soy food intake and breast cancer survival. *JAMA*, 302(22), pp. 2437–2443. Available at: https://doi.org/10.1001/JAMA.2009.1783.

Shultz, S.J. *et al.* (2005) Sex differences in knee joint laxity change across the female menstrual cycle. *The Journal of Sports Medicine and Physical Fitness*, 45(4), p. 594. Available at: https://doi.org/10.1249/00005768-200405001-00719.

Si, X.W., Yang, Z.K. and Feng, X. (2024) A meta-analysis of the intervention effect of mindfulness training on athletes' performance. *Frontiers in Psychology*, 15, 1375608. doi: 10.3389/fpsyg.2024.1375608. PMID: 38939219.

Sims, S.T. and Heather, A.K. (2018) Myths and methodologies: Reducing scientific design ambiguity in studies comparing sexes and/or menstrual cycle phases. *Experimental Physiology*, 103(10), pp. 1309–1317. Available at: https://doi.org/10.1113/EP086797.

Sims, S.T. and Yeager, S. (2022) *Next Level: Your Guide to Kicking Ass, Feeling Great, and Crushing Goals Through Menopause and Beyond*. Rodale Books.

Sims, S.T. *et al.* (2023) International society of sports nutrition position stand: Nutritional concerns of the female athlete. *Journal of the International Society of Sports Nutrition*, 20(1). Available at: https://doi.org/10.1080/15502783.2023.2204066.

Singh, M. (2012) Early age of natural menopause in India, a biological marker for early preventive health programs. *Climacteric: The Journal of the International Menopause Society*, 15(6), pp. 581–586. Available at: https://doi.org/10.3109/13697137.2011.643514.

Singh, V. *et al.* (2023) Dietary regulations for microbiota dysbiosis among post-menopausal women with type 2 diabetes. *Critical Reviews in Food Science and Nutrition*, 63(29), pp. 9961–9976. Available at: https://doi.org/10.1080/10408398.2022.2076651.

Sinha-Hikim, I. *et al.* (2006) Effects of testosterone supplementation on skeletal muscle fiber hypertrophy and satellite cells in community-dwelling older men. *The Journal of Clinical Endocrinology and Metabolism*, 91(8), pp. 3024–3033. Available at: https://doi.org/10.1210/jc.2006-0357.

Sirard, J.R., Pfeiffer, K.A. and Pate, R.R. (2006) Motivational factors associated with sports program participation in middle school students. *The Journal of Adolescent Health: Official Publication of the Society for Adolescent Medicine*, 38(6), pp.

696–703. Available at: https://doi.org/10.1016/J.JADOHEALTH.2005.07.013.

Sitruk-Ware, R. et al. (2024) Regulatory challenges of new male contraceptive methods. Andrology [Preprint]. Available at: https://doi.org/10.1111/ANDR.13720.

Skinner, B., Moss, R. and Hammond, L. (2020) A systematic review and meta-analysis of the effects of foam rolling on range of motion, recovery and markers of athletic performance. Journal of Bodywork and Movement Therapies, 24(3), pp. 105–122. Available at: https://doi.org/10.1016/j.jbmt.2020.01.007.

Skovlund, C.W. et al. (2016) Association of hormonal contraception with depression. JAMA Psychiatry, 73(11), pp. 1154–1162. Available at: https://doi.org/10.1001/JAMAPSYCHIATRY.2016.2387.

Skovlund, C.W. et al. (2018) Association of hormonal contraception with suicide attempts and suicides. American Journal of Psychiatry, 175(4), pp. 336–342. Available at: https://doi.org/10.1176/APPI.AJP.2017.17060616.

Smekal, G. et al. (2007) Menstrual cycle: No effect on exercise cardiorespiratory variables or blood lactate concentration. Medicine and Science in Sports and Exercise, 39(7), pp. 1098–1106. Available at: https://doi.org/10.1249/MSS.0B013E31805371E7.

Smith, G.I. et al. (2014) Testosterone and progesterone, but not estradiol, stimulate muscle protein synthesis in postmenopausal women. The Journal of Clinical Endocrinology and Metabolism, 99(1), pp. 256–265. Available at: https://doi.org/10.1210/JC.2013-2835.

Smith, M.J. et al. (2002) Effects of ovarian hormones on human cortical excitability. Annals of Neurology, 51(5), pp. 599–603. Available at: https://doi.org/10.1002/ANA.10180.

Smith, N.K., Jozkowski, K.N. and Sanders, S.A. (2014) Hormonal contraception and female pain, orgasm and sexual pleasure. The Journal of Sexual Medicine, 11(2), pp. 462–470. Available at: https://doi.org/10.1111/JSM.12409.

Smolensky, I. et al. (2023) Sex-specific differences in metabolic hormone and adipose tissue dynamics induced by moderate low-carbohydrate and ketogenic diet. Scientific Reports, 13(1), pp. 1–10. Available at: https://doi.org/10.1038/s41598-023-43587-9.

Soares, C.N. (2019) Depression and menopause: An update on current knowledge and clinical management for this critical window. The Medical Clinics of North America, 103(4), pp. 651–667. Available at: https://doi.org/10.1016/J.MCNA.2019.03.001.

Soares, C.N. and Zitek, B. (2008) Reproductive hormone sensitivity and risk for depression across the female life cycle: A continuum of vulnerability? Journal of Psychiatry and Neuroscience, 33(4), pp. 331–343.

Soleymani, M. et al. (2019) Dietary patterns and their association with menopausal symptoms: A cross-sectional study. Menopause (New York, N.Y.), 26(4), pp. 365–372. Available at: https://doi.org/10.1097/GME.0000000000001245.

Soliman, A.M. et al. (2021) Impact of endometriosis on fatigue and productivity impairment in a cross-sectional survey of Canadian women. Journal of Obstetrics and Gynaecology Canada; Journal d'Obstetrique et Gynecologie du Canada, 43(1), pp. 10–18. Available at: https://doi.org/10.1016/J.JOGC.2020.06.022.

Solli, G.S. et al. (2020) Changes in Self-Reported Physical Fitness, Performance, and Side Effects Across the Phases of the Menstrual Cycle Among Competitive Endurance Athletes. Int J Sports Physiol Perform. 21;15(9):1324–1333. doi: 10.1123/ijspp.2019-0616. PMID: 32957079.

Somboonwong, J., Chutimakul, L. and Sanguanrungsirikul, S. (2015) Core temperature changes and sprint performance of elite female soccer players after a 15-minute warm-up in a hot-humid environment. Journal of Strength and Conditioning Research, 29(1), pp. 262–269. Available at: https://doi.org/10.1519/01.JSC.0000491321.12969.1D.

Sommer, B. et al. (2023) Phytoestrogen-based hormonal replacement therapy could benefit women suffering late-onset asthma. International Journal of Molecular Sciences, 24(20). Available at: https://doi.org/10.3390/IJMS242015335.

Sons, A. and Eckhardt, A.L. (2021) Health literacy and knowledge of female reproduction in undergraduate students. Journal of American College Health, pp. 1–8. Available at: https://doi.org/10.1080/07448481.2021.1909034.

De Souza, M.J. et al. (1990) Effects of menstrual phase and amenorrhea on exercise performance in runners. Medicine and Science in Sports and Exercise, 22(5), pp. 575–580. Available at: https://doi.org/10.1249/00005768-199010000-00006.

Soyka, L.A. et al. (2002) Abnormal bone mineral accrual in adolescent girls with anorexia nervosa. Journal of Clinical Endocrinology & Metabolism, 87(9), pp. 4177–4185. Available at: https://doi.org/10.1210/jc.2001-011889.

Spiegel, K., Leproult, R. et al. (2004) Leptin levels are dependent on sleep duration: Relationships with sympathovagal balance, carbohydrate regulation, cortisol, and thyrotropin. The Journal of Clinical Endocrinology and Metabolism, 89(11), pp. 5762–5771. Available at: https://doi.org/10.1210/JC.2004-1003.

Spiegel, K., Tasali, E. et al. (2004) Brief communication: Sleep curtailment in healthy young men is associated with decreased leptin levels, elevated ghrelin levels, and increased hunger and appetite. Annals of Internal Medicine, 141(11), pp. 846–850. Available at: https://doi.org/10.7326/0003-4819-141-11-200412070-00008.

Stachenfeld, N.S. (2014) Hormonal changes during menopause and the impact on fluid regulation. *Reproductive Sciences (Thousand Oaks, Calif.)*, 21(5), pp. 555–561. Available at: https://doi.org/10.1177/1933719113518992.

Stanczyk, F.Z., Matharu, H. and Winer, S.A. (2021) Bioidentical hormones. *Climacteric*, 24(1), pp. 38–45. Available at: https://doi.org/10.1080/13697137.2020.1862079.

Stanford, J.B. (2019) Big data meets the menstrual cycle. *Fertility and Sterility*. United States, pp. 464–465. Available at: https://doi.org/10.1016/j.fertnstert.2019.05.035.

Stecco, A. *et al.* (2023) From muscle to the myofascial unit: Current evidence and future perspectives. *International Journal of Molecular Sciences*, 24(5). Available at: https://doi.org/10.3390/lJMS24054527.

Stecco, C. *et al.* (2018) Update on fascial nomenclature. *Journal of Bodywork and Movement Therapies*. United States, p. 354. Available at: https://doi.org/10.1016/j.jbmt.2017.12.015.

Steinberg, F.M. *et al.* (2011) Clinical outcomes of a 2-y soy isoflavone supplementation in menopausal women. *The American Journal of Clinical Nutrition*, 93(2), pp. 356–367. Available at: https://doi.org/10.3945/AJCN.110.008359.

Stepto, N.K. *et al.* (2020) Exercise and insulin resistance in PCOS: Muscle insulin signalling and fibrosis. *Endocrine Connections*, 9(4), pp. 346–359. Available at: https://doi.org/10.1530/EC-19-0551.

Stevens-Lapsley, J.E. and Kohrt, W.M. (2010) Osteoarthritis in women: Effects of estrogen, obesity and physical activity. *Women's Health*, 6(4), pp. 601–615. Available at: https://doi.org/10.2217/WHE.10.38.

St-Onge, M.P. (2016) Impact of sleep duration on food intake regulation: Different mechanisms by sex? *Obesity (Silver Spring, Md.)*, 24(1), p. 11. Available at: https://doi.org/10.1002/OBY.21374.

Stromberg, S.E., Russell, M.E. and Carlson, C.R. (2015) Diaphragmatic breathing and its effectiveness for the management of motion sickness. *Aerospace Medicine and Human Performance*, 86(5), pp. 452–457. Available at: https://doi.org/10.3357/AMHP.4152.2015.

Stuenkel, C.A. (2021) Compounded bioidentical menopausal hormone therapy: A physician perspective. *Climacteric: The Journal of the International Menopause Society*, 24(1), pp. 11–18. Available at: https://doi.org/10.1080/13697137.2020.1825668.

Suchomel, T.J. *et al.* (2018) The importance of muscular strength: Training considerations. *Sports Medicine (Auckland, N.Z.)*, 48(4), pp. 765–785. Available at: https://doi.org/10.1007/S40279-018-0862-Z.

Sullivan, B.E. *et al.* (2009) Effect of acute resistance exercise and sex on human patellar tendon structural and regulatory mRNA expression. *Journal of Applied Physiology (Bethesda, Md.: 1985)*, 106(2), pp. 468–475. Available at: https://doi.org/10.1152/JAPPLPHYSIOL.91341.2008.

Sunderland, C. and Nevill, M. (2003) Effect of the menstrual cycle on performance of intermittent, high-intensity shuttle running in a hot environment. *European Journal of Applied Physiology*, 88(4–5), pp. 345–352. Available at: https://doi.org/10.1007/S00421-002-0722-1.

Sundgot-Borgen, J. *et al.* (2019) Elite athletes get pregnant, have healthy babies and return to sport early postpartum. *BMJ Open Sport & Exercise Medicine*, 5(1), p. e000652. Available at: https://doi.org/10.1136/BMJSEM-2019-000652.

Sung, E. *et al.* (2014) Effects of follicular versus luteal phase-based strength training in young women. *SpringerPlus*, 3(1). Available at: https://doi.org/10.1186/2193-1801-3-668.

Svensson, R.B. *et al.* (2016) Effect of aging and exercise on the tendon. *Journal of Applied Physiology (Bethesda, Md.: 1985)*, 121(6), pp. 1353–1362. Available at: https://doi.org/10.1152/JAPPLPHYSIOL.00328.2016.

Swarup, S. *et al.* (2024) Metabolic Syndrome. StatPearls Publishing. www.ncbi.nlm.nih.gov/books/NBK459248.

Szymanski, L.M. and Satin, A.J. (2012) Strenuous exercise during pregnancy: Is there a limit? *American Journal of Obstetrics and Gynecology*, 207(3), pp. 179.e1–179.e6. Available at: https://doi.org/10.1016/J.AJOG.2012.07.021.

Taim, B.C. *et al.* (2023) The prevalence of menstrual cycle disorders and menstrual cycle-related symptoms in female athletes: A systematic literature review. *Sports Medicine (Auckland, N.Z.)*, 53(10), pp. 1963–1984. Available at: https://doi.org/10.1007/S40279-023-01871-8.

Takeda, T. (2023) Premenstrual disorders: Premenstrual syndrome and premenstrual dysphoric disorder. *The Journal of Obstetrics and Gynaecology Research*, 49(2), pp. 510–518. Available at: https://doi.org/10.1111/JOG.15484.

Taku, K. *et al.* (2012) Extracted or synthesized soybean isoflavones reduce menopausal hot flash frequency and severity: Systematic review and meta-analysis of randomized controlled trials. *Menopause (New York, N.Y.)*, 19(7), pp. 776–790. Available at: https://doi.org/10.1097/GME.0B013E3182410159.

Tan, T.W. (2023) Effect of non-pharmacological interventions on the prevention of sarcopenia in menopausal women: A systematic review and meta-analysis of randomized controlled trials. *BMC Women's Health*, 23(1). Available at: https://doi.org/10.1186/S12905-023-02749-7.

Taraborrelli, S. (2015) Physiology, production and action of progesterone. *Acta Obstetricia et Gynecologica*

Scandinavica, 94 Suppl 161, pp. 8–16. Available at: https://doi.org/10.1111/aogs.12771.

Taylor, T.R. *et al.* (2018) A restorative yoga intervention for African-American breast cancer survivors: A pilot study. *Journal of Racial and Ethnic Health Disparities*, 5(1), pp. 62–72. Available at: https://doi.org/10.1007/S40615-017-0342-4.

Teede, H.J. *et al.* (2023) Recommendations from the 2023 international evidence-based guideline for the assessment and management of polycystic ovary syndrome. *Fertility and Sterility*, 120(4), pp. 767–793. Available at: https://doi.org/10.1016/j.fertnstert.2023.07.025.

Tenforde, A.S. *et al.* (2015) Running habits of competitive runners during pregnancy and breastfeeding. *Sports Health*, 7(2), pp. 172–176. Available at: https://doi.org/10.1177/1941738114549542.

Tenforde, A.S. *et al.* (2017) Association of the Female Athlete Triad Risk Assessment Stratification to the Development of Bone Stress Injuries in Collegiate Athletes. *American Journal of Sports Medicine*, 45(2), pp. 302–310. Available at: https://doi.org/10.1177/0363546516676262.

Teychenne, M. and York, R. (2013) Physical activity, sedentary behavior, and postnatal depressive symptoms: A review. *American Journal of Preventative Medicine*, 45(2), pp. 217–227. Available at: https://doi.org/10.1016/j.amepre.2013.04.004.

The 2023 nonhormone therapy position statement of The North American Menopause Society (2023) *Menopause (New York, N.Y.)*, 30(6), pp. 573–590. Available at: https://doi.org/10.1097/GME.0000000000002200.

The Lancet (2024) Time for a balanced conversation about menopause. *The Lancet*, 403(10430), p. 877. Available at: https://doi.org/10.1016/S0140-6736(24)00462-8.

The North American Menopause Society (2019) *Menopause Practice Textbook: A Clinician's Guide*. Sixth edition. Edited by C. Crandall. Pepper Pike, Ohio. Available at: https://menopause.org/publications/professional-publications/em-menopause-practice-em-textbook (Accessed: 10 June 2024).

Thomas, D.R. (2007) Loss of skeletal muscle mass in aging: Examining the relationship of starvation, sarcopenia and cachexia. *Clinical Nutrition (Edinburgh, Scotland)*, 26(4), pp. 389–399. Available at: https://doi.org/10.1016/J.CLNU.2007.03.008.

Thompson, B. *et al.* (2020) The effect of the menstrual cycle and oral contraceptives on acute responses and chronic adaptations to resistance training: A systematic review of the literature. *Sports Medicine (Auckland, N.Z.)*, 50(1), pp. 171–185. Available at: https://doi.org/10.1007/S40279-019-01219-1.

Thompson, B.M. *et al.* (2021) The effect of the menstrual cycle and oral contraceptive cycle on muscle performance and perceptual measures. *International Journal of Environmental Research and Public Health*, 18(20). Available at: https://doi.org/10.3390/IJERPH182010565.

Thompson, C. *et al.* (2023) Restorative yoga therapy for third-year medical students in pediatrics rotation: Working to improve medical student well-being. *Journal of Education and Health Promotion*, 12(1). Available at: https://doi.org/10.4103/JEHP.JEHP_1027_22.

Thurston, R.C. *et al.* (2009) Gains in body fat and vasomotor symptom reporting over the menopausal transition: The study of women's health across the nation. *American Journal of Epidemiology*, 170(6), pp. 766–774. Available at: https://doi.org/10.1093/AJE/KWP203.

Thurston, R.C. *et al.* (2015) Behavioral weight loss for the management of menopausal hot flashes: A pilot study. *Menopause (New York, N.Y.)*, 22(1), pp. 59–65. Available at: https://doi.org/10.1097/GME.0000000000000274.

Thurston, R.C., Santoro, N. and Matthews, K.A. (2011) Adiposity and hot flashes in midlife women: A modifying role of age. *The Journal of Clinical Endocrinology and Metabolism*, 96(10). Available at: https://doi.org/10.1210/JC.2011-1082.

Tiidus, P.M., Deller, M. and Liu, X.L. (2005) Oestrogen influence on myogenic satellite cells following downhill running in male rats: A preliminary study. *Acta Physiologica Scandinavica*, 184(1), pp. 67–72. Available at: https://doi.org/10.1111/J.1365-201X.2005.01427.X.

Toma, M. (2015) Missed shots at the free-throw line: Analyzing the determinants of choking under pressure. *Journal of Sports Economics*, 18(6), pp. 539–559. https://doi.org/10.1177/1527002515593779 (Original work published 2017).

Torres-Tamayo, N. *et al.* (2018) 3D analysis of sexual dimorphism in size, shape and breathing kinematics of human lungs. *Journal of Anatomy*, 232(2), pp. 227–237. Available at: https://doi.org/10.1111/JOA.12743.

Tounsi, M. *et al.* (2018) Soccer-related performance in eumenorrheic Tunisian high-level soccer players: Effects of menstrual cycle phase and moment of day. *The Journal of Sports Medicine and Physical Fitness*, 58(4), pp. 497–502. Available at: https://doi.org/10.23736/S0022-4707.17.06958-4.

Tourny, C. *et al.* (2023) Endometriosis and physical activity: A narrative review. *International Journal of Gynaecology and Obstetrics: The Official Organ of the International Federation of Gynaecology and Obstetrics*, 163(3), pp. 747–756. Available at: https://doi.org/10.1002/IJGO.14898.

Travlos, A.K. and Marisi, D.Q. (1996) Perceived exertion during physical exercise among individuals high and low in fitness. *Perceptual and Motor Skills*, 84(2), pp. 419–424. Available at: https://doi.org/10.2466/PMS.1996.82.2.419.

Tricco, A.C. *et al.* (2017) Comparisons of interventions for preventing falls in older adults: A systematic review and meta-analysis. *JAMA*, 318(17), pp. 1687–1699. Available at: https://doi.org/10.1001/JAMA.2017.15006.

Tsai, S.Y. (2016) Effect of yoga exercise on premenstrual symptoms among female employees in Taiwan. *International Journal of Environmental Research and Public Health*, 13(7). Available at: https://doi.org/10.3390/IJERPH13070721.

Tsampoukos, A. *et al.* (2010) Effect of menstrual cycle phase on sprinting performance. *European Journal of Applied Physiology*, 109(4), pp. 659–667. Available at: https://doi.org/10.1007/S00421-010-1384-Z.

Tschon, M. *et al.* (2021) Gender and sex are key determinants in osteoarthritis not only confounding variables: A systematic review of clinical data. *Journal of Clinical Medicine*, 10(14). Available at: https://doi.org/10.3390/JCM10143178.

Tsekoura, M. *et al.* (2017) Sarcopenia and its impact on quality of life. *Advances in Experimental Medicine and Biology*, 987, pp. 213–218. Available at: https://doi.org/10.1007/978-3-319-57379-3_19.

Turan, V. *et al.* (2015) Benefits of short-term structured exercise in non-overweight women with polycystic ovary syndrome: A prospective randomized controlled study. *Journal of Physical Therapy Science*, 27(7), p. 2293. Available at: https://doi.org/10.1589/JPTS.27.2293.

Turnock, L.A. (2021) "There's a difference between tolerance and acceptance": Exploring women's experiences of barriers to access in UK gyms. *Wellbeing, Space and Society*, 2, p. 100049. Available at: https://doi.org/10.1016/J.WSS.2021.100049.

Van Uffelen, J.G.Z., Khan, A. and Burton, N.W. (2017) Gender differences in physical activity motivators and context preferences: A population-based study in people in their sixties. *BMC Public Health*, 17(1). Available at: https://doi.org/10.1186/S12889-017-4540-0.

United Nations, D. of E. and S.A.P.D. (2019) *Contraceptive Use by Method 2019: Data Booklet (ST/ESA/SER.A/435)*.

Upchurch, D.M. and Johnson, P.J. (2019) Gender differences in prevalence, patterns, purposes, and perceived benefits of meditation practices in the United States. *Journal of Women's Health*, 28(2), p. 135. Available at: https://doi.org/10.1089/JWH.2018.7178.

Utian, W.H. (2005) Psychosocial and socioeconomic burden of vasomotor symptoms in menopause: A comprehensive review. *Health and Quality of Life Outcomes*, 3. Available at: https://doi.org/10.1186/1477-7525-3-47.

Vahdat, H.L. *et al.* (2024) The role of advocacy in sustaining male contraceptive research and development. *Andrology* [Preprint]. Available at: https://doi.org/10.1111/ANDR.13721.

Vaiksaar, S. *et al.* (2011) No effect of menstrual cycle phase and oral contraceptive use on endurance performance in rowers. *Journal of Strength and Conditioning Research*, 25(6), pp. 1571–1578. Available at: https://doi.org/10.1519/JSC.0B013E3181DF7FD2.

Vannuccini, S. *et al.* (2020) Dysmenorrhea and heavy menstrual bleeding in elite female athletes: Quality of life and perceived stress. *Reproductive Sciences (Thousand Oaks, Calif.)*, 27(3), pp. 888–894. Available at: https://doi.org/10.1007/S43032-019-00092-7.

Vannuccini, S. *et al.* (2022) Hormonal treatments for endometriosis: The endocrine background. *Reviews in Endocrine & Metabolic Disorders*, 23(3), pp. 333–355. Available at: https://doi.org/10.1007/S11154-021-09666-W.

Vidic, Z. (2024) Gender differences on coping, stress, resilience and mindfulness within an academic course intervention with a mindfulness meditation component. *Current Psychology 2024*, pp. 1–11. Available at: https://doi.org/10.1007/S12144-024-06395-6.

Vigil, P. *et al.* (2017) Ovulation, a sign of health. *The Linacre Quarterly*, 84(4), pp. 343–355. Available at: https://doi.org/10.1080/00243639.2017.1394053.

Vizza, L. *et al.* (2016) The feasibility of progressive resistance training in women with polycystic ovary syndrome: A pilot randomized controlled trial. *BMC Sports Science, Medicine and Rehabilitation*, 8(1). Available at: https://doi.org/10.1186/S13102-016-0039-8.

Vladutiu, C.J., Evenson, K.R. and Marshall, S.W. (2010) Physical activity and injuries during pregnancy. *Journal of Physical Activity & Health*, 7(6), pp. 761–769. Available at: https://doi.org/10.1123/JPAH.7.6.761.

Van Vliet, H.A.A.M. *et al.* (2006) Biphasic versus triphasic oral contraceptives for contraception. *The Cochrane Database of Systematic Reviews*, 2006(3). Available at: https://doi.org/10.1002/14651858.CD003283.PUB2.

Vogel, K. *et al.* (2023) Female athletes and the menstrual cycle in team sports: Current state of play and considerations for future research. *Sports (Basel, Switzerland)*, 12(1). Available at: https://doi.org/10.3390/SPORTS12010004.

Vokes, T.J. *et al.* (1988) Osmoregulation of thirst and vasopressin during normal menstrual cycle. *The American Journal of Physiology*, 254(4 Pt 2). Available at: https://doi.org/10.1152/AJPREGU.1988.254.4.R641.

Volpi, E., Nazemi, R. and Fujita, S. (2004) Muscle tissue changes with aging. *Current Opinion in Clinical Nutrition and Metabolic Care*, 7(4), p. 405. Available at:

https://doi.org/10.1097/01.MCO.0000134362.76653.B2.

Voogt, J.L. *et al.* (2001) Regulation of prolactin secretion during pregnancy and lactation. *Progress in Brain Research*, 133, pp. 173–185. Available at: https://doi.org/10.1016/S0079-6123(01)33013-3.

Wagenmaker, E.R. and Moenter, S.M. (2017) Exposure to acute psychosocial stress disrupts the luteinizing hormone surge independent of estrous cycle alterations in female mice. *Endocrinology*, 158(8), pp. 2593–2602. Available at: https://doi.org/10.1210/EN.2017-00341.

Waghmare, S.V. and Shanoo, A. (2023) Polycystic ovary syndrome: A literature review with a focus on diagnosis, pathophysiology, and management. *Cureus*, 15(10). Available at: https://doi.org/10.7759/CUREUS.47408.

Walker, V.R. and Korach, K.S. (2004) Estrogen receptor knockout mice as a model for endocrine research. *ILAR Journal/National Research Council, Institute of Laboratory Animal Resources*, 45(4), pp. 455–461. Available at: https://doi.org/10.1093/ILAR.45.4.455/2/ILAR-45-4-455IGF2.GIF.

Wallace, J.P. and Rabin, J. (1991) The concentration of lactic acid in breast milk following maximal exercise. *International Journal of Sports Medicine*, 12(3), pp. 328–331. Available at: https://doi.org/10.1055/s-2007-1024691.

Wang, F.J., Hsiao, C.H. and Hsiung, T.T. (2022) Marketing strategies of the female-only gym industry: A case-based industry perspective. *Frontiers in Psychology*, 13. Available at: https://doi.org/10.3389/FPSYG.2022.928882.

Wang, M. *et al.* (2022) Menopausal status, age at natural menopause and risk of diabetes in China: A 10-year prospective study of 300,000 women. *Nutrition & Metabolism*, 19(1). Available at: https://doi.org/10.1186/S12986-022-00643-X.

Wang, Y. *et al.* (2022) Prevalence of Achilles tendinopathy in physical exercise: A systematic review and meta-analysis. *Sports Medicine and Health Science*, 4(3), pp. 152–159. Available at: https://doi.org/10.1016/J.SMHS.2022.03.003.

Wang, Y., Nicholes, K. and Shih, I.M. (2020) The origin and pathogenesis of endometriosis. *Annual Review of Pathology*, 15, pp. 71–95. Available at: https://doi.org/10.1146/ANNUREV-PATHMECHDIS-012419-032654.

Warner, P.E. *et al.* (2004) Menorrhagia I: Measured blood loss, clinical features, and outcome in women with heavy periods: A survey with follow-up data. *American Journal of Obstetrics and Gynecology*, 190(5), pp. 1216–1223. Available at: https://doi.org/10.1016/J.AJOG.2003.11.015.

Watkins, A. (2021) Reevaluating the grandmother hypothesis. *History and Philosophy of the Life Sciences*, 43(3). Available at: https://doi.org/10.1007/S40656-021-00455-X.

Wattanapermpool, J. and Reiser, P.J. (1999) Differential effects of ovariectomy on calcium activation of cardiac and soleus myofilaments. *The American Journal of Physiology*, 277(2). Available at: https://doi.org/10.1152/AJPHEART.1999.277.2.H467.

Weber, D.D., Aminazdeh-Gohari, S. and Kofler, B. (2018) Ketogenic diet in cancer therapy. *Aging*, 10(2), pp. 164–165. Available at: https://doi.org/10.18632/AGING.101382.

Weina, S.U. (2006) Effects of pregnancy on the Army Physical Fitness Test. *Military Medicine*, 171(6), pp. 534–537. Available at: https://doi.org/10.7205/MILMED.171.6.534.

Weiss, G. *et al.* (2004) Menopause and hypothalamic-pituitary sensitivity to estrogen. *JAMA*, 292(24), pp. 2991–2996. Available at: https://doi.org/10.1001/JAMA.292.24.2991.

Wells, G. *et al.* (2002) V. Meta-analysis of the efficacy of hormone replacement therapy in treating and preventing osteoporosis in postmenopausal women. *Endocrine Reviews*, 23(4), pp. 529–539. Available at: https://doi.org/10.1210/ER.2001-5002.

Wells, K.R. *et al.* (2020) The Australian Institute of Sport (AIS) and National Eating Disorders Collaboration (NEDC) position statement on disordered eating in high performance sport. *British Journal of Sports Medicine*, 54(21), pp. 1247–1258. Available at: https://doi.org/10.1136/bjsports-2019-101813.

White, E., Pivarnik, J. and Pfeiffer, K. (2014) Resistance training during pregnancy and perinatal outcomes. *Journal of Physical Activity and Health*, 11(6), pp. 1141–1148. Available at: https://doi.org/10.1123/JPAH.2012-0350.

Whiteman, M.K. *et al.* (2003) Risk factors for hot flashes in midlife women. *Journal of Women's Health*, 12(5), pp. 459–472. Available at: https://doi.org/10.1089/154099903766651586.

Wickham, K.A. *et al.* (2021) Sex differences in the physiological responses to exercise-induced dehydration: Consequences and mechanisms. *Journal of Applied Physiology*, 131(2), pp. 504–510. Available at: https://doi.org/10.1152/JAPPLPHYSIOL.00266.2021.

Wieloch, N. *et al.* (2022) Sport and exercise recommendations for pregnant athletes: A systematic scoping review. *BMJ Open Sport & Exercise Medicine*, 8(4), p. e001395. Available at: https://doi.org/10.1136/BMJSEM-2022-001395.

Wiepjes, C.M. *et al.* (2020) Fracture risk in trans women and trans men using long-term gender-affirming hormonal treatment: A nationwide cohort study.

Journal of Bone and Mineral Research, 35(1), pp. 64–70. Available at: https://doi.org/10.1002/JBMR.3862.

Wierckx, K., Elaut, E., Declercq, E., Heylens, G. *et al.* (2013) Prevalence of cardiovascular disease and cancer during cross-sex hormone therapy in a large cohort of trans persons: A case-control study. *European Journal of Endocrinology*, 169(4), pp. 471–478. doi: 10.1530/EJE-13-0493.

Wiewelhove, T. *et al.* (2019) A meta-analysis of the effects of foam rolling on performance and recovery. *Frontiers in Physiology*, p. 376. Available at: https://doi.org/10.3389/fphys.2019.00376.

Wikström-Frisén, L., Boraxbekk, C.J. and Henriksson-Larsén, K. (2017) Effects on power, strength and lean body mass of menstrual/oral contraceptive cycle based resistance training. *The Journal of Sports Medicine and Physical Fitness*, 57(1–2), pp. 43–52. Available at: https://doi.org/10.23736/S0022-4707.16.05848-5.

Wilcox, A.J., Dunson, D. and Baird, D.D. (2000) The timing of the "fertile window" in the menstrual cycle: Day specific estimates from a prospective study. *BMJ (Clinical Research Ed.)*, 321(7271), pp. 1259–1262. Available at: https://doi.org/10.1136/bmj.321.7271.1259.

Wilke, J. *et al.* (2019) Fascia thickness, aging and flexibility: Is there an association? *Journal of Anatomy*, 234(1), pp. 43–49. Available at: https://doi.org/10.1111/JOA.12902.

Wilke, J. *et al.* (2020) Acute effects of foam rolling on range of motion in healthy adults: A systematic review with multilevel meta-analysis. *Sports Medicine (Auckland, N.Z.)*, 50(2), pp. 387–402. Available at: https://doi.org/10.1007/s40279-019-01205-7.

Wilkinson, M. and Brown, R.E. (2015) *An Introduction to Neuroendocrinology*. Second edition. Cambridge, UK: Cambridge University Press.

Williams, D.M. (2008) Exercise, affect, and adherence: An integrated model and a case for self-paced exercise. *Journal of Sport and Exercise Psychology*, 30(5), pp. 471–496. Available at: https://doi.org/10.1123/JSEP.30.5.471.

Van Wingen, G.A. *et al.* (2008) Progesterone selectively increases amygdala reactivity in women. *Molecular Psychiatry*, 13(3), pp. 325–333. Available at: https://doi.org/10.1038/SJ.MP.4002030.

Van Wingen, G.A. *et al.* (2011) Gonadal hormone regulation of the emotion circuitry in humans. *Neuroscience*, 191, pp. 38–45. Available at: https://doi.org/10.1016/J.NEUROSCIENCE.2011.04.042.

Wirth, J.C. and Lohman, T.G. (1982) The relationship of static muscle function to use of oral contraceptives. *Medicine and Science in Sports and Exercise*, 14(1), pp. 16–20. Available at: https://doi.org/10.1249/00005768-198201000-00003.

Witkowski, S. *et al.* (2023) Physical activity and exercise for hot flashes: Trigger or treatment? *Menopause (New York, N.Y.)*, 30(2), pp. 218–224. Available at: https://doi.org/10.1097/GME.0000000000002107.

Witten, T. *et al.* (2024) Nonhormonal pharmacotherapies for the treatment of postmenopausal vasomotor symptoms. *Cureus*, 16(1). Available at: https://doi.org/10.7759/CUREUS.52467.

Wójcik, M., Szczepaniak, R. and Placek, K. (2022) Physiotherapy management in endometriosis. *International Journal of Environmental Research and Public Health*, 19(23). Available at: https://doi.org/10.3390/IJERPH192316148.

Wolfe, L.A. *et al.* (1998) Acid-base regulation and control of ventilation in human pregnancy. *Canadian Journal of Physiology and Pharmacology*, 76(9), pp. 815–827. Available at: https://doi.org/10.1139/CJPP-76-9-815.

Wong, C. *et al.* (2018) Mindfulness-Based Stress Reduction (MBSR) or psychoeducation for the reduction of menopausal symptoms: A randomized, controlled clinical trial. *Scientific Reports*, 8(1). Available at: https://doi.org/10.1038/S41598-018-24945-4.

Woodward, A., Klonizakis, M. and Broom, D. (2020) Exercise and polycystic ovary syndrome. *Advances in Experimental Medicine and Biology*, 1228, pp. 123–136. Available at: https://doi.org/10.1007/978-981-15-1792-1_8.

Worsley, R. *et al.* (2017) Moderate-severe vasomotor symptoms are associated with moderate-severe depressive symptoms. *Journal of Women's Health (2002)*, 26(7), pp. 712–718. Available at: https://doi.org/10.1089/JWH.2016.6142.

Wright, V.J. *et al.* (2024) The musculoskeletal syndrome of menopause. *Climacteric* [Preprint]. Available at: https://doi.org/10.1080/13697137.2024.2380363.

Wu, J. *et al.* (2023) Sarcopenia: Molecular regulatory network for loss of muscle mass and function. *Frontiers in Nutrition*, 10. Available at: https://doi.org/10.3389/FNUT.2023.1037200.

Xu, H. *et al.* (2023) Effectiveness of aerobic exercise in the prevention and treatment of postpartum depression: Meta-analysis and network meta-analysis. *PLOS One*, 18(11), p. e0287650. Available at: https://doi.org/10.1371/JOURNAL.PONE.0287650.

Yan, H. *et al.* (2019) Estrogen improves insulin sensitivity and suppresses gluconeogenesis via the transcription factor foxo1. *Diabetes*, 68(2), p. 291. Available at: https://doi.org/10.2337/DB18-0638.

Yan, H., Ding, Y. and Guo, W. (2021) Suicidality in patients with premenstrual dysphoric disorder—A systematic review and meta-analysis. *Journal of Affective Disorders*, 295, pp. 339–346. Available at: https://doi.org/10.1016/j.jad.2021.08.082.

Yonkers, K.A. and Simoni, M.K. (2018) Premenstrual disorders. *American Journal of Obstetrics and Gynecology*, 218(1), pp. 68–74. Available at: https://doi.org/10.1016/j.ajog.2017.05.045.

Yovich, J.L. *et al.* (2020) Pathogenesis of endometriosis: Look no further than John Sampson. *Reproductive Biomedicine Online*, 40(1), pp. 7–11. Available at: https://doi.org/10.1016/J.RBMO.2019.10.007.

Yu, J.-L. *et al.* (2022) Tracking of menstrual cycles and prediction of the fertile window via measurements of basal body temperature and heart rate as well as machine-learning algorithms. *Reproductive Biology and Endocrinology*, 20(1), p. 118. Available at: https://doi.org/10.1186/s12958-022-00993-4.

Yu, R. (2015) Choking under pressure: The neuropsychological mechanisms of incentive-induced performance decrements. *Frontiers in Behavioral Neuroscience*, 9(FEB). Available at: https://doi.org/10.3389/FNBEH.2015.00019.

Yumuk, V. *et al.* (2015) European guidelines for obesity management in adults. *Obesity Facts*, 8(6), pp. 402–424. Available at: https://doi.org/10.1159/000442721.

Zaccaro, A. *et al.* (2018) How breath-control can change your life: A systematic review on psycho-physiological correlates of slow breathing. *Frontiers in Human Neuroscience*, 12, p. 353. Available at: https://doi.org/10.3389/FNHUM.2018.00353/FULL.

Zadek, F. *et al.* (2022) Cerebrospinal fluid and arterial acid–base equilibria in spontaneously breathing third-trimester pregnant women. *British Journal of Anaesthesia*, 129(5), p. 726. Available at: https://doi.org/10.1016/J.BJA.2022.07.048.

Zalewska, O. *et al.* (2024) Women's awareness of reproductive health. *Medicina*, 60(1), p. 158. Available at: https://doi.org/10.3390/MEDICINA60010158.

Zhang, L. *et al.* (2020) Menopausal symptoms and associated social and environmental factors in midlife Chinese women. *Clinical Interventions in Aging*, 15, pp. 2195–2208. Available at: https://doi.org/10.2147/CIA.S278976.

Zhang, Z. *et al.* (2017) Effects of slow and regular breathing exercise on cardiopulmonary coupling and blood pressure. *Medical & Biological Engineering & Computing*, 55(2), pp. 327–341. Available at: https://doi.org/10.1007/S11517-016-1517-6.

Zhao, L. *et al.* (2012) Effects of progressive muscular relaxation training on anxiety, depression and quality of life of endometriosis patients under gonadotrophin-releasing hormone agonist therapy. *European Journal of Obstetrics, Gynecology, and Reproductive Biology*, 162(2), pp. 211–215. Available at: https://doi.org/10.1016/J.EJOGRB.2012.02.029.

Zhu, J.W., Reed, J.L. and Van Spall, H.G.C. (2022) The underrepresentation of female athletes in sports research: Considerations for cardiovascular health. *European Heart Journal*, 43(17), pp. 1609–1611. Available at: https://doi.org/10.1093/EURHEARTJ/EHAB846.

Zondervan, K.T. *et al.* (2022) Endometriosis classification systems: An international survey to map current knowledge and uptake. *Journal of Minimally Invasive Gynecology*, 29(6), pp. 716–725.e1. Available at: https://doi.org/10.1016/J.JMIG.2022.01.014.

Zuraikat, F.M. *et al.* (2021) Sleep and diet: Mounting evidence of a cyclical relationship. *Annual Review of Nutrition*, 41, pp. 309–332. Available at: https://doi.org/10.1146/ANNUREV-NUTR-120420-021719.

Zwickl, S. *et al.* (2024) Persistent menstruation in transgender people using testosterone gender-affirming hormone therapy. *International Journal of Transgender Health* [Preprint]. Available at: https://doi.org/10.1080/26895269.2024.2403140.

Zwingerman, R., Chaikof, M. and Jones, C. (2020) A critical appraisal of fertility and menstrual tracking apps for the iPhone. *Journal of Obstetrics and Gynaecology Canada; Journal d'Obstetrique et Gynecologie du Canada*, 42(5), pp. 583–590. Available at: https://doi.org/10.1016/j.jogc.2019.09.023.

Subject Index

Author Index